YOUR CHILD'S HEALTH

YOUR CHILD'S HEALTH
Answers to parents' questions

IVAN BLUMENTHAL
MB, ChB, MRCP(UK), DCH

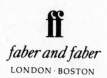

faber and faber
LONDON · BOSTON

First published in 1987
by Faber and Faber Limited
3 Queen Square, London WC1N 3AU

Photoset and Printed in Great Britain by
Redwood Burn Limited
Trowbridge, Wiltshire
All rights reserved

British Library Cataloguing in Publication Data

Blumenthal, Ivan
    Your child's health.
    1. Children—Diseases
    I. Title
    618.92′000240431   RJ61
ISBN 0–571–14707–0

To my wife Liz, Morris and Toby

Contents

Preface ix

Acknowledgements x

1 Growth and Development 1
   Short child; Failure to thrive; Physical
   development; Normal sexual development;
   Dental development; Mental development

2 Behaviour and Learning Problems 36
   Common behaviour problems; Sleep
   problems; Habit spasms (tics); Hyperactive
   child; School refusal; Dyslexia; Autism

3 Fever; Infectious Disease; Immunisations 58

4 Nutrition 85
   Infant feeding; Iron deficiency anaemia;
   Rickets; Obesity; Anorexia nervosa

5 The Diabetic Child 103

6 Alimentary Tract Problems 121
   Coeliac disease; Cystic fibrosis;
   Gastroenteritis; Toddler diarrhoea; Gastro-
   oesophageal reflux; Pyloric stenosis;
   Constipation and encopresis; Infantile colic;
   Periodic syndrome; Threadworms

7 Miscellaneous Abdominal Problems 155
   Appendicitis; Inguinal hernia; Umbilical
   hernia; Hydrocele

8 Kidney and Genitalia Problems 160
   Nephrotic syndrome; Urinary infections;
   Undescended testis; Torsion of the testis;
   Hypospadias; Circumcision; Vaginal
   discharge

9 Enuresis 173
10 Heart and Chest Problems 182
Common heart murmurs; Asthma;
Bronchiolitis; Pneumonia
11 Ear, Nose, Throat and Eye Problems 213
Otitis media; Glue ear; Nose bleeds; Sinusitis;
Sore throat; Croup; Squint; Sticky eye;
Conjunctivitis; Styes; Allergic rhinitis
12 Skin Problems 236
Eczema; Scabies; Lice; Spots and rashes;
Warts; Mouth conditions
13 Bone and Joint Problems 256
Growing pains; Arthritis; Unstable hip;
Talipes; 'Pigeon' toes; Knock knee; Flat feet;
Congenital torticollis; Scoliosis
14 Neurological Problems 276
Epilepsy; Febrile convulsions; Migraine;
Meningitis; Cerebral palsy; Muscular
dystrophy
15 Jaundice and other Blood Disorders 308
16 Some Birth Abnormalities 317
Spina bifida; Cleft lip and palate; Down's
syndrome
17 Miscellaneous Problems 337
Accidental poisoning; Cot (crib) death;
Enlarged glands
Useful addresses 350
Selected Reading 359
Index 363

Preface

Shortly after starting work with children and their parents it became apparent to me that communication could be improved if instructions or information were given in both oral and written form. As an aid to communication in my everyday practice I started writing a series of leaflets on common conditions affecting children. The encouraging response from parents together with frequent requests for leaflets from nurses, medical students and health education departments prompted me to update them and gather them together in the form of a book.

I have tried to write this book in a way that could easily be understood by both the layman and the professional. If information on a particular topic is omitted or not sufficiently detailed I would suggest that further information be obtained by using the 'useful addresses' section of the book. In Britain the Health Education Authority provides well written and beautifully illustrated material free of charge on a wide range of subjects such as pregnancy, infant feeding and accident prevention.

Throughout the text I have used the word paediatrician: a paediatrician is a doctor who has specialised in diseases of children. In accordance with convention, in the greater part of the text the child has been referred to as 'he', but could equally have been called 'she'.

I hope that this book will be helpful in removing some of the mysticism and confusion of paediatrics.

September, 1986

Acknowledgements

I should like to thank my secretary, Mrs Jennifer Holden, for her patience and the many hours she spent typing the manuscript, not to mention the innumerable spelling mistakes she corrected. I am indebted to Miss P. A. Downie, Medical and Nursing Editor, Faber and Faber, for her invaluable help and advice in bringing this book to fruition.

Others to whom I am grateful for assisting me or providing material are Lynne Ainsworth, Jean Muskett, John Fallows, David Smith, Colgate Palmolive and N. H. Eastwood and Son.

I am particularly grateful to those parents and their children who have helped me by allowing the use of photographs to illustrate some sections. To Mrs A. Besterman I am indebted for the line drawings.

Lastly, but not least, I thank my wife for her encouragement and help.

Chapter 1

Growth and Development

THE SHORT CHILD

Most children with short stature are referred to a paediatrician for one of three reasons:

1. Parents notice that the child is shorter than his contemporaries and become concerned that he may be too short.
2. The child may be teased and becomes shy, self-conscious or withdrawn and parents seek advice.
3. At a school medical or some other medical review it is noted that the child is short or is not growing as well as he should.

The vast majority of children referred to a paediatrician are short because their parents are short and/or they are 'late developers'. The latter comprise children whose sexual development occurs later than average. Investigations are seldom necessary. On seeing a short child a paediatrician is required to determine whether a problem exists and, if so, whether it can be remedied. This task has become very much easier as a result of the many growth charts which are now available. These charts, which express a year in decimals (Figs. 1/1, 1/2), are divided into 'centiles'; each represents a percentage of the normal population. For example, a height on the 50th centile for a particular age means that half the children of that age will be above and half below that height. There are many reasons why a child may be short and the diagnostic approach adopted by most paediatricians requires that a number of pertinent questions about the child and his family be asked.

1. Is he abnormally small?

The answer can be obtained from charts in Figures 1/1 and 1/2. Short

1

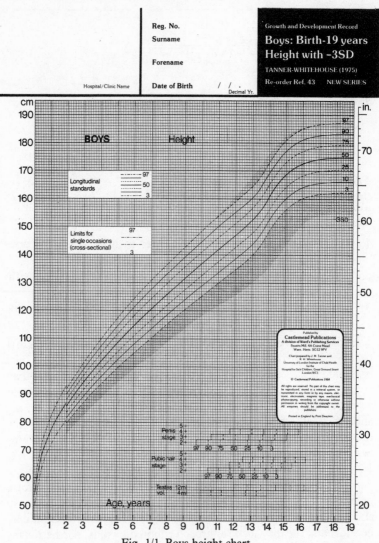

Fig. 1/1 Boys height chart

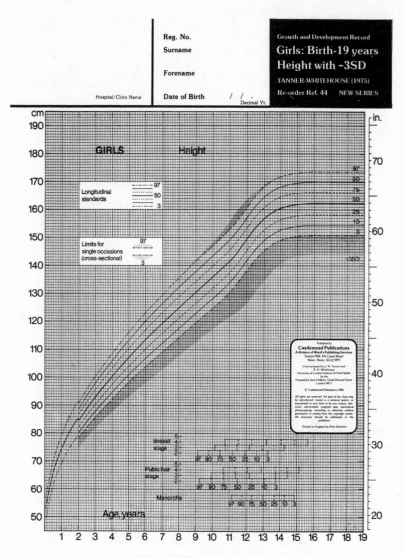

Fig. 1/2 Girls height chart

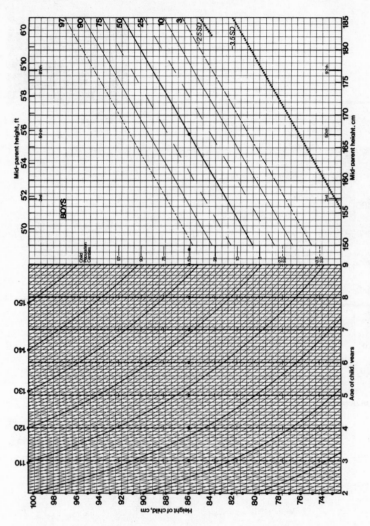

Fig. 1/3 Boys height chart allowing for parents' height

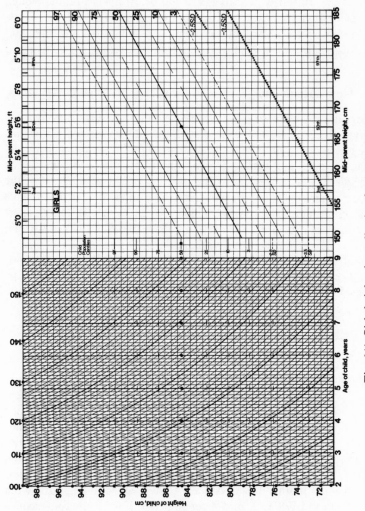

Fig. 1/4 Girls height chart allowing for parents' height

stature is arbitrarily defined as a height below the 3rd centile though by definition 3% of the population are normal. The 3SD line is the line above which 100% of the population should fall and any child with a height below this line is abnormal and requires investigation.

2. How does the height compare with that of his parents?

For children between 2–9 this answer can be obtained from charts in Figures 1/3 and 1/4. On the left the child's age is plotted against height. At the point where the age and height lines meet, a horizontal line is drawn and extended across the right side of the chart. The child's height in relation to the parents' height is indicated at the point where the mid-parent height (the sum of the parents' heights halved) intersects the horizontal line. All children with genetic short stature (short parents) have a height above the –3.5SD line. A height below this line or between –2.5 and –3.5SD lines strongly suggests another cause for the short stature and requires further investigation.

Because of the variation in growth above age 9 it has not been possible to compile charts, and judgement must be based on common sense.

3. What is his adult height likely to be?

By plotting the parents' height on charts in Figures 1/1, 1/2 it is possible to predict the child's adult height. In the case of a boy 13cm should be added to the mother's height before it is plotted, while for a girl 13cm should be subtracted from the father's height. The midpoint of the distance between the parents' heights is called the mid-parental height: 95% of children will have an adult height 8.5cm on either side of this point. For example, a girl whose father measures 185cm and mother 168cm is likely to have an adult height between 161.5cm and 178.5cm (mid-parental height 170cm). By comparing a child's current height with his predicted adult height it should soon become clear which children are shorter than would be expected on the basis of their parental height.

4. Is he growing at a normal rate?

The answer to this question can only be accurately obtained by taking

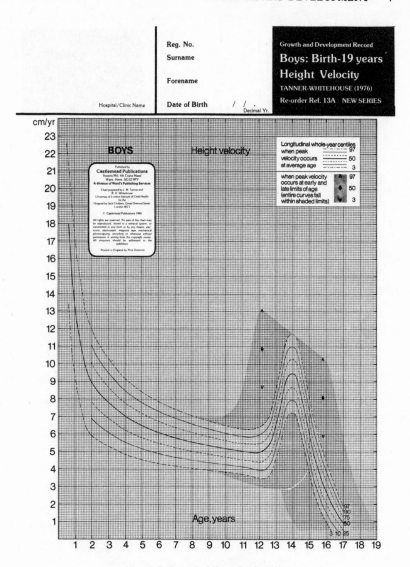

Fig. 1/5 Boys height velocity chart

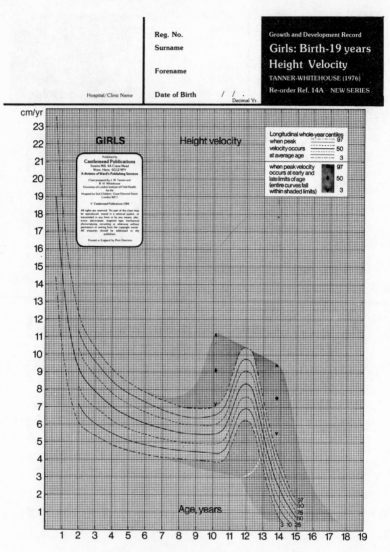

Fig. 1/6 Girls height velocity chart

repeated measurements over a period of at least a year so that the number of centimetres gained per year can be calculated. Between 3 and onset of puberty the *variation* in centimetres (cm) gained each year is seldom more than 2. The number of cm gained per year is called the growth velocity and should be plotted on charts in Figures 1/5, 1/6. For example, heights measured at 4 and 6 years show a difference of 12cm. Velocity is 6cm/year which should be plotted at age 5. The growth spurt is related to sexual development, the earlier the development the greater the spurt. The shaded part of the chart allows for both early and late developers. A growth velocity below the 25th centile in children with a height between the 3rd centile and 3SD line on charts in Figures 1/1, 1/2, requires further investigation.

5. At what stage is his sexual development or is there a family history of late onset of puberty?

See sexual development (p. 17). A short child who is a 'late developer' may appear much shorter than his peers who are having a growth spurt in the early teens. This can cause short children very much unhappiness. The time of onset of puberty is in part genetically determined. In a short child who is seen before puberty a history of late onset of menstruation in the mother or a late growth spurt and delayed need to shave in the father would suggest that the child is likely to be a 'late developer'.

6. Does he look normal?

Short children who look abnormal can be divided into two groups; those with abnormal body proportions (shortening or lengthening of trunk or limbs) and those who have a 'syndrome' (abnormal physical features). Charts are available for determining normal body proportions and bone x-rays help with the diagnosis of these conditions. Syndromes can usually be identified by the physical appearance of the child.

7. Has he always been a healthy child?

Events before birth can influence subsequent growth. There are various reasons why a baby may not grow normally in the womb. A small percentage of 'undergrown' babies continue their slow growth throughout childhood. Heart, lung and kidney disease and thyroid deficiency can cause stunting of growth, as can malabsorption and malnutrition.

8. What are his home conditions like?

Children who are unhappy and emotionally deprived do not grow normally. Although the reason is not clear, it would seem that diminished food intake contributes to their growth failure. Studies have shown that social deprivation is the commonest cause of short stature in the United Kingdom.

These questions having been asked, the paediatrician will have made a decision about which children should be investigated and which should continue to be observed. The investigations selected will depend on what is considered to be the most likely cause for the short stature. For example, if kidney disease or thyroid deficiency are suspected tests will be arranged to exclude them. In girls with unexplained short stature a genetic blood (chromosome) test is usually done.

An x-ray of the left wrist may be taken so that 'bone age' can be estimated. Throughout childhood bones are maturing and when they are fully developed in the late teens growth ceases. The rate at which bones mature varies considerably; it is not uncommon for a 12-year-old 'late developer' to have a bone age of a 9- or 10-year-old. The main advantage in knowing the extent to which the bones have matured is that it assists the paediatrician in predicting the child's eventual height.

Growth hormone tests: About 1 in 5000 children are born with growth hormone deficiency. There are numerous tests to detect growth hormone deficiency; all stimulate the brain to produce a rise in growth hormone to a level more than 15mU/1, without which the child cannot be passed as normal. The tests can be divided into those producing a rise in growth hormone by a natural stimulus or a drug. Natural stimulus tests consist of taking blood for growth hormone during deep sleep or after strenuous exercise. The drugs most commonly used to stimulate a rise in growth hormone are clonidine, arginine and insulin.

If growth hormone deficiency is diagnosed early (before school age) treatment with growth hormone can restore the child to his expected height. Late treatment, say at about 9, restores only two-thirds of the height loss. Until very recently growth hormone required extraction from the human brain at post-mortem and consequently was in short supply. This limited supply was only sufficient to provide for the needs of those children with proven growth hormone deficiency. Growth hormone is now manufactured and has become widely available. In 1985 treatment with human growth hormone was stopped in Britain and the USA after reports of a rare dementing brain disease in young persons previously treated with growth hormone. There are some children who are short and grow slowly yet have normal growth hormone tests. There is now good evidence that some of these children despite normal tests do benefit from growth hormone. Unfortunately, at present there is no way of knowing which children are likely to respond, the only way of finding out is to give a course of growth hormone and gauge the response. Not yet knowing the percentage likely to respond, such an approach could be regarded as an expensive gamble in view of the high cost of the hormone.

Children who are genetically short and are late developers sometimes become miserable and very concerned about their height in the early teens. Steroid hormones are drugs which are used to bring on the growth spurt and temporarily improve the height, however they have the disadvantage of causing a reduction in final height. This is a serious drawback which has greatly limited their use. Although there is some recent evidence that low doses would be more acceptable, it would seem much more sensible to attend to the psychological needs of these children rather than give them hormones.

Finally, height is but one of many attributes of the child; those who are short are compensated in a variety of other ways.

FAILURE TO THRIVE

About 1 in 20 hospital admissions are for failure to thrive. Put simply, failure to thrive means that the child is not gaining weight as well as he should, or he is losing weight.

What is the 'normal' rate at which a baby should gain weight?

After birth many babies lose as much as 10% of birth weight. By 7–10 days this is regained and thereafter there should be a steady increase. Weight charts should be available at all community clinics where each child should be weighed naked and his weight plotted at regular intervals to determine whether he is thriving. Two such charts, which are suitable for premature babies and children up to 2 are shown in Figures 1/7 and 1/8. The numbers on the right (3–97) represent the percentage of the normal population. Information about the use of decimal age is shown in Figure 1/9.

Why do some infants not thrive?

There are many reasons why a child does not thrive, the most common being that he is not getting enough nourishment. The reason why he is not getting enough most often relates to feeding and/or social problems. Other common causes for failure to thrive are illness and loss of nourishment through vomiting or malabsorption.

Children who get enough food but do not retain it can usually be identified by a history of diarrhoea or vomiting. Those who get enough and retain it but do not thrive 'burn up' energy at an increased rate. Chronic infections, heart, liver or kidney disease all cause excess energy to be burned up.

Certain infants who are undergrown at birth, particularly those with genetic abnormalities, may continue to gain weight at a slow rate throughout childhood. The reason for this is not clear.

The social problems are many and varied. They may be associated with difficulties in the family, the mother or child. Some of the more common maternal causes are illness, depression, anxiety, physical or emotional exhaustion. Illness in the child, particularly where there has been a prolonged separation between mother and child, may produce bonding difficulties and failure to thrive. Of the family problems the two which stand out are marital conflict and stress – financial, unemployment or whatever.

What does the paediatrician do?

He should take a detailed medical, feeding and social history. A thorough examination will be made to exclude any physical abnormality. To highlight when the problem originated parents should give him all the weight measurements since birth together with the relevant dates. Usually there is no obvious cause and the paediatrician will arrange for the child to be admitted to hospital.

What happens in hospital?

This depends on whether the mother stays with the child. If the

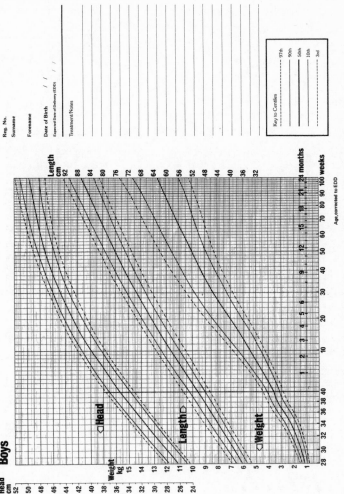

Fig. 1/7 Boys: Preterm to 2 years, length, weight and head circumference

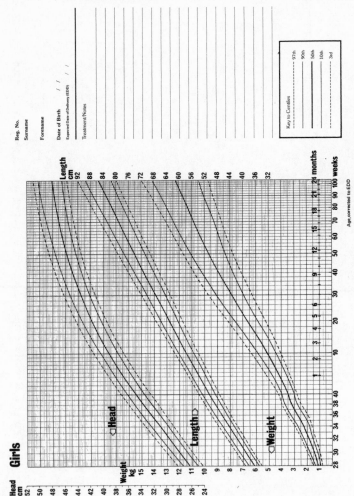

Fig. 1/8 Girls: Preterm to 2 years, length, weight and head circumference

TABLE OF DECIMALS OF YEAR

	1 JAN.	2 FEB.	3 MAR.	4 APR.	5 MAY	6 JUNE	7 JULY	8 AUG.	9 SEPT.	10 OCT.	11 NOV.	12 DEC.
1	000	085	162	247	329	414	496	581	666	748	833	915
2	003	088	164	249	332	416	499	584	668	751	836	918
3	005	090	167	252	334	419	501	586	671	753	838	921
4	008	093	170	255	337	422	504	589	674	756	841	923
5	011	096	173	258	340	425	507	592	677	759	844	926
6	014	099	175	260	342	427	510	595	679	762	847	929
7	016	101	178	263	345	430	512	597	682	764	849	932
8	019	104	181	266	348	433	515	600	685	767	852	934
9	022	107	184	268	351	436	518	603	688	770	855	937
10	025	110	186	271	353	438	521	605	690	773	858	940
11	027	112	189	274	356	441	523	608	693	775	860	942
12	030	115	192	277	359	444	526	611	696	778	863	945
13	033	118	195	279	362	447	529	614	699	781	866	948
14	036	121	197	282	364	449	532	616	701	784	868	951
15	038	123	200	285	367	452	534	619	704	786	871	953
16	041	126	203	288	370	455	537	622	707	789	874	956
17	044	129	205	290	373	458	540	625	710	792	877	959
18	047	132	208	293	375	460	542	627	712	795	879	962
19	049	134	211	296	378	463	545	630	715	797	882	964
20	052	137	214	299	381	466	548	633	718	800	885	967
21	055	140	216	301	384	468	551	636	721	803	888	970
22	058	142	219	304	386	471	553	638	723	805	890	973
23	060	145	222	307	389	474	556	641	726	808	893	975
24	063	148	225	310	392	477	559	644	729	811	896	978
25	066	151	227	312	395	479	562	647	731	814	899	981
26	068	153	230	315	397	482	564	649	734	816	901	984
27	071	156	233	318	400	485	567	652	737	819	904	986
28	074	159	236	321	403	488	570	655	740	822	907	989
29	077		238	323	405	490	573	658	742	825	910	992
30	079		241	326	408	493	575	660	745	827	912	995
31	082		244		411		578	663		830		997

Fig. 1/9 Decimal table. In this table decimal age has been used. The year is divided into 10, not 12. Each date in the calendar is marked (from the table) in terms of thousandths of the year. Thus January 7th 1962 is 62.016. The child's birth date is similarly recorded, e.g. a child born on June 23rd 1959 has the birth day 59.474. Age at examination is then obtained by simple subtraction, e.g. 62.016 − 59.474 = 2.542, and the last figure is rounded off. This system greatly facilitates the computing of velocities, since the proportion of the year between 2 examinations is easily calculated

child is fed by the mother nursing staff will closely supervise feeding, alternatively nurses will feed the child. Weight measurements will be regularly recorded. A breast-feeding mother may be convinced that her infant is not getting enough. Insufficient breast milk as a cause for failure to thrive is indeed rare but does occur. When this situation arises I have found three ways of dealing with it:

1. The easiest is to give bottle (formula) feeds and stop breast feeding.
2. Continue breast feeding but 'top up' with the bottle (formula) after each feed.
3. Express breast milk and feed it by bottle temporarily (a day or two) to prove that the volume is sufficient.

'Test feeds' (weighing before and after breast feeds) require weighing at each feed over a 24-hour period. I seldom recommend this because it only serves to increase maternal anxiety and, furthermore, heightened anxiety may itself cause less milk to be produced.

What tests are done in hospital?

Only very basic investigations are done; blood and urine tests to screen for anaemia, kidney disease and infection. Tests for malabsorption (sweat test and intestinal biopsy) are sometimes required (see pp. 122, 125). These tests cause no discomfort. A sweat test involves collecting sweat on a piece of paper after which it is analysed. During an intestinal biopsy a small capsule attached to a thin feeding tube is swallowed, then a small part of the lining of the bowel is sucked into the capsule. The capsule is withdrawn and the lining (mucosa) is examined in the laboratory.

What is the further management?

Some children still do not gain weight while in hospital and after being fully investigated are discharged. Although the reason may not be found and may be social, parents at least have the satisfaction of knowing that there is no physical cause. Where a physical abnormality or malabsorption are found the infant is given the appropriate treatment.

Most children gain weight on the ward and continue to gain weight after discharge. These children require no more than a few weight measurements over the following months.

When children gain weight in hospital but fail to do so after discharge then family help is required. The type of help depends on the nature of the problem, which is almost always social. Besides the family doctor and the paediatrician the family may require help from other professionals such as dietitians, health visitors, social workers, psychiatrists or psychologists.

In conclusion, in Britain, where food is plentiful, failure to thrive accounts for about 5% of hospital admissions. It is seldom a serious problem and the cause is mostly of a social nature.

PHYSICAL DEVELOPMENT

Size at birth depends on sex, birth sequence and mother's size. In general boys are bigger than girls, second and subsequent births are bigger than the first-born child in a family. The father's genetic influence on size comes into effect towards the second birthday, the ultimate size being equally influenced by father and mother.

The normal rate of growth (height and weight) throughout childhood is shown in Figures 1/1, 1/2, 1/10, 1/11. Figures 1/7 and 1/8 show normal growth of a premature baby and also include the normal rate of head growth in the first two years.

The head contains two dimples (fontanelles), the back one closes at about 2–3 months and the front one at about 18 months, closure may occur much earlier or later. Occasionally children have a third fontanelle between the front and back. It is quite common to see flattening of one side of the head and bulging of the opposite side, particularly in premature infants. This worries parents: it is caused by the baby's lying with his head predominantly on one side. The head assumes a normal shape between the first and second year. When assessing the size of a baby's head it is always important to take into consideration the size of the baby and the parents' head size. A big baby will obviously have a big head, while the opposite applies to a small baby. If a parent has an unusually large or small head the child could quite naturally be expected to have a very big or very small head.

NORMAL SEXUAL DEVELOPMENT

The various stages of puberty have been standardised by Professor J. M. Tanner and co-workers at the Hospital for Sick Children, London. These standards which are now used internationally are described below. Figure 1/12 shows the ages at which the stages of pubertal development are attained together with testicular size, age of menstruation and peak height velocity (fastest rate of growth). The size of the testes is expressed as a volume (ml). In order to estimate accurately the size, paediatricians use a string of plastic models of different sizes for comparison.

Parents may be concerned when breast development is more advanced on one side; this does occasionally happen but is quite normal. Boys at the time of puberty often have some breast enlargement and tenderness. This may cause anxiety; reassurance is all that is required. Puberty which occurs too early or unduly late requires referral to a paediatrician.

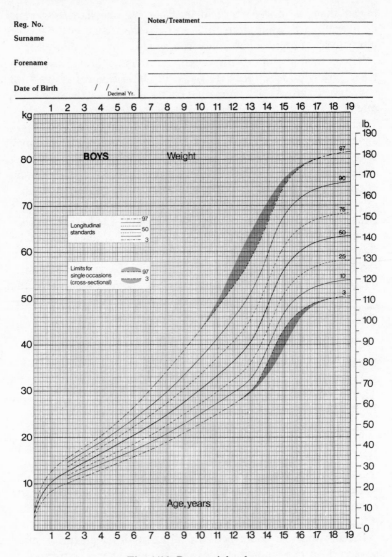

Fig. 1/10 Boys weight chart

Reg. No.

Surname

Forename

Date of Birth   /   /   .
                         Decimal Yr.

Notes/Treatment _____

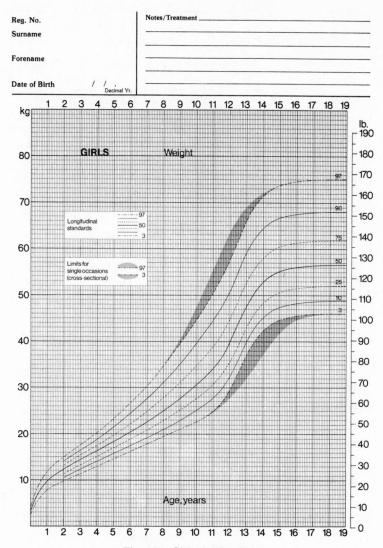

Fig. 1/11 Girls weight chart

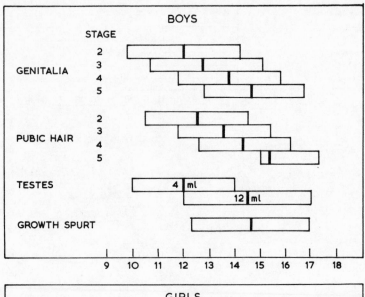

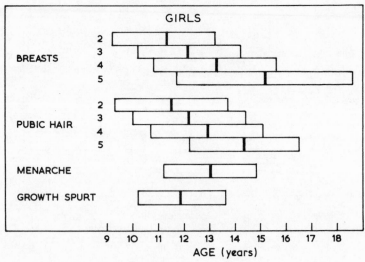

Fig. 1/12 Timing of events in puberty

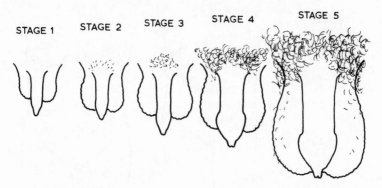

Fig. 1/13 Stages of pubic hair and genital development in boys

BOYS: GENITAL DEVELOPMENT (Fig. 1/13)

Stage 1. Pre-adolescent: the testes, scrotum and penis are of about the same size and proportions as in early childhood.

Stage 2. Enlargement of the scrotum and testes. The skin of the scrotum reddens and changes in texture. Little or no enlargement of the penis.

Stage 3. Lengthening of the penis. Further growth of the testes and scrotum.

Stage 4. Increase in breadth of the penis and development of the glans. The testes and scrotum are larger; the scrotum darkens.

Stage 5. Adult.

BOYS: PUBIC HAIR (Fig. 1/13)

Stage 1. Pre-adolescent: no pubic hair.

Stage 2. Sparse growth of slightly pigmented downy hair chiefly at the base of the penis.

Stage 3. Hair darker, coarser and more curled, spreading sparsely over the junction of the pubes.

Stage 4. Hair adult in type, but covering a considerably smaller area than in the adult. No spread to the inner surface of the thighs.

Stage 5. Adult quantity and type with distribution of a horizontal pattern and spread to the inner surface of the thighs. Spread up the lower abdomen is late and rated Stage 6.

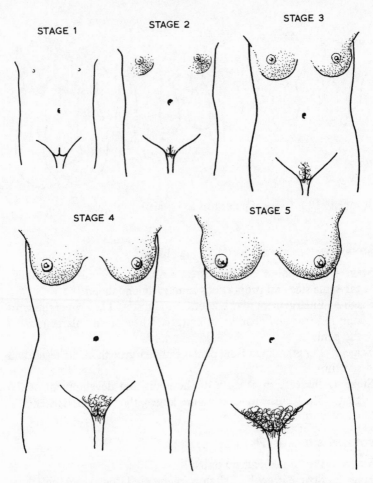

Fig. 1/14 Stages of breast and pubic hair development in girls

GIRLS: BREAST DEVELOPMENT (Fig. 1/14)

Stage 1. Pre-adolescent: elevation of the papilla (nipple) only.

Stage 2. Breast bud stage. Elevation of the breast and papilla as a small mound. Enlargement of the areola (darkened ring around the nipple) diameter.

Stage 3. Further enlargement and elevation of the breast and areola, with no separation of their contours.

Stage 4. Projection of the areola and papilla above the level of the breast.

Stage 5. Mature stage, projection of the papilla alone due to recession of the areola.

GIRLS: PUBIC HAIR (Fig. 1/14)

Stage 1. Pre-adolescent: no pubic hair.

Stage 2. Sparse growth of slightly pigmented downy hair chiefly along the labia.

Stage 3. Hair darker, coarser and more curled, spreading sparsely over the junction of the pubes.

Stage 4. Hair adult in type, but covering a considerably smaller area than in the adult. No spread to the inner surface of the thighs.

Stage 5. Adult quantity and type with distribution of a horizontal pattern and spread to the inner surface of the thighs. Spread up the lower abdomen is late and rated Stage 6.

DENTAL DEVELOPMENT

Dental development is similar to other development in that it shows a wide range of variation and is more advanced in girls. Those primary teeth which erupt first are usually the first to fall out: the first and second incisors (A and B) generally erupt between 6–13 months and are followed by the first premolar (C) between 12 and 15 months. Canines (D) erupt between 16–18 months and second premolars (E) between 2–3 years when primary dentition (20 teeth) is complete (Fig. 1/15). Starting at about 6 the permanent teeth begin to appear. The first molars are usually the first to appear and, as they appear behind the premolars (primary teeth) and do not replace any teeth, they are often mistaken for primary teeth. Most children have 28 permanent teeth by age 13. The third molars (wisdom teeth) erupt from age 17 onwards giving a full complement of 32 permanent teeth (Fig. 1/16).

Are babies born with teeth?

Yes, about 1 in 2000 are born with incisors. If these teeth are firm they should not be removed. Removal is required for loose teeth so that they are not inhaled by the baby.

How can we help the teething baby?

Teething causes discomfort which produces irritability and crying. It does little else, so if your child is unwell do not blame it on teething without first obtaining medical advice. Painful gums may be helped if

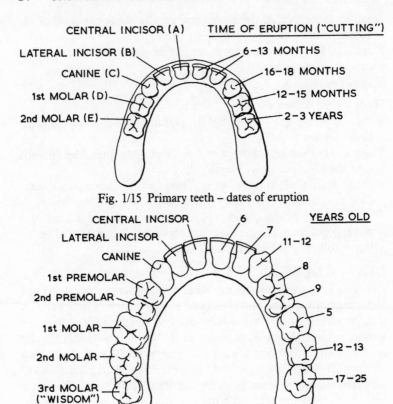

Fig. 1/15 Primary teeth – dates of eruption

Fig. 1/16 Permanent teeth

the child sucks a firm, hard object such as a plastic ring or sugar-free rusk. Gum applications are not very helpful for they provide temporary relief only, they are soon washed away by the baby's saliva. Sugar-free paracetamol (acetominophen (USA)) given from time to time does seem to provide the most effective pain relief.

MENTAL DEVELOPMENT

Development is a continuous process from conception to maturity, being more rapid in females. At birth it is never possible to be certain that a child will not have a mental or physical handicap. Only by monitoring the child's development with time can doctors and health visitors be sure that he is normal. For this purpose developmental screening charts have been devised. Besides innate ability the rate at which a normal child develops depends on both familial factors and his environment.

Most schemes for the assessment of development are divided into 4 categories:

1. Posture and large movements
2. Vision and fine movements
3. Hearing and speech
4. Social behaviour and play

A categorised chart enables the examiner to highlight quickly specific areas of development delay. It is important to realise that the child who is mentally subnormal is late in *all* categories, except occasionally in posture and large movements (sitting and walking). A delay of only or mainly movement (large and fine) suggests a defect of the movement part of the brain, a condition known as cerebral palsy (spasticity) (see p. 297).

The developmental charts provided on the following pages are based on the average age of attainment of each skill. For example, the average age of walking alone is 13 months; this means that at that age as many as 50% will be able to walk alone.

The sequence of development is the same for all children, but the rate varies from child to child. When assessing a child's development due consideration should always be given to the wide range of normal variation. The average child of 8 months sits without support, however, sitting alone at 5 months or 12 months may both be normal. How then do we define normal? There is no fine line which enables one to distinguish normal from abnormal, suffice to say that the farther away from the average the more likely to be abnormal. Development is not necessarily a smooth continuous process. There may be lulls and spurts with different skills developing at different rates. A 2-year-old who runs, builds a tower of 6–7 bricks, puts on his shoes and socks yet utters no more than 2–3 words may be quite normal. How does prematurity affect development: will a child born 3 months early remain 3 months behind? These questions are often asked by parents. Given the wide normal variation in development plus the marked difference in exposure to stimuli before and after birth the child's development may or may not be appropriate for the age *since birth*. A child born 3 months early and seen at 9 months may have developed to a level compatible with 6 or 9 months; both are normal. After the first 12–18 months the effect of prematurity pales into insignificance.

Development charts are *not* a test of the child's IQ (intelligence quotient); they are merely screening tests to detect a physical or mental handicap so that appropriate help can be given to the child and his family as early as possible. The charts which have been constructed here are based on studies of British children by the late Dr Mary Sheridan. There is no pass or fail; the average child should be able to perform two thirds of the skills at each age.

When assessing a child the performance may be affected by factors such as tiredness, hunger, separation from parents, strange surroundings or illness. At times some children are just awkward and refuse to co-operate. For these reasons paediatricians prefer to make assessments in an unhurried relaxed atmosphere in surroundings which are as natural as possible. A 5-minute assessment in a noisy outpatient clinic is often a fruitless exercise. Assessments are most reliable when made on a few occasions over a number of months.

What is the Denver Developmental Screening Test?

It is a screening test that was produced in America in the 1960s and is now widely used by child health clinics and paediatricians throughout the world. It is very easy to apply and unlike the Sheridan method used in these tables, it has the advantage of showing the percentage of children attaining each skill at a particular age. A revised version which is even simpler to use has recently been produced. In the UK copies of the test may be obtained from:

The Test Agency, Cournswood House, North Dean, High Wycombe, Bucks; telephone: 024024 3384.

When should the child be toilet trained?

Most children can be toilet trained between 18 months and 2½ years. Bowel control is usually achieved earlier than bladder control. There is no simple rule about when to start, each child is different. The following three guidelines should be considered before starting:
1. The child should be physically mature enough to feel when he needs to go and should be capable of controlling himself. This is seldom possible much before 18 months.
2. The child should be mentally mature enough to communicate his need to go.

3. The child should be emotionally mature enough to want to please and to revel in praise.

Toilet training should be undertaken in a relaxed, patient manner. Be lavish with your praise when he performs in the potty. Be prepared for accidents; when they occur you may feel frustrated, but try not to become exasperated. A child who senses your annoyance for something he really cannot help may become upset and refuse to co-operate.

6 WEEKS

Posture and Large Movements
When lifted or pulled to sit, head falls loosely backwards.
Held sitting, head falls forward, with back in one complete curve.
When lying on front, chin intermittently lifted off couch.

Vision and Fine Movements
Turns head and eyes towards light.
Follows with eyes through range of about a quarter of circle.

Hearing and Speech
Startled by loud noises.
Movements momentarily stopped in response to noise such as ringing of a bell.

Social Behaviour and Play
Smiles in response to overtures from the mother.

3 MONTHS

Posture and Large Movements
Held sitting, back nearly straight, head erect and steady for several seconds before bobbing forward.
When lying on front, takes weight on forearms and lifts upper part of chest off couch.

Vision and Fine Movements
Moves eyes from side to side through half a circle.
Watches movements of hands.

Hearing and Speech
Sudden loud noises still cause distress, causing blinking, screwing up of eyes or crying.

May turn eyes and head towards sound.

Social Behaviour and Play
Holds objects for a few moments when placed in hands.

6 MONTHS

Posture and Large Movements
Held sitting, head is firmly erect and back quite straight.
When lying on front lifts head and chest well up, supporting himself
    on extended arms.
Rolls over, front to back (sometimes back to front).

Vision and Fine Movements
Moves head and eyes eagerly in every direction.
When toys fall out of sight forgets them.
Follows adults' movements across room.

Hearing and Speech
Turns immediately to mother's voice across room.
Laughs, chuckles and squeals aloud in play.
Turns to minimal sound (e.g. rattle) at ear level.
Vocalises well 'words' such as ba, ka, muh, goo, der, adah.

Social Behaviour and Play
Reaches out for objects and puts everything in mouth.
Puts hands to bottle and pats it when feeding.
Feeds self a biscuit.
Not yet shy with strangers.
Likes to be picked up and played with.

9 MONTHS

Posture and Large Movements
Sits alone.
Moves about by rolling or squirming.
Tries to crawl, may succeed.
Pulls to stand holding on to support for a few moments, but cannot
    lower himself. Falls backwards with bump.

Vision and Fine Movements
Pokes at small sweet with index finger and beginning to point at more
    distant objects with same finger.

Picks up small sweet between finger and thumb with pincer grip.
Searches in correct direction for toys which have fallen out of sight
  (e.g. over edge of table or cot).

Hearing and Speech
Vocalises deliberately by imitating speech sounds – sounds repeated
  e.g. ma-ma, da-da, ba-ba.
Shouts for attention, listens, then shouts again.
Responds to minimal sound both below and above the level of the
  ear.
Understands 'no-no' and 'bye-bye'.

Social Behaviour and Play
Holds, bites and chews a biscuit.
Now quite aware of strangers who make him feel frightened or shy.
  He may cling to his parents and hide his face.
Plays peek-a-boo and imitates hand clapping.
Works for toy out of reach.
Resists when toy is taken away.

12 MONTHS

Posture and Large Movements
Crawls rapidly on all fours.
Holding onto furniture pulls to standing and lets himself down
  again.
Stepping sideways, cruises around furniture.
Walks with one or both hands held.
May stand alone for a few seconds.
May walk alone.

Vision and Fine Movements
Picks up small objects, e.g. raisin or sweet, with very precise pincer
  grasp of thumb and index finger.
Starts casting, drops and throws toys deliberately and watches them
  fall to the ground.
Points with index finger at objects which he wants or which interest
  him.
Prolonged intent regard for people, animals and cars.
Bangs 2 bricks together.

Hearing and Speech
Knows and immediately turns to own name.

Understands simple instructions associated with gesture such as 'say
   bye-bye', 'clap hands', 'give it to Mummy', 'come to Daddy'.
Demonstrates definition-by-use of everyday objects, e.g. combs hair
   with comb, or rubs shoes with shoe brush.

Social Behaviour and Play
Drinks from cup with little assistance.
Holds spoon but cannot yet use it by himself.
Helps with dressing by holding out arm for sleeve and foot for shoe.
Stops 'mouthing' objects.
Quickly finds brick hidden under cup while watching.
Says 'bye-bye' on request, sometimes spontaneously.

15 MONTHS

Posture and Large Movements
Walks alone (about 10% of children never crawl, and walk late. At
   the usual age of walking these children shuffle on their hands and
   bottoms and are known as 'shufflers'. Shuffling commonly runs in
   families).
Creeps upstairs safely, and sometimes gets downstairs backwards,
   slowly.

Vision and Fine Movements
Builds tower of 2 bricks.
Looks with interest at pictures in book and pats page.

Hearing and Speech
Speaks 3 or more recognisable words (other than 'Mummy' or
   'Daddy').
Points to familiar persons, animals, toys when requested.

Social Behaviour and Play
Holds spoon, brings it to mouth and licks it, but cannot prevent it
   from turning over.
Physically restless and intensely curious.
Needs constant supervision to protect from danger.

18 MONTHS

Posture and Large Movements
Walks well with feet only slightly apart, starts and stops safely.
Pushes and pulls large toys and boxes round floor.

Walks upstairs and sometimes downstairs with helping hand.
Runs carefully 2–3 metres.
Climbs on to chairs.

Vision and Fine Movements
Scribbles to and fro.
Builds tower of 3 bricks.
Beginning to show preference for one hand.
Enjoys simple picture books, often recognising and putting finger on
    boldly-coloured items on page.
Turns pages several at a time.

Hearing and Speech
Points to eyes, mouth and nose.
Uses more than 6 recognisable words and understands many more.
Enjoys nursery rhymes and tries to join in.
Obeys simple commands such as 'shut the door', 'get Teddy', 'fetch
    shoes'.

Social Behaviour and Play
Holds spoon and gets food safely to mouth.
Holds cup between both hands, drinks without much spilling.
Takes off shoes, socks and hat, but cannot replace.
Casting objects to floor now much less, mainly in anger or play.
Emotionally still very dependent upon familiar adult, especially
    mother.

2 YEARS

Posture and Large Movements
Runs safely, starting and stopping and avoiding obstacles.
Walks upstairs and (often) down, holding on to rail or wall; two feet
    to a step.
Throws small ball forwards overhand without falling.
Walks into large ball when trying to kick it.
Sits on small bicycle, but unable to use pedals. Pushes forward with
    feet on floor.

Vision and Fine Movements
Builds a tower of 6 or 7 bricks.
Hand preference now obvious.
Imitates vertical line.

Enjoys picture books, recognising fine details in favourite pictures.
Turns book pages singly.

Hearing and Speech
Uses 50 or more recognisable words.
Puts 2 or more words together to form simple sentences.
Refers to self by name.
Talks to self as he plays, but much still incomprehensible to others.
Constantly asking names of objects and people.
Joins in nursery rhymes and songs.

Social Behaviour and Play
Asks for food and drink.
Able to put on shoes, socks and hat.
Imitates domestic activities, e.g. ironing.
Clings tightly in affection, fatigue or fear.
Resistive and rebellious when thwarted.
Has, as yet, no idea of sharing toys or adults' attention.
Plays happily near other children, but not with them.

2½ YEARS

Posture and Large Movements
Walks upstairs confidently and (usually) downstairs holding rail, 2
    feet to step.
Can jump with 2 feet together from low step.
Throws hand ball somewhat stiffly at body level. Kicks large ball, in
    a gentle and lopsided fashion.
Pushes and pulls large toys with some skill.

Vision and Fine Movements
Recognises minute details in picture books.
Picks up 'hundreds and thousands'.
Draws horizontal line.

Hearing and Speech
Uses 200 or more recognisable words. Now able to use plurals.
Knows full name.
Continually asking questions beginning 'what', 'who'.
Uses pronouns, I, me and you, correctly.
Thoughts may come quicker than he can say them, causing him to
    stutter or stammer.

Social Behaviour and Play
Eats skilfully with spoon and fork.
Washes and dries hands under supervision.
Pulls down pants at toilet but seldom able to pull them up again.
Active and curious with little notion of common dangers.
Engages in simple make-believe play.
Enjoys picture books and stories.

3 YEARS

Posture and Large Movements
Walks alone upstairs with alternating feet and downstairs two feet to
    a step.
Able to give broad jump over length of adult shoes.
Can stand and walk on tiptoe.
Stands on 1 foot for 1 second.
Rides tricycle using pedals.

Vision and Fine Movements
Builds tower of 9 bricks.
Copies circle.
Draws man with head and usually indication of one or two other fea-
    tures or parts.
Matches 2–3 colours.
May know names of colours.

Hearing and Speech
Gives full name, sex and sometimes age.
Carries on simple conversations and verbalises past experiences in 4–
    5 word sentences.
Asks many questions beginning 'what', 'where', 'who'.

Social Behaviour and Play
Dresses with supervision. Can pull pants down and up but needs help
    with fastenings. Puts on shoes and socks.
Goes to toilet alone.
Starts playing with and not alongside other children.
Understands sharing playthings and sweets.
Shows appreciation of present and past and a need to defer satisfac-
    tion of wishes to future.

4 YEARS

Posture and Large Movements
Walks alone up and downstairs, 1 foot per step.
Climbs ladders, trees and slide.
Stands on 1 foot for 3–4 seconds.
Hops on 1 foot.

Vision and Fine Movements
Builds tower of 10 or more bricks.
Builds bridges and steps from bricks.
Copies cross.
Draws a man with head, legs and trunk, and (usually) arms and fingers.

Hearing and Speech
Speech grammatically correct and completely intelligible.
Pronunciation may show substitution of the following groups r – l – w – y – or p – th – f – s or k – t.
Comprehends prepositions, 'under, on, in front of, behind'.
Asks questions beginning with 'why', 'when', 'how'.
Listens to and tells long stories, sometimes confusing fact with fantasy.
Counts to 10 or more.

Social Behaviour and Play
Dresses without supervision, but usually has difficulty with shoe laces and ties.
Washes and dries hands without supervision.
Understands taking turns as well as sharing.
Well aware of past, present and future time.

5 YEARS

Posture and Large Movements
Walks easily on narrow line.
Can stand on 1 foot for 8–10 seconds with arms folded.
Hops 2–4 metres forward on each foot.
Bounces and catches ball.

Vision and Fine Movements
Copies square and triangle.

Good control of pencil when writing or drawing.
Draws recognisable man with head, trunk, limbs and features.
Draws a house with door, windows, roof and chimney.

Hearing and Speech
Speech fluent, however may still confuse s, f, th.
Delights in reciting or singing rhymes and jingles.
Gives full name, age and address and sometimes birthday.
Defines words, e.g. 'banana is fruit'.

Social Behaviour and Play
General behaviour more sensible, controlled and independent.
Comprehends need for order and tidiness, but needs constant reminders.
Chooses own friends.
Becomes aware of clock time.
Begins to understand need for rules and fair play.
Tender and protective to younger children and pets.

ACKNOWLEDGEMENT

Figures 1/1 to 1/11 are all reproduced by permission of the copyright holders Castlemead Publications, Ware, Hertfordshire SG12 9PY. (Chart reference numbers are GPB2, GPG2, 11A, 12A, 13A, 14A, 15, 16, 43, 44.) The author and publishers acknowledge with thanks this permission: for charts GPB2, GPG2 Drs Douglas Gairdner and Julie Pearson and Professor J. M. Tanner for the remainder.

Chapter 2

Behaviour and Learning Problems

COMMON BEHAVIOUR PROBLEMS

All parents experience some type of behaviour problem in their children. The severity of the problem and the ability to cope depend on the psychological make-up of the child and parents. The ability to cope is strongly influenced by social factors, the commonest being stress, unemployment, poor housing and marital problems. In our society for most families the brunt of the responsibility for child care falls on the mother while the father goes out to work. This constant care of a difficult child (or children) may take its toll and eventually the mother becomes both physically and mentally exhausted.

The tired, emotionally drained mother becomes irritable and less tolerant, while the child, not understanding reason, senses his mother's low ebb and becomes more demanding. A vicious circle is thus established. The message is clear – every mother requires a break from her children. Most behaviour problems can be helped by having one or two nights out each week. More often than not a relative or friend will be willing to help out.

Other than sleep problems and colic the commonest behaviour problems seen by paediatricians are feeding problems, temper tantrums and screaming, breath-holding attacks and head banging. Each of these will be discussed separately.

Feeding problems

These cause parents much anxiety and frustration. There are two types, both frequently co-exist. The first is the child who refuses to eat his meals, the second, the child who dawdles or plays with his food. Most children are between 6 months and 3 years. There is nothing more disheartening for the mother who slaves away in the kitchen preparing Toby's favourite food only to have him turn his nose up at it, smear it in his hair or feed it to the dog. Even more so when she finds that he always eats for mother-in-law (granny).

A child is a small adult and has a personality which can be strong willed. No amount of persuasion, coercion or punishment will make him eat when he does not want to. Like all of us he likes to be the centre of attention and any attention he derives from not eating or dawdling is used to his advantage. Like an adult his appetite varies and when he is hungry he will eat. The difference between the child and adult is that the appetite of a child varies with age. A child of 8 months does not gain weight as rapidly as the child of 3 months and can be expected to have a diminished appetite even though food consumption may actually be more. He eats more because he is bigger rather than hungrier.

All good mothers are naturally concerned about their child's food consumption and weight. It is overconcern that creates a problem. Children with feeding problems always eat when hungry and consequently gain weight at a normal rate for their age. The fact that weight gain is *normal* should allay parental concern but this seldom happens. Instead, mealtimes become a battleground or circus with mum or dad doing all sorts of tricks to get Toby to eat. This is clearly a behaviour problem, the child reacting to the parents' overconcern. No drugs or 'tonics' are of any use. Attention to the following points will improve the problem considerably.

1. Establish a mealtime routine – the child should always be given meals in a set place at roughly the same time. Although not always possible it is best for all the family to eat together, particularly in the evening. This gives father a good opportunity of talking to the child about his day.
2. Do not let the child choose the menu. Cook a meal of your choice, but remember variety is the spice of life. Most children like sweet, colourful food which is easily chewed. If the child does not want the food tell him there is nothing else. Never cook an alternative for it will show him that he can get what he wants.
3. Between meals do not give him snacks, sweets or biscuits. If he does require a drink give him water or a *low calorie* fruit drink. Milk should be avoided because it contains calories and is filling, thereby reducing appetite at mealtimes.

4. Do not feed him if he wants to feed himself. Let him have his independence. This may be messy and time consuming but cannot be helped.
5. Do not start the child with too much – let him have small portions. He may ask for more.
6. Do not insist on a strict order of courses. If he wants to eat his pudding first and then his meat that is all right.
7. If he refuses to eat or dawdles do not make a fuss. After a *reasonable* time remove the food. He may scream but ignore it. If he again refuses to eat at the next meal he certainly will eat at the one after.
8. Never try to persuade the child to eat or force feed him.

Temper tantrums and screaming

These occur mainly between 1 and 3. They represent the clash of the developing personality of the child with the will of those caring for him. The child strives for attention or self-gratification and any frustration of these desires leads to a tantrum or screaming. Parental attitude is very important. Too rigid control makes matters worse by limiting the child's freedom and provoking a reaction. On the other hand a parent who does not control the child encourages his actions. He realises he can get what he wants by having a tantrum and manipulates the situation to his advantage. To avoid this, parents need to adopt a 'team' approach to discipline and should be consistent. What is unacceptable to one parent on one day should be unacceptable to the other parent on another day. When attempting to discipline a child who cannot reason it is sometimes very difficult to strike the right balance between firmness and what is reasonable. An exhausted mother may find it hard to be reasonable when the child is behaving so 'unreasonably'. In these circumstances it can be very helpful to separate mother and child by admitting the child to the children's ward for a few days. Many mothers are very grateful for the rest and seem to cope so much better afterwards.

The following are suggestions for dealing with temper tantrums and screaming:

1. Keep the child occupied – it keeps him out of mischief and avoids parental rebuke. Admission to a nursery school is an ideal way of

keeping a child occupied. He should also be encouraged to play with children of his own age.

2. Keep dangerous objects or valuables well out of his way. Children have inquisitive minds and quite naturally want to explore. It is a sign of developing intelligence. Removal of these objects is preferable to watching over him and continually saying 'no', thereby provoking a reaction.

3. Reduce opportunities for resistance – decide on a course of action rather than ask the child. For example, 'We are going home now' rather than, 'Shall we go home now?' Make reasonable requests and, if necessary, assist him. For example, when asked to put away his toys mother should help him.

4. Ignore the tantrums – perhaps easier said than done, but essential. Smacking, scolding or trying to reason with the child will only encourage further tantrums. Under no circumstances should you give him what he wants. He will soon realise that tantrums achieve nothing and stop having them.

Breath-holding attacks

They affect as many as 5% of children. One in four have another member of the family who also suffered from breath-holding attacks. Attacks can start as early as the first weeks of life but are usually first seen between 7 and 12 months. Frequency varies considerably from attacks occurring at weekly or monthly intervals to numerous attacks each day. Breath holding can be divided into two types (Blue and White), depending on the colour of the child during the attack. The Blue type accounts for more than half while a small number of children have both Blue and White attacks.

What are breath-holding attacks?

Characteristically breath-holding attacks follow an orderly sequence and may be interrupted at any point along the sequence.

In the *Blue type* the child cries loudly for about 15 seconds, breathes out and holds his breath. He then becomes blue and passes out, only to awaken within seconds. If he continues holding his breath he will not awaken but instead will become stiff, extend his arms and arch his back. He then becomes limp and awakens with gasping breaths. Most children hold their breath for less than 30 seconds and when longer there may be a convulsion (shaking of limbs) followed by a limp phase before wakening. After a short period of confusion the child then resumes normal activity. It is rare for a child to be drowsy after a breath-holding attack.

The *White type* is similar, except that he passes out sooner, before he has had much chance to give a yelp. During the episode he looks pale (white) and a convulsion may develop after a shorter time.

What is the cause of breath-holding attacks?

The causes of the Blue and White type appear to be different. The Blue attack is a behaviour problem like a temper tantrum. It is the *immediate* response of the child to anger or frustration. It is also an attention-seeking device, attacks predictably being brought on by certain patterns of behaviour. For example, removing his favourite toy, shouting at or smacking him may bring on an attack. These children are often 'difficult' and may have a low frustration tolerance.

The White attack is not caused by a behaviour problem. The cause seems to be similar to the cause of fainting attacks in the older child; in both there is a slowing of the heart rate during the attack. White attacks are the *immediate* response to sudden fright and minor injuries, especially bumps on the head during a fall. Various names are used by doctors to describe White attacks, the most common being 'pallid syncope', 'reflex anoxic seizures' and 'vagal attacks'.

How are breath-holding attacks diagnosed?

The only way is by a careful and accurate history.

What conditions may be confused with a breath-holding attack?

It is common for loss of consciousness to be confused with epilepsy. There is, however, *no* connection. The blue colour has sometimes erroneously been confused with heart disease. Almost all children with breath-holding attacks have a normal heart.

Do breath-holding attacks cause brain damage?

Brain damage *never* occurs.

Will he grow out of breath-holding attacks?

Yes, 90% disappear spontaneously by 6 years, most going within 4. A few children with the White type develop fainting attacks in their teens.

What should be done when an attack occurs?

Other than remaining calm and not making a fuss nothing need be done. Most parents like to do something and a firm pat on the back does no harm.

Is there any treatment for breath-holding attacks?

These attacks are harmless and eventually go. It would therefore seem undesirable to give drugs every day to prevent such attacks. Although many parents find breath holding frightening, and may be embarrassed by the attacks, almost all seem to cope with reassurance only. When drug treatment is used it is for White attacks and mainly because parents are very anxious and find it difficult to cope. The drug used is atropine, which may be very helpful in reducing the number of attacks.

Head banging

This is a common problem affecting about 7 in 100 children. It usually starts after 6 months and stops spontaneously between 2–3 years but may persist into school age. Banging usually occurs in the evening before the child falls asleep, but sometimes occurs during sleep. The head is banged incessantly against the mattress, cot sides or walls and banging may last from a few minutes to several hours. Many head bangers can be identified by large bruises on the forehead.

The cause of head banging is not known. It occurs in both normal and mentally-retarded children. It may be a sign of insecurity and be used as an attention-seeking device. It is said to be more common in children who are under stimulated and emotionally deprived. Physical discomfort such as teething, ear pain or a wet nappy has also been incriminated as a cause. Other than rare reports of cataracts in persistent head bangers, head banging is harmless and should be ignored. For the child who always has a bruised forehead from banging against the cot sides, a soft, plastic covered foam can be purchased for the cot from shops selling baby products.

Head rolling or head nodding

These habits are common in the child under 3. The child may roll his head to such a degree that an area of baldness appears over the back of the head. When head nodding is accompanied by head tilting and lateral movement of the eye (nystagmus) the habit is called spasmus nutans. These habits are harmless and should be ignored.

Cot (crib) rocking

This usually starts after the age of 6 months. The child rocks to and fro in the cot, often much to the irritation of his parents. This habit cannot be stopped, it should be ignored until it eventually goes.

Tooth grinding (bruxism)

This occurs both day and night, but mainly at night. Daytime tooth grinding is more common in retarded children. It is usually short-lived and best ignored.

Nail biting, nail picking and hair-plucking

These habits offer a release from tension; trying to stop them may make the habit worse. In some children they persist throughout childhood and sometimes into adulthood.

Thumb or finger sucking

This habit is so common in the pre-school child as to be regarded as a passing phase in the child's development. The habit is innocuous and should be ignored. In the case of the school-age child the position is different, permanent damage to the teeth and shape of the face may occur. Every effort should be made to persuade the child to stop sucking his thumb.

Masturbation

It is a gratifying habit which is both normal and natural. All children (and adults) have masturbated at some time. Masturbation should be ignored; on finding the child flushed and excited you should pretend you have not noticed.

Stammering (stuttering)

About 1 in 20 pre-school children have a mild stammer. It is normal and arises because the child is unable to express his thoughts as quickly as they occur. By school age a stammer is found in about 1 in 100 children, more commonly in boys than girls. It seems as if the tendency to stammering runs in families. Many children who stammer are nervous or tense, probably best described as 'highly strung'. There is no doubt that the more fuss that is made, the more likely the problem will become worse.

If the stammer is mild, worrying as it is, you should try not to comment on it. By pretending you have not noticed it you will best help the child. The child with a severe stammer should be referred to a speech therapist. This is often helpful; she will try to get him to relax and will show him ways of overcoming the problem.

Most children with stammers overcome the difficulty by the time they reach their early teens, however, a few persist into adult life.

SLEEP PROBLEMS

Parents report two main problems about their child's sleep in the early years of life. The first is difficulty in getting the child to go to bed although he sleeps on subsequently through the night. The second is the child who goes to bed and then wakes during the night. The two, of course, frequently co-exist. These problems are common (about 20% in the first 5 years) and I have every sympathy for the mother who feels at her wits' end. She has discovered that smacking is useless and drugs are ineffective. She cannot reason with him because he does not understand. Exhausted and longing for sleep she is unable to leave him to cry because the neighbours may complain or he makes himself sick.

Most children with sleep problems are *not* naughty and do not have a medical reason for their problem. They are often 'difficult' children and a history of colic in the first months of life is common. The sleep problem is best regarded as a behaviour problem, the child having acquired a bad habit. Breaking the habit is easy provided both parents modify their behaviour towards the child in a consistent manner. The following suggestions are a guide to the correct management:

1. Establish a routine – under normal day-to-day circumstances try to put your child to bed at the same time. If possible both mother

and father should take turns in putting the child to bed. Bedtime crying is worst in both a wide-awake child or one who is over-tired. To avoid both these, the child should be allowed to sleep during the day but should be wakened so that the amount of day-time sleep is not excessive.

2. Give him a warm bath. This is best done about a half-hour before bedtime. Most children enjoy playing in the bath and it tires them. This is a good task for fathers. It gives them the oppor-tunity to play with the child after work and gives the mother a break.

3. Go through your regular bedtime routine – story, drinks, kisses, etc. Although not always possible, it is always best for the child to sleep in a separate room from the parents.

4. Place your child in his cot or bed and say goodnight. Tell him you will see him in the morning and turn off the light. Leave the room and close the door (optional). In cold weather a bed first warmed with a hot water bottle is comforting for the child. A night light or subdued lighting are preferred by most children. If your child will not remain in the bedroom a chain catch should be fitted to the bedroom door so that the door can be opened but not sufficiently wide for the child to get through.

5. Do not go back into the room. The child will probably cry and this will distress you, a perfectly natural feeling, but you must not give in. Most children do not cry for more than half an hour, but some may cry for 1–2 hours when it may be extremely diffi-cult to resist going to him. If you go to him it teaches him that if he cries long enough he will eventually get his own way. Fortu-nately the time he spends crying will become shorter each night and after 4 or 5 nights the habit will be broken.

6. Having broken the habit you may find he still cries briefly when put to bed. This is quite normal and if the crying continues it is all right to go into the bedroom to check all is well. Do not talk to him or pick him up.

7. During the night, if he awakens and cries, attend to him. Do not pick him up or put him in your bed.

8. A child who gets out of bed should immediately be given a spank and put back to bed. Make this as matter-of-fact as possible. Show him you mean it.

9. Continue doing this each time he gets up. You may be surprised how often he gets up the first night or two but don't be discour-

aged as he is testing to find out whether or not you really mean it. *Do not give up.*

10. In the morning praise him for staying in his bed and reward him with his favourite cereal.

The night chosen to start this regimen requires some thought. It is best to choose a night when neither parent is required to work the following day. A Friday or Saturday night may be most suitable. You may find it heavy going but do persevere for the desired effect will soon be achieved.

Another method which can be very effective is to admit the child to a children's ward; the child usually sleeps through the first night, much to the mother's embarrassment. Hospital admission is good for the mother who has not slept for days and is at the end of her tether. It is also particularly helpful for single-parent families and in homes with marital stress. Although uncommon, discharge from the ward is sometimes followed by a relapse, which can easily be corrected by a behaviour modification programme supervised by a clinical psychologist.

What about drugs?

Although widely used, I believe they have little value. Most parents have tried drugs before referral to a paediatrician and invariably have discontinued them because they did not work. Trying to break a bad sleeping habit with a drug is like trying to stop smoking with a drug – it is useless.

Many parents are concerned that the child's 'lack of sleep' may cause intellectual impairment. There should be no need for concern; if a child is not getting enough sleep he will nap quite oblivious of the time of day or his surroundings. Furthermore, some comfort can be derived from the fact that most paediatricians feel that the more intelligent child tends to sleep *less* than the less intelligent.

Other night time problems in children include:

1. *Sleep rituals.* About the age of 2 most children develop some sort of sleep ritual, demanding this, that and the other before going to sleep. He may demand a drink, ask for his teddy to be placed next to him or ask for the door to be left open a specific width. These are all devices to delay mother's departure from the bedroom. Within reason it is best to do as he asks and by school age most children cease to have sleep rituals.

2. *'Delaying tactics'*. These are common in school age children. The child will try every conceivable trick to avoid going to bed. The time interval from when he is told to go to bed until he actually gets into bed may be as long as an hour. Parents who have had a hard day at work and want to sit and relax in the evening become short tempered with such a child. It is a frequent source of friction between parents and their children and sometimes difficult to handle. This problem is best managed by a certain amount of tolerance and firmness by the parents.

3. *Night terrors*. These occur commonly between 4–8 years, usually in the first hours of sleep as deep sleep changes to light sleep. The child awakens terrified and screaming in a state of clouded consciousness, not recognising his parents or familiar surroundings. He may get out of bed and wander about. During the episode he will look frightened; he will have a racing pulse, deep breathing, wide pupils and may sweat profusely. The episode usually lasts a few minutes but may last 15–20 minutes. He is unable to recall his bad dream and the next morning has no recollection of the previous evening's events. Parents are often alarmed at the child's 'strange' behaviour and need to be reassured. The problem eventually stops and the child usually requires no treatment. When night terrors are very frequent and cause a lot of family distress diazepam 5–10mg at bedtime is usually very helpful.

4. *Nightmares*. These occur commonly between 8–10 years. The child awakens terrified, with a clear recollection then and the next morning.

5. *Sleep walking*. This commonly arises between 11–14 years. A child who is not fully conscious rises from his bed and walks about without any subsequent memory of the night's events.

How much sleep is normal?

There is a wide individual variation. A newborn sleeps about 20 hours each day taken mainly as a series of naps, but by the time he is a year old this has fallen to 12 hours. The need for sleep continues to fall slowly throughout early childhood until adolescence when the fall is more rapid. The length of time spent sleeping in the day and night is similar in the first 3–4 months after which night-time sleeping predominates.

HABIT SPASM (TIC)

Habit spasms or tics are common, affecting as many as 12% of children, boys more than girls. They are a major source of parental anxiety and occur at any age from 2 onwards, developing most commonly about 7. Children with tics are often sensitive, obsessional and 'highly strung'.

What is a tic?

It is an involuntary, purposeless movement of interconnected muscles, eye blinking being the most frequent tic in childhood. Other common movements are shaking of the head, shrugging of one or both shoulders, grunting, sniffing and coughing. Although kicking movements of the legs and flexion movements of the arms may occur, these are unusual. Most movements involve muscles of the face, head or shoulders. Children are prefectly aware of what they are doing, find it senseless and distressing, but have no control over the movements. When a child is asked why he blinks his eye he will reply 'I can't help it, something makes me do it.' The movements usually occur irregularly and may last less than a second or they occur repetitively and last over several minutes. The tic is worse when the child is anxious, self-conscious, emotionally upset or excited. They are reduced by distracting the child and always disappear during sleep. Sometimes a tic follows on purposeful movements; for example, throat clearing while the throat is infected may continue well after the infection has subsided.

Will the tic go?

Yes, in nearly half it will completely disappear. This may occur within days, weeks or years, most rapid improvement seems to occur in those aged between 6 and 8. Of those that persist the vast majority show improvement, usually in late adolescence.

What is the treatment?

There is no treatment as such. The best way to help the child is to disregard the tic completely. Any attempt to get the child to desist from making the movements is pointless. Indeed, it is harmful; it draws attention to the problem and consequently the child is put under stress. Mimicry by other children at school sometimes happens. Dealing with the perpetrators draws attention to the problem, making it worse. It may be better to encourage the child to ignore the mimicry.

These measures are all that are required for most children. However, some who are experiencing stress or anxiety in the home or at school can be helped further by expert psychological help from a clinical psychologist or child psychiatrist.

What is Tourette syndrome?

It is the most severe form of habit spasm, affecting 2–3% of the general population – about 100 000 Americans have it – and starts before 15 years. There are many different types, which are always accompanied by involuntary noises such as grunting, throat clearing or shrieking; eventually the noises are followed by utterances of inappropriate or obscene words. Symptoms wax and wane over 3–4 month periods; old symptoms may disappear to be replaced by new ones, or new symptoms may be added to existing symptoms. Stress makes symptoms worse. The child who may be grunting, blinking his eyes, grimacing and making jerky movements of his head and arms has too often in the past been misdiagnosed as a 'psychiatric case'. It is in fact nothing of the sort; the cause is not known for certain but is probably a chemical imbalance in the brain. Many children have learning difficulty and educational problems. The illness is permanent, although some children do have long remissions. There are two drugs, haloperidol and pimozide, which are highly effective in relieving symptoms so that these children can lead normal lives.

What is a psychogenic cough?

It is a habit or tic. There are few children's conditions that can cause more disruption in the home or classroom than psychogenic cough. Parents become very anxious when the family doctor has tried umpteen antibiotics or cough suppressants without any response, matters usually become worse when the hospital doctor orders a number of elaborate tests to no avail.

It affects children over 6 and often starts with a trivial upper respiratory infection and cough, which progresses over several weeks and months to an explosive barking cough. The noise has been likened to the call of the Canada goose and most appropriately these children are named 'honkers'. A very frequent sign of psychogenic cough is the chin on chest posture which is adopted during coughing. The most important clues to the diagnosis are the fact that coughing disappears during sleep, and that the cough can be produced on request. Prolonged absence from school is common because of disruption or concern about the infectivity of the cough.

The outlook is excellent, the cough eventually disappears, often soon after the child and parents have been told that there is nothing seriously wrong and that it is a habit. A mild tranquilliser may sometimes be helpful. When reassurance fails or there are other obvious behaviour problems the help of a child psychiatrist or psychologist is worthwhile.

THE HYPERACTIVE CHILD

Most parents of a hyperactive child are bewildered at the 'strange' way he behaves. Many feel guilty or are ashamed of the fact that they are unable to control his behaviour. These feelings of bewilderment and shame commonly cause despair, particularly after much gratuitous advice from well-meaning neighbours and friends has proved to be of no avail.

What is the cause?
We do not know. What we do know is that it is not caused by brain damage. The tendency for the brain to function differently is probably inherited from both parents in the same way as size or intelligence.

How common is hyperactivity in children?
In the USA it is said to affect between 4–10% of school age children, boys more than girls. In Britain, the incidence appears to be very much less. The reason for this marked difference could, for the most part, be explained by a difference in definition and its interpretation. The child with 'classical' hyperactivity is quite definitely different and there is unlikely to be any dispute about the diagnosis. On the other hand, large numbers of 'hyperactive' children display behaviour which is very difficult to distinguish from normal childhood behaviour. The crux of the matter would appear to be that 'hyperactivity' means different things to different mothers, teachers and doctors. What may be normal to one is abnormal to another. There is no definitive test for hyperactivity, the diagnosis is therefore highly subjective.

What is a 'hyperactive child'?
The difference between the normal and the hyperactive child is the intensity, persistence and clustering of his symptoms. These symp-

toms are always apparent before age 7. The three cardinal symptoms are inattention, impulsivity and movement abnormality. Each will be discussed in more detail.

Inattention. Children are unable to concentrate for any length of time. Mothers often say 'He does not finish what he starts.' In extreme instances he is described as rushing from one activity to another. At school teachers describe him as having a short 'concentration span' unless in a one-to-one situation. They say he is easily distracted and needs a calm, quiet atmosphere or he is unable to work or concentrate. Teachers frequently say 'He hears but does not seem to listen and is always asking for things to be repeated.'

Impulsivity. This means that the child has little control over his impulses. It causes much distress to both parents and teachers and is expressed differently at various ages; a toddler may have difficulty with toilet training while an older child may have difficulty in refraining from frequent temptations such as playing with matches, stealing or lying. These children have a low frustration tolerance, are excitable and have difficulty in waiting their turn. At school they call out in class, talk excessively, make noises and are generally disruptive.

Movement abnormality commonly takes two forms: hyperactivity and clumsiness. The hyperactive child is always on the go; he would rather run than walk. When he is not actively engaged in something he will fidget, tap, kick or display some other form of 'irritating' behaviour. He may stand out in a crowd because of his noisy behaviour. Hyperactive toddlers commonly climb on to things and open and close doors and, for this reason, are particularly prone to accidents. More than half are clumsy. Common difficulties encountered are fastening buttons or zips, tying shoe laces, throwing or catching a ball, riding a bicycle.

What other problems may a hyperactive child have?
1. Learning difficulties and educational problems are common and are the main cause for referral of these children to educational psychologists.
2. Difficulty with interpersonal relations. Parents are unable to discipline him and his 'antisocial' behaviour alienates his siblings and peers. For actions which he cannot help or control he is constantly criticised, chastised or punished. The feeling of constantly being picked on and made to feel unwelcome may have a profound

effect on the child's developing personality. He is commonly moody and easily riled. Parents sometimes refer to the child as having a 'low boiling point' or a 'short fuse'. To vent their frustration many children behave in an aggressive way.

What happens to the hyperactive child?
The hyperactivity diminishes with time and by puberty has all but disappeared. However, it is unfortunate that other symptoms may persist. A small number will always be 'underachievers', will have difficulty with social adjustment and may fall foul of the law. It is believed by many experts that early, effective intervention may greatly reduce the chances of these unpleasant consequences.

How should the hyperactive child be managed?
Each child or family is different and management will vary. Many families have disturbed relationships and marital problems caused by feelings of guilt and hostility to the child. For the most part effective management requires a 'team' approach. The team usually comprises a paediatrician/psychiatrist together with a clinical/educational psychologist and a health visitor/social worker. The team makes ongoing assessments of the child's health, personality, physical and intellectual abilities. Team members will liaise with the family and school and attempt to iron out problems as they arise. Not only will they provide support, but will also take a firm hand in advising parents, family members and teachers on how to deal with the child. Such a team approach, providing support and effective counselling of marital, family and educational problems may be all that is required.

What about drugs?
Attentional difficulties in particular are greatly benefited by the use of drugs, which may result in improved academic performance. Paradoxically, the most effective and widely used drug, methylphenidate (Ritalin), is a stimulant. Because stimulants are most active in improving attentional difficulties they are mostly used for this reason rather than as a means of reducing hyperactivity, which gradually improves without treatment.

Does drug treatment have side-effects?
Insomnia or sleep disturbances and decreased appetite are the most frequently observed side-effects of stimulants, with weight loss, irritability and abdominal pains almost as common. These and a host of other less frequent side-effects (e.g. headaches, nausea, dizziness,

dry mouth, constipation) usually disappear as the child becomes tolerant to the drug, or resolve if the dose is reduced.

While these side-effects are not serious, of more concern is evidence that growth may be suppressed. This seems to occur when high doses are used for a prolonged period. The risk can be considerably reduced by using small doses and omitting the drug when away from school, during school holidays and over weekends.

What is the Feingold diet?

In the early 1970s Dr Ben Feingold obtained much publicity when he stated that many hyperactive children could be dramatically improved by removing colouring agents and certain food additives from the diet. Despite a lack of scientific proof, this theory soon gained wide acceptance and the diet became known as the 'Feingold diet'. There have since been a few controlled studies which have looked at Feingold's theory. Although the results have been conflicting, it would be fair to say that the bulk of evidence is against any dietary cause for hyperactivity. Nevertheless, trying the Feingold diet does no harm provided it is supervised by a dietitian. I usually do not dissuade parents from trying the diet as they need to assess any benefit for themselves. I have found that there is sometimes a short-term benefit. The fact that improvement did not persist suggests to me that any benefit may have been due to a 'psychological' effect rather than the diet itself. Ultimately, if some benefit does accrue, for whatever reason, then the diet has been worth trying.

Is there a support group for parents?

Yes, the address is shown on page 352. Much of the information provided by the British Support Group is of a highly controversial nature. Having a hyperactive child is not easy, most parents are prepared to try anything even if there is only a remote possibility of some benefit. Parents would be well advised to seek the advice of their child's paediatrician before acting on any information provided by the group.

SCHOOL REFUSAL

There are four common reasons for school absenteeism:

1. Absence because of illness.

2. Truancy – this is a behaviour problem. These children often engage in other forms of delinquent behaviour.
3. Parental indifference – these children stay off school because their parents are ineffectual and do not really care. Some actually connive with their children to stay off school. This is mainly a problem of the socially deprived.
4. School refusal – the child has an emotional cause for staying away.

School refusal is a common problem seen by both paediatricians and child psychiatrists. It affects boys and girls equally and can affect any school-age child. In Britain, most are teenagers while in the USA it is more prevalent among younger children.

It usually starts over a period of several weeks with the child's getting emotionally upset whenever it is time to go to school. In some children the onset may be sudden, often following absence from school for an illness or holiday. The child's emotional upset may cause him to have physical symptoms such as loss of appetite, nausea, vomiting, diarrhoea or frequent urge to urinate. Some children look pale, tremble, and may complain of headaches. Others who do not look anxious may appear miserable and tearful.

While the basic problem is school refusal it is frequently not recognised by parents or their doctors because the physical symptoms masquerade as a variety of illnesses. It is quite common to find these children suffering from prolonged episodes of 'migraine', 'glandular fever', 'viral illness', 'colitis', 'hepatitis'. Invariably physical examination and blood tests do not reveal any abnormality. Not surprisingly the 'illness' often shows improvement in the evening and over weekends.

School refusal can occur in any child, but most could best be described as loners; they do not like going out and do not mix well with other children. Some have had difficulty settling down when they first started school or when they changed schools. They are often wilful and domineering at home but timid outside. Many are over-dependent on their mothers and very clingy, frequently following their mother around the house like a toddler. Virtually all studies show that the parents, particularly the mother, are overanxious and overprotective. Many do things for their children which the children are perfectly capable of doing for themselves; their reluctance to untie the apron strings discourages the child from developing a sense of independence. The child with school refusal does not seem to have any more problems within the school than any other child. There is, however, an occasional child whose ability is overstretched, school refusal arising as a sign of his inability to cope. For the vast majority changing schools will not make the slightest difference.

Children are best managed by a child psychiatrist or psychologist. He will work closely with the child, his parents, and the school. For the problem to be overcome most speedily it is essential that parents accept that this is an emotional problem. Because there are physical symptoms, parents often find it hard to accept and seek second or third opinions. Generally schools are very helpful and their co-operation can usually be relied upon.

The psychiatrist tries to establish a relationship with the child. Although some difficulty may be encountered initially, this usually does not take long. In consultation with the child a plan for a return to school will be drawn up. This plan will need to be strictly enforced by the parents and the school. Occasionally children may be given a mild tranquilliser as a temporary measure. Exclusion for a short while from some feared activity at the school may also help. With the support of parents and the school a return is usually possible within a few weeks. A few children with school refusal do have emotional problems in adult life, the most common being agoraphobia (a fear of going out).

DYSLEXIA

About 10% of children have a learning difficulty. Although they are of normal intelligence they have difficulty with a specific aspect of learning. The most usual difficulties encountered are with reading, spelling, writing and arithmetic. Of these the best known is the difficulty with reading and spelling known as dyslexia. While large numbers of children experience greater difficulty with reading and spelling than would be expected from their level of intelligence, the term dyslexia is usually reserved for the few in whom the difficulty is most marked and very obvious.

It affects boys more frequently than girls, and often runs in families. The cause is not known but is thought to be due to an inherited abnormality in brain function. The child has 'word blindness': although he sees perfectly normally he cannot interpret the letters he sees into meaningful words, hence his reading difficulty. Similarly, his brain is unable to translate what he hears into meaningful written words, hence his inability to spell. He may write the letters in the wrong order, for example cat may be written as 'tca'. Mirror reversal of letters or numbers is commonly seen, for example, d is written for b, q for p. Many children without dyslexia also go through a stage of doing this when they learn to write.

Children with dyslexia have a good grasp of spoken language, they are able to talk fluently and have a large vocabulary. Almost all have difficulty in distinguishing left from right. This problem causes difficulty with telling the time. In common with other learning problems they have an increased frequency of emotional problems, clumsiness and untidy handwriting. The emotional problems vary considerably and may range from occasional mood changes to violent outbursts of temper. It is probable that they arise from frustration. The child who has normal or high normal intelligence is likely to be baffled and frustrated when he is unable to perform 'simple' tasks his contemporaries or juniors are able to do. The situation becomes even less tolerable when his parents or teachers are forever calling him 'lazy' or 'stupid' and he may even be punished.

After the child and parents are told the diagnosis they usually breathe a sigh of relief on learning that there is an explanation for his perplexing difficulty, which hitherto had been quite inexplicable. Parents are advised to try to develop the child's non-literary talents. The child is usually referred to an educational psychologist who will assess the child and will then make arrangements for his special educational needs. Because letters and words cannot easily be recognised they need to be learned by rote. A trick for memorising right and left has also to be devised. When emotional problems are severe the educational psychologist will give advice about these. There has been a recent report that a few dyslexics may benefit from using only one eye when reading.

Some children do improve in their teens although most dyslexics remain hampered by their disability all their lives. When choosing a career the dyslexic should choose one which does not involve much writing or reading.

AUTISM

About 1 in 2500 children is autistic, numbering in England and

Wales about 3000. Boys are affected more than girls. About half the children with autism also have some other obvious condition affecting the brain, such as cerebral palsy (p. 297) or epilepsy; careful examination of the remainder often shows minor abnormalities suggesting an abnormality of brain function.

What is autism?

The autistic child usually looks normal and can only be distinguished by his 'odd' behaviour. There are many abnormalities of behaviour; these are best categorised under three headings:

1. *An inability to socialise.* The child seems to lack an awareness of other human beings as the most important and interesting features of the environment. He pays more attention to objects than to people. His behaviour could best be described as aloof and indifferent. Common descriptions given by parents are that he is 'self-sufficient', 'like in a shell', 'happiest when left alone' and 'acts as if people weren't there'. Because of his indifference to humans, there is little eye-to-eye contact when trying to communicate with him.

2. *An inability to communicate.* He is unable to show any form of communication. Unlike the child with aphasia who cannot speak but can communicate in other ways, the autistic child is unable to demonstrate any form of communication. About half do not develop any form of spoken language. Those who do speak often have a curiously distinctive pitch to their speech. They have odd speech patterns, often echoing what is said to them or confusing pronouns. For example, they may refer to themselves as 'you' or 'he' instead of 'I'.

3. *An inability to use their imagination.* This creates what can sometimes be described as bizarre behaviour. They tend to engage in repetitive activities and routines and resist change. They may pass their time twisting and turning objects, opening and closing doors, arranging objects in meaningless patterns or just aimlessly wandering. Because their world is confusing it is not surprising that they resist change by clinging to the few things they understand. Trying to change their routine brings about screaming and trantrums. In their strange world they are often frightened of harmless objects but are quite indifferent to real danger. Although

it is very difficult to test intelligence, tests have shown that only a fifth have an IQ (intelligence quotient) in the normal range.

What is the cause?

The cause is not known, but is most likely an abnormality of the brain. Although the cause may be genetic there is no real risk for subsequent children.

What can be done?

There is no specific treatment. The type of schooling required will depend on the child's intelligence and his ability to communicate. As learning is normally achieved through communication, teaching an autistic child who is unable to communicate and is usually retarded is doubly difficult. The child can be greatly helped if both the school and the parents work closely with a psychologist or child psychiatrist. Not only will this provide insight into the child's thought processes but it will allow those caring for the child to adopt a consistent approach to teaching him and controlling his behaviour. In Britain parents can obtain some useful information which is well written and presented by contacting The National Society for Autistic Children (p. 351).

Chapter 3

Fever; Infectious Disease; Immunisations

THE CHILD WITH A TEMPERATURE

Contrary to the belief of large numbers of parents a high temperature is harmless. The body copes by producing sweat, which causes cooling when it evaporates. With the rare exception of children with abnormal sweat glands all children are able to sweat and do tolerate a high temperature; all that is required is extra fluid to replace sweat loss. Fever causes many children to become delirious, during which they talk a lot of gibberish. On finding a child talking nonsense and who does not appear fully conscious, parents not surprisingly become frightened and alarmed. Besides causing delirium, fever also has an effect on other body functions, for example, it is quite common to find protein or sugar in the urine during episodes of high temperature.

What causes a high temperature?

Children who have been well who suddenly develop a high temperature do so because they have acquired an infection. In most cases the infection is caused by a virus.

Is it necessary to know whether a child has a temperature?

Children with a fever usually have signs or symptoms of an infection, the fact that they have a high temperature only confirms what is already self-evident. Knowing whether a child has a high temperature may, however, assist the management of febrile convulsions (see p. 285) or help in the diagnosis of urinary infections where fever may be the only clue to the diagnosis. Children with a high temperature are hot and flushed, leaving their parents with little doubt about their fever. Although there is little to be gained by recording the temperature many parents do like to measure it.

How should the temperature be taken?

The accuracy of temperature taking depends on the type of thermometer, the site where the temperature is taken and the time allowed for the thermometer to heat up. Before using a mercury thermometer always check that the mercury has been shaken down to the minimum level. After use the thermometer should be cleaned by allowing it to stand in a cold antiseptic solution for a few minutes.

Taking the temperature in the armpit (axilla) is the most safe, hygienic and accurate method in both premature and mature babies in the first weeks of life. The bulb of the thermometer is placed high in the armpit, the shaft projecting forward while the arm is held firmly against the side of the chest. The thermometer should be left in position for 5–7 minutes before the temperature is read.

The child below 3 or 4 is usually too young for a thermometer to be placed in the mouth safely. After the first weeks of life, the most accurate but hazardous way of taking the temperature is by placing the thermometer in the back passage (rectum) (Fig. 3/1) to a depth of 4–5 cm and left in place for 3 minutes. Great care should be taken to hold the child firmly. If the child is able to wriggle free there is a risk the thermometer may break in the rectum.

A child older than 4 is usually mature enough to have his temperature taken in the mouth. For most accuracy the bulb of the thermometer should be held for 10 minutes under the tongue with the mouth closed. Needless to say, the temperature is likely to be inaccurate if the child has just had a hot drink, a hot bath or been exercising.

What about plastic strip thermometers?

These are disposable but may be re-used. Temperature is recorded by placing the strip on the forehead for 1 minute. A recent development is a plastic strip which is placed under the tongue for 1 minute. Strip thermometers contain crystals which glow or change colour at the appropriate temperature. They are safe, cheap, convenient, but inaccurate. Their inaccuracy must, however, be balanced against the fact that in the 'real world' temperature taking with glass thermometers is seldom performed with any degree of precision by most parents. For those parents who favour convenience more than precision, strip thermometers are more than adequate.

What is the normal temperature?

Body temperature is not static; it varies slightly throughout the day. It is usually highest in the late afternoon and lowest between 3

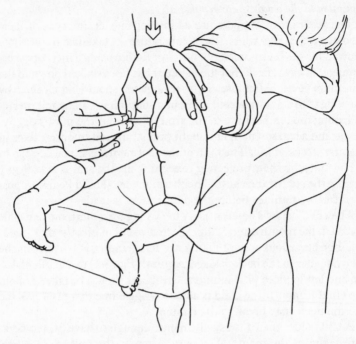

Fig. 3/1 Taking a rectal temperature. The child is placed on a bed or his mother's lap. He is immobilised by applying firm pressure to the buttocks or back

and 5 in the morning. The average temperature is 37°C (98.6°F); a variation of 1°C (2°F) is normal. For practical purposes fever should be regarded as a temperature greater than 38°C (100.6°F). Temperature also varies slightly at different sites, but the variation is so slight that for practical purposes it can be ignored. Most thermometers in the USA are on the Fahrenheit scale. Formulae for conversion of thermometer scales are:

$$\text{Degrees C} = \frac{\text{Degrees F} - 32}{1.8}$$

$$\text{Degrees F} = (\text{Degrees C} \times 1.8) + 32$$

How should a fever be treated?
As mentioned previously, all that is required is extra fluid to

replace sweat loss; the type of fluid is of little importance. Because many parents and doctors believe that children feel more comfortable without fever, treatment is given. Paracetamol (acetominophen (USA)) is the treatment of choice. See page 288 for information on aspirin. Sponging the child with tepid water is a practice widely used by both parents and hospitals in the belief that it lowers the temperature. Although the water feels warm, it may cause discomfort to a feverish child to whom it feels cold. When combined with paracetamol, tepid sponging is no more effective than paracetamol alone and should be abandoned.

When should the doctor be called?

It is probably advisable to have all children with a high temperature checked by a doctor. It is particularly important in the young child who is unable to communicate. The doctor will examine the child in an attempt to identify the part of the body which has become infected. Where treatment is needed this will be provided early in the illness.

COMMON INFECTIOUS DISEASES

Most of the infections I shall be describing produce a temperature. Many parents (and some doctors) suffer from 'fever phobia'. This means that any temperature in the child causes them to panic. Before reading about these illnesses I should like to emphasise that fever is *not* harmful and itself does not require treatment.

Measles (rubeola). In the developed countries measles is not a serious illness. It is mainly a childhood disease, starting from 6 months onwards. In Britain it occurs mainly in winter and spring. The main features are fever, rash, cough, running nose and sore eyes. The incubation period (time from exposure to start of illness) is usually about 10 days.

The sequence of events is illustrated in Figure 3/2. The illness starts with a fever which usually rises slowly to reach a maximum in 4–5 days, after which it suddenly falls. Cough, runny nose and sore eyes develop with the onset of fever. The child will be irritable, unwell, will not want to eat and may object to light.

After the fever has been present for 2 days, white spots (Koplick's spots) appear inside the cheek. On the 4th day the rash develops fol-

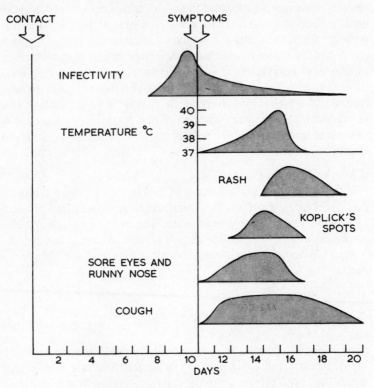

Fig. 3/2 Sequence of events in measles

lowing which the Koplick's spots start to disappear so that by the third day of the rash they are gone. Measles is diagnosed by seeing Koplick's spots or the characteristic rash. The rash is purple red and may be slightly itchy. It first appears on the forehead, behind the ears and on the upper part of the neck. There is a gradual spreading downwards until it reaches the feet by the third day, at which time the more extensively involved upper part of the body begins to fade. A brownish discolouration appears over the area where the rash was and may last a few weeks. By the time it has faded the child should be well and eating normally. Coughing commonly persists for a further week.

A temperature which persists or one that starts to rise again suggests that an ear infection or pneumonia are present. Older children with ear infection usually complain of pain. About 1 in 1000 children develop encephalitis (inflammation of the brain); in a small number it may be serious.

There is no treatment for measles. The ear infection and pneumonia which occur following measles are frequently caused by bacteria. When these complications arise antibiotics are usually prescribed. Measles is contagious from the 7th day after exposure to the 5th day after the rash appears. It is most infectious immediately before the rash appears.

German measles (rubella). The main symptoms are a feeling of being unwell, enlarged glands (nodes) and a rash. The symptoms are very mild; large numbers of children have German measles without ever knowing. If it were not for the fact that German measles could be very harmful to the unborn baby when acquired in pregnancy, we should not be concerned about it. Infection acquired in the early weeks of pregnancy can cause brain damage, blindness or deafness in the baby. Outbreaks of German measles usually occur in spring. The incubation period is 14–21 days and the child is infectious 7 days before to 4 days after the onset of the rash.

Unlike teenagers and adults, children do not feel unwell 3–4 days before the rash but do develop enlarged glands. The glands may be tender and those in the neck, at the back of the skull and behind the ears are most commonly enlarged. Occasionally red eyes and runny nose may accompany the rash. The rash is pink red, starts on the face and rapidly spreads to the rest of the body usually lasting 1–5 days (average 3). The temperature may be normal or slightly elevated (Fig. 3/3).

No treatment is needed. Rare complications of German measles are arthritis, encephalitis and an abnormality of blood clotting (thrombocytopenia). These are not serious and usually settle without any treatment.

There are several viruses which can cause signs and symptoms like rubella so that the diagnosis should always be made with reservation. It is possible to confirm the diagnosis with specialised laboratory tests, but in practice this is seldom done or indeed necessary in children. Even if your doctor has diagnosed German measles, because of the uncertainty your daughter should still be immunised. (This is the advice for Britain and Australia; in the USA both boys *and* girls are immunised.) Rashes similar to German measles can also be caused by drugs and roseola infantum.

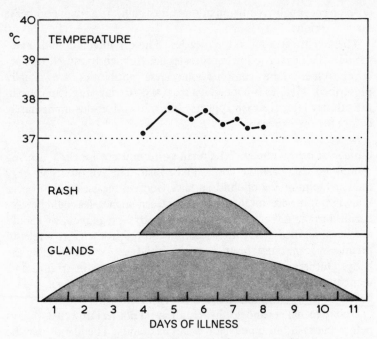

Fig. 3/3 Sequence of events in German measles

Roseola infantum (xanthum subitum) is probably caused by a virus and affects pre-school children, especially infants. Although the rash is similar to German measles it can be distinguished by the temperature which is higher and usually lasts 3–4 days during which the child is irritable. The rash, which seldom lasts more than 24 hours, develops *after* the temperature and irritability have settled (Fig. 3/4). Like German measles there is no treatment.

Erythema infectiosum (fifth disease). This is a common contagious illness in children which is caused by parvovirus. Epidemics occur in late winter and spring. The incubation period is about 10 days. The characteristic feature is the rash besides which there are usually no other symptoms. A few children do, however, develop sore joints. The rash typically starts on the face giving the so-called 'slapped cheek appearance'. It then spreads to the trunk and limbs, the distinguishing feature of the body rash is its 'lacy' appearance. The rash usually fades within a week but may recur periodically in the follow-

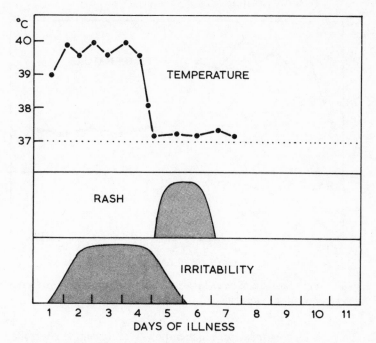

Fig. 3/4 Sequence of events in roseola infantum

ing weeks after the child has had a hot bath. No treatment is required.

Chicken-pox. The virus which causes chicken-pox is called varicella. It can also cause a skin infection, shingles (herpes zoster), in adults many years after the attack of chicken-pox. Varicella infections can occur at any age and are most prevalent in the autumn, winter and spring. The incubation period is 14–16 days.

The day before the rash starts the child may have a headache, feel unwell and be off his food. The rash starts as red blotches which develop into clear fluid blisters so that they look like teardrops. Within 6–8 hours the fluid becomes cloudy, the blister dries out leaving a dimple and then a scab. The scabs usually fall off in 1–3 weeks leaving pink areas on the skin. The rash develops in crops over 3–4 days so that blisters (vesicles) and scabs will be present at the same time. The trunk and upper legs and arms are mainly involved; it may be very itchy. Small white ulcers also develop in the mouth. There is a rise in temperature which parallels the outbreak of the rash; the more severe the rash the higher the fever (Fig. 3/5).

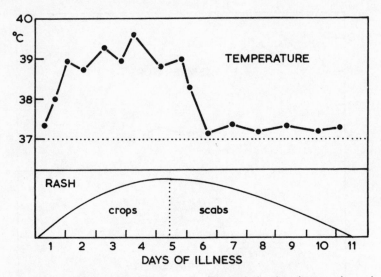

Fig. 3/5 Typical pattern of chicken pox. The rash develops in crops (waves) each ending with scab formation

There is no treatment for chicken-pox. Itching can be controlled by applying calamine lotion or taking antihistamine medication. The fingernails should be kept short and clean so that scratching does not cause infection of the skin. Chicken-pox is a benign illness: all children make a complete recovery. It is, however, a serious illness in newborns, adults and children on steroids or those with an impaired ability to fight infection. In such children the infection can be prevented or considerably modified if an injection (zoster immune globulin) is given within 72 hours of exposure. An effective chicken-pox vaccine has been developed, but because of the benign nature of the illness and concern about the long-term effects it is currently not used in Britain.

A child with chicken-pox is infectious from about 5 days before onset of the rash until the scabs are completely dry (about 5–10 days). The illness is spread both by direct contact and air infection.

Whooping cough. In young children, particularly those under a year, whooping cough is a potentially serious illness. It can occur throughout the year and usually starts in the spring and continues into the early part of winter. Whooping cough is caused by a bacterium called 'pertussis'. The incubation period is usually 7–10 days and the illness can be divided into 3 phases:

1. A 'cold' phase during which the child has symptoms like a common cold. The main symptoms are a slight fever, runny nose, red eyes and mild cough mainly at night. This phase lasts 1–2 weeks and whooping cough is seldom suspected. This is followed by:

2. A phase of coughing spasms lasting 2–4 weeks or longer. The number of spasms varies but may be as many as 40 in a day in severe illness. Between the spasms the child is well. Each coughing spasm consists of 5–10 short expiratory coughs followed by a whoop (crowing sound) as the child gasps for breath. During the spasm the face may go red or blue, the eyes bulge or stream with tears and the tongue protrudes. The mouth may contain a large amount of mucous and saliva. At the end of the spasm children frequently vomit, they are exhausted and appear dazed; a few have convulsions. Repeated vomiting causes weight loss. Bouts of coughing may be triggered by yawning, sneezing, eating and drinking and exercise. Many children have whooping cough without a whoop. This is particularly common in the first year of life. The phase of coughing spasms is followed by:

3. The recovery phase which lasts 1–2 weeks during which the symptoms gradually decrease in frequency and severity. During the next year or two when the child gets a respiratory infection the coughing spasms and vomiting may temporarily return.

The diagnosis of whooping cough may be made by hearing the whoop. A blood test during the coughing spasm phase may show changes in the blood (lymphocytosis) which would strongly support the diagnosis. The best and only way to confirm the diagnosis is to grow (culture) the *pertussis* in the laboratory. This is possible in the 'cold' phase and early in the coughing spasm phase provided no treatment has been given. The bacteria are grown by taking a pernasal swab; a fine flexible wire with cotton wool at the tip is passed through the nostrils to the back of the nose causing little discomfort.

About 10 children die annually from whooping cough in England and Wales: three-quarters in their 1st year. A few survivors develop permanent lung damage (bronchiectasis). Most deaths are caused by pneumonia which is the commonest complication. Each year as thousands of unimmunised children are affected it becomes a major source of distress to young children and a cause of anxiety in their parents. Hundreds of children are admitted to hospital.

The treatment of whooping cough varies according to the severity. Most children can be nursed at home under the supervision of the family doctor. The most severe, together with those with pneumonia or convulsions, are usually treated in hospital. Hospital treatment may require the use of oxygen, and clearing of throat and chest secretions by intermittent suction and physiotherapy. In young children tube feeding or small frequent feeds are often needed. A variety of medicines may be used to control the cough, none of which appears very effective. The most commonly used medicines are phenobarbitone, salbutamol, promethazine and atropine.

The antibiotic of choice is erythromycin estolate, which is most effective when given for 14 days. Unfortunately, erythromycin has no effect on the illness when given during the phase of coughing spasms, which is when the diagnosis is most likely to be made. Why then is erythromycin prescribed? It helps to reduce the spread of the illness in the community. By freeing the child of pertussis bacteria it becomes safe to expose the child to other susceptible children after 7 days. It is also possible that erythromycin may help prevent the onset of pneumonia. Erythromycin given in the 'cold' phase usually reduces the severity or stops the disease progressing. It is used preventively when an older child develops whooping cough and there is an unimmunised baby in the home. The untreated child is infective for 7 days after exposure to 3 weeks from the start of coughing spasms.

Mumps. Mumps occurs all year round, but is most common in winter and spring. The incubation period is 16–18 days. It is often very mild, about 30–40% of children have mumps without ever knowing. The illness starts with a child who feels unwell, is off his food, has a headache and a temperature, which may last a few days. Starting within a day of his symptoms he complains of soreness at the back of the jaw which is worse when he chews. Within hours he is noticed to have a swelling below or in front of the ear lobe on one or both sides. This swelling is caused by a salivary (spit) gland called the parotid. It reaches its maximum size in 1–3 days and then shrinks back to its unsual size in a further 3–7 days, occasionally longer. The swollen parotid is tender and causes the ear lobe to be pushed up and outwards, it is quite different from enlarged neck glands. One side usually enlarges a day or two before the other and salivary glands below the jaw may also become enlarged. Redness and swelling are commonly present in the mouth around the opening of the tube which leads from the affected gland.

Mumps virus can affect many organs, but produces few serious effects. The most frequent complications are inflammation of the brain and surrounding membranes (meningo-encephalitis) and inflammation of the testis (orchitis) in post-pubertal boys. Meningo-encephalitis is benign, the child making a complete recovery within a few days. Despite popular belief that orchitis results in impotence or sterility, this almost never happens.

There is no treatment of mumps. When discomfort is severe pain relief with paracetamol (acetominophen) may be required. Mumps vaccine is very effective; it is given at 15 months in the USA, but is not used in Britain. A child with mumps is infectious from 3 days before until 7 days after the start of the swelling.

Glandular fever (infectious mononucleosis). This illness is caused by a virus known as Epstein–Barr virus. The incubation period is thought to be 4–14 days. This may not be very accurate, however, because it is usually very difficult to determine both the source of infection and the time of contact. Glandular fever may start slowly or suddenly and the severity of the illness is very variable. Generally, the younger the child the milder the symptoms; large numbers of children have glandular fever without ever knowing. The typical story is that of headache and fever in a child who is unwell and off his food. The fever may last a few days to a fortnight. Sore throat and generalised glandular enlargement soon follow, glands at the back of the neck being particularly severely involved. Other signs which are sometimes present are swelling of the eyelids, red spots on the roof of the mouth and a rash. Interestingly, if the antibiotic, ampicillin, is given for the sore throat then almost all children develop a rash.

While the diagnosis of glandular fever is common in children, confirmation of the diagnosis is less frequent. There are characteristic blood changes (atypical lymphocytes) in glandular fever. Two other infections (cytomegalovirus and toxoplasmosis) produce an identical illness with similar blood changes. The diagnosis can be confirmed by blood tests specific for glandular fever. The two most commonly used in laboratories in Britain are Paul Bunnell and Monospot tests. These tests may take a few weeks to become positive and many children and about 10% of adolescents with glandular fever (proven Epstein–Barr virus infection) never have positive tests.

There is no specific treatment. Glandular enlargement gradually subsides over days or weeks. Discomfort from sore throat or tender glands may require treatment with paracetamol. Almost all children make a complete recovery, but a few children do feel unwell, tired and depressed for several months.

After recovery the virus remains in the saliva for many months. The disease is spread by exchange of saliva from child to child on contaminated objects or by kissing between parents and children or kissing among young adults.

Herpes. There are two types of herpes, Herpes 1 and Herpes 2. Herpes 2 has received much attention in the media because it causes a venereal infection with a rapidly rising incidence. Childhood infections are almost exclusively caused by Herpes 1.

There are 2 common forms of Herpes 1 in children:

1. Herpetic gingivostomatitis – inflammation and ulceration of the mouth and lips.
2. Herpes labialis – recurrent sores on the lips and skin of the face commonly known as 'cold sores'.

In the first 4 years of life most children are infected with herpes virus. About 90% show no evidence of the infection, the remainder become ill and at times ill enough to warrant admission to hospital.

The average incubation period for herpetic gingivostomatitis is 6 days (range 2–12). The child develops a high fever, sore throat, becomes very irritable, refuses to eat, salivates, and may have difficulty in speaking. Small blisters form in the mouth and on the lips, they rapidly break up to form shallow grey ulcers with red margins. The gums become red and swollen and bleed easily. Neck glands become enlarged and tender. Improvement usually occurs in 5–10 days. Most children can be treated at home, but some require hospital admission for intravenous fluids (a drip). Pain relief is provided with paracetamol. Local anaesthetic paste or lozenges may also be helpful. Iced drinks, ice cream and jelly are usually accepted when other foods are refused.

Other parts of the body that may be affected by herpes are the genitalia in girls (herpetic vulvovaginitis) and the eyes (herpetic keratoconjunctivitis). 'Cold sores' are not caused by a new herpes infection but rather a reactivation of the previous infection, 90% of which were asymptomatic. Following the herpes infection the virus remains permanently dormant in the nerves of the mouth. In some individuals certain 'trigger factors' can activate the virus so that it produces sores on the lips and skin of the face. Repetitive triggers may cause a problem of recurrent cold sores. The sores start as blisters which produce a feeling of pain, tingling or itching. They soon progress to ulcers and crusting forms in 3–4 days. Healing usually occurs within 5–12 days. Common trigger factors are fever, sunshine, emotional upset or stress, menstruation and gastroenteritis. There is no treatment for cold sores. They may be helped by applying a drying agent such as calamine lotion.

Herpes infections are generally benign but may be serious in new borns and in children with eczema. The recent discovery of acyclovir, a drug extremely effective against herpes, has dramatically improved the outlook, but acyclovir cream applied to cold sores has not been shown to promote faster healing.

Herpes appears to be spread by close bodily contact. The virus is present in the saliva, sores on the lips and skin, urine and faeces, all of which are a potential course of infection. It can be spread from cold sores to the genitals or eyes. Small children particularly are fond of stuffing their hands in their mouths, and are less inhibited about touching their genitals, so can easily self-infect themselves. They need careful observation while the sores are obvious, and encouragement to be thorough in hand washing.

Viral hepatitis (inflammation of the liver). It is caused by a virus known as hepatitis A virus. The incidence shows a wide geographical variation: it is uncommon in Britain and the USA but very common in some Third World countries. The incubation period is 15–40 days (average 30). The severity of the illness may vary from the child with few symptoms to the one who is very ill. It starts with the child feeling nauseated, tired and off his food, sometimes complaining of an intermittent dull ache in the upper part of the abdomen. The older child may have a fever and headache while the young child may have loose stools and fail to gain weight. Examination may show enlarged lymph glands and enlargement of the liver and spleen. Finger pressure over the liver (upper part of the abdomen on right) may be painful.

In many children the illness progresses no further than this stage, but in others, jaundice (a yellow colour of the skin and eyes) develops. The onset of jaundice may be associated with an improvement in symptoms. Parents will notice that the child's urine is much darker and the stools may look pale. The skin, which is often itchy, regains its normal colour after a week; rarely, jaundice may persist for a few months.

Almost all children make a complete recovery and can be looked after at home. If the child feels well he need not rest in bed. No special diet is required; let the child eat or drink whatever he likes. In the early stages when he may be vomiting make sure that he gets plenty of fluid so that he does not become dehydrated.

The infection is spread by the oral faecal route (like gastroenteritis); spread can best be eliminated by careful attention to hand washing after toileting or nappy changes. Great care should be taken in the handling and disposal of a young child's stools. Feeding utensils which are handled by the child and also used by other members of the family should where possible be boiled after use. The child remains infectious for one week after the onset of jaundice and if he is well enough he may then return to nursery or school.

Gamma globulin is a protective blood product which will modify or prevent the illness when given before its onset, particularly early in the incubation period. It may be given to close family contacts, and is also given to children travelling to 'high risk' areas when they are likely to stay for an extended period.

Scarlet fever. Scarlet fever, which was very common 50 years ago, is now rare. When I see a child with a temperature and rash parents, particularly grandparents, do occasionally ask 'Could it be scarlet fever'? I have included some information about this condition so that they might realise that whatever the cause might be it is probably not scarlet fever.

It is caused by bacteria known as streptococci. After an incubation period of 2–4 days the child develops fever, headache, vomiting and a sore throat; some have abdominal pain. The throat is red and the palate may have red spots. The tongue becomes white and furred with projecting red areas ('white strawberry tongue') and later changes to a red colour ('red strawberry tongue'). Within 12–48 hours the rash appears: it starts as pinhead red spots which give the skin a sandpaper-like texture and looks like sunburn with goose-pimples. It is usually not present on the face, which is flushed except for the area around the mouth. After a week when the temperature has settled and the child is feeling better the skin starts to peel, the head and face first then spreading to the rest of the body so that the hands and feet peel after 2–3 weeks. The diagnosis is sometimes made by finding a child with a peely skin who gives a history of a sore throat 2–3 weeks previously. The child is infectious for 10–21 days after onset of the rash or for 1 week after the start of treatment with penicillin. In the old days scarlet fever was an illness greatly feared because it was often followed by rheumatic fever or nephritis.

Table 3/1 Summary of incubation periods and infectivity

Disease	Incubation period (days)	Infectivity
Measles	10–15	5 days before to 5 days after onset of rash
German measles	14–21	7 days before to 4 days after onset of rash
Roseola	7–17 (usually 10)	Unknown
Erythema infectiosum	10	Unknown
Chicken-pox	14–16	About 5–10 days after onset of rash
Whooping cough	7–10	7 days before until 3 weeks after onset of coughing or 1 week after the start of treatment
Mumps	16–18	3 days before to 7 days after onset of swelling
Glandular fever	?4–14	Unknown
Hepatitis	15–40 (average 30)	Up to 1 week after onset of jaundice
Scarlet fever	2–4	10–21 days after onset of rash or one week after start of treatment

IMMUNISATIONS

To appreciate the need for immunisation it is necessary to know something about the illnesses it is hoped to prevent. Information about each of these illnesses is presented below or elsewhere in the book.

Diphtheria begins just like a sore throat but quickly develops into a serious illness which can last for weeks. It blocks the nose or throat, making it difficult and sometimes impossible for the child to breathe. It also produces a poison which gets into the child's bloodstream and attacks the heart and nervous system. Diphtheria is now very rare in Britain, but it is still a disease that can kill.

Tetanus is caught when germs from the soil get into an open wound. It produces a poison which attacks the nervous system, causing painful muscle spasms. These spasms can happen in any muscle in the body but often they are in the jaw and neck, which is why tetanus used to be called 'lockjaw'. Tetanus is rare, but there's still a real chance of getting it and it can be fatal.

Poliomyelitis usually called polio, now only occurs occasionally, but it is still a real risk. It attacks the nervous system and this can cause paralysis of the muscles. It can affect any muscle in the body. If it affects the breathing muscles, a child may have to be helped to breathe artificially, and even then may die. If it affects the legs, they can become weak or even paralysed, and sometimes this is permanent.

Tuberculosis is a serious disease which can affect many parts of the body. In children it commonly causes pneumonia and infection around the brain (meningitis). Despite an effective vaccine and treatment, a few children in the United Kingdom continue to die from tuberculosis each year. In the USA probably well over a 1000 children die each year from tuberculosis.

When should children in Britain be immunised?

A scheme commonly used in Britain is shown below. If this schedule becomes interrupted the remaining doses should be given as if there had been no break:

At birth many hospitals give BCG (tuberculosis immunisation) to Asian babies and any others likely to come into contact with tuberculosis.

Table 3/2 Recommended childhood immunisation schedule for Britain

Age	Immunisation
From 3 months	Diphtheria ⎫ Whooping cough ⎬ single injection known as 'triple vaccine' Tetanus Oral polio ⎭
5–6 months	Diphtheria Whooping cough Tetanus Oral polio
9–11 months	Diphtheria Whooping cough Tetanus Oral polio
15–24 months	Measles
About 5 years	Diphtheria (booster) Tetanus (booster) Oral polio (booster)
Girls aged 10–14	Rubella (German measles)
Girls and boys at about 13 years	Tuberculosis (BCG)
15–19 years (leaving school)	Tetanus Oral polio

When should children in the USA be immunised?

The scheme recommended by the American Academy of Pediatrics is shown below. The schemes in Australia and Canada are broadly the same, the notable exception being rubella vaccine in Australia, which is given only to girls as in the British scheme. At present haemophilus vaccine is recommended routinely only in the USA.

Why should children be immunised?

Immunisation protects children against these illnesses. It is highly

Table 3/3 Recommended childhood immunisation schedule for the USA

Age	Immunisation
2 months	Diphtheria Whooping cough Tetanus Oral polio } also known as DTPT
4 months	Diphtheria Whooping cough Tetanus Oral polio
6 months	Diphtheria Whooping cough Tetanus Oral polio
12 months	BCG (tuberculosis vaccine)
*15 months	Mumps Measles Rubella (German measles)
*18 months	Diphtheria Whooping cough Tetanus Oral polio
2 years	Haemophilus vaccine
4–7 years	Diphtheria Whooping cough Tetanus Polio
14–16 years	Tetanus Diphtheria

* These can be given at the same time (recommendation of Advisory Committee on Immunisation Practices).

effective and on rare occasions when the illness is not prevented it is much milder. Immunisation not only protects the child who is immunised, but will also reduce risk within your family later, if you have another child. A new baby is always at risk from germs carried by older children. If the older children are immunised, then the baby is less at risk. In the case of girls vaccination against German measles protects future children.

What are the side-effects?

There are few serious side-effects of vaccination. Most children do however show a slight reaction to the triple vaccine. Within 48 hours they may become feverish, miserable and off their food. There may also be some redness and swelling at the site of the injection. Very rarely the fever may cause a convulsion (febrile convulsion) which does not have any harmful efffects. The frequency of these effects is higher with the USA vaccine.

With the exception of the child who has had a convulsion, these *minor* reactions should *not* be used as a contra-indication to further 'triple' (DTP) injections. In the case of a convulsion, *only* whooping cough should be omitted on future occasions.

Can whooping cough vaccine cause brain damage?

Yes, it may, but so can whooping cough. The number of children suffering brain damage is estimated at 1 in 310 000 immunisations. If *all* the children in Britain were immunised each year about 2 would be brain damaged. Is it worth taking the risk? Yes, the risk is small when compared with the fact that in the last major whooping cough epidemic in Britain in 1982 involving 66 000 children, 13 died. This equation of course does not take into account the fact that there are children who survive with permanent lung damage (bronchiectasis). The risk given above is based on the most comprehensive British study which was conducted between 1976 and 1979. In a study of 1000 children there were 4 in whom no obvious cause for their brain damage could be found. Because these children had been immunised prior to the onset of the brain damage the cause was attributed to whooping cough vaccine. There are many experts who regard this evidence as highly speculative and doubt whether there is any risk at all.

Is whooping cough vaccine effective?

Extremely, studies show that the efficacy varies between 80–90%.

What are the contra-indications?

There are *no* scientifically validated reasons for not giving whooping cough vaccine, but it would be foolhardy to give the vaccine to a child who convulsed after a previous vaccination or any child who has a fever. Minor infections without fever or being generally unwell even if on an antibiotic are not reasons for delaying immunisation. This is particularly true for those babies who always seem snuffly or chesty.

After a thorough review of the medical literature, Illingworth (1984), a leading British paediatrician recently wrote the following about whooping cough vaccine, 'I was unable to determine the evidence on which it is said by some that epilepsy (in the child or a near or distant relative), developmental delay, perinatal hypoxia, cerebral irritation in the newborn, neurological disease, family history of central nervous system disorders or any other condition increase the risk of brain damage as a result of the vaccine.' In recent years there has been much confusion about the indications and contra-indications of whooping cough vaccine. For example, in Britain it has been the practice to withhold the vaccine from any child with brain damage, while the French have taken the opposite view and actively encouraged vaccine uptake in these children.

Should a child over 3 be given whooping cough vaccine?

Yes, although three-quarters of the deaths and much of the persisting illness occur in children under 1 year, it is considered worthwhile to have these children immunised. The reason is more for the protection of other younger children than the vaccinated child. An unvaccinated 4-year-old may pass whooping cough on to a newborn baby with disastrous consequences.

Does a smaller dose make it safer?

There is no evidence that a smaller dose is safer and it will almost certainly be less effective.

Which are 'live' vaccines?

These are polio, mumps, measles, rubella (German measles) and the BCG (tuberculosis). Although these vaccines contain a living virus or bacterium (BCG), they can safely be given to children when their mothers are pregnant.

Can more than one 'live' vaccine be given at the same time?

Yes, but if one has been given separately, a gap of 3 weeks is required before the next should be given. This is not because there is any danger, but unless they are given simultaneously one may stop the other's working.

Which children should not be given 'live' vaccine?

There are a few rare conditions which cause a lowered immunity (resistance) to infections. Children with these illnesses should not have live vaccine. Your family doctor or paediatrician will be able to advise you about these illnesses. Children on *oral* steroids may have a lowered immunity and should also not receive live vaccine.

Is measles vaccine completely safe?

No, but much safer than measles itself. The risk of getting encephalitis (inflammation of the brain) after the vaccine is at least 20 times less than the risk of encephalitis after measles itself. Furthermore, encephalitis after the vaccine is usually milder and recovery is complete. About 15% of children have a fever 7–10 days after the vaccine and about 1 in 1000 has a 'febrile' convulsion. The risk of a convulsion is nearly 10 times less than having a convulsion during measles itself.

One death occurs in every 3–5000 reported cases of measles, yet in Britain only about 60% of children are immunised against measles. In the USA where almost all children are immunised the number of cases of measles has fallen from 400 000 annually before the vaccine was licensed in 1963 to as few as 3000 in 1981.

Are there any contra-indications to measles vaccination?

None, other than those mentioned for live vaccines, but if *the child* suffers from febrile convulsions or epilepsy it would be reasonable to give 'human measles immunoglobulin' at the same time. Two injections are given at different sites. This reduces the fever but still seems to provide adequate protection. Because the protection is not as good as when the vaccine is given without immunoglobulin, the American Academy of Pediatrics does not recommend the use of immunoglobulin in this way. Children at risk from fever should take paracetamol (acetominophen) at the first sign.

Can measles vaccine be given to children with egg allergy?

Yes, despite early fears it was soon realised that egg allergy was *not* a contra-indication. This question no longer arises because nowadays measles vaccine is not grown on eggs; it is grown in chicken cell embryos.

Should measles vaccine be given if the child has just been in contact with measles?

Yes, the vaccine may be effective in preventing measles even if given within 3 days of exposure. An alternative way of preventing or modifying measles is to give measles immunoglobulin within 6 days of exposure. If measles does not develop the vaccine should then be given only after 3 months.

Is it harmful to give measles or whooping cough vaccine to a child who has already had the illness?

No, it is not. Parents often incorrectly think the child has had measles or whooping cough and if there is the slightest doubt the child should be immunised. In the same way, children who have been previously immunised can be safely immunised again. This often happens when a child moves from one country to another and the immunisation records are lost.

Is polio vaccine safe?

Yes, but about once in every 3 million doses the vaccinated child or close contacts will develop a paralytic illness like polio. Because of this it is important for the mother or father who are not already immunised to be immunised at the same time as their child.

Does it matter if the baby vomits after the polio vaccine?

Yes, it does. If a child vomits within an hour then the dose should be repeated.

What about the German measles (rubella) vaccine?

It is safe, but should *not* be given if there is the slightest possibility that the young girl is pregnant. Pregnancy should also be delayed for 3 months after vaccination. Vaccination early in pregnancy may expose the developing fetus to the risk of being damaged, but, in practice, studies of pregnant vaccinated women have shown this risk to be negligible. German measles is very difficult to diagnose and the diagnosis is frequently wrong. Even if you feel your child has had German measles, it would be best if she were immunised. This is the only sure way of protecting her future children. After German measles vaccination a small number of children develop fever and joint pains.

If a mother is pregnant is it safe for her child to have German measles vaccination?

It is perfectly safe. There is no evidence to suggest that the virus can be transferred from child to mother.

Is BCG (tuberculosis vaccination) safe?

Yes, sometimes a local reaction occurs at the injection site which may cause an abscess or scarring. These are more common when the injection has been given under rather than into the skin and also when a jet injector has been used. The abscess may persist for a number of months. BCG need not be given to all teenage children; only those with no immunity (resistance) to tuberculosis are given the vaccine in Britain. Before BCG is given the state of immunity is first determined by a skin test (tuberculin test).

Where should BCG be given?

The lower part of the outer aspect of the arm is usually the injection site chosen. No matter how carefully BCG is given a small percentage of children do end up with an ugly scar. If your doctor discusses the injection site with you or the child I should recommend that you ask him to give the injection on the inner aspect of the upper arm; the chance of scarring is less than on the outer aspect and the site concealed.

How effective is BCG?

Most studies in the Western world suggest that BCG provides 75–80% protection against tuberculosis. The protective effect of BCG is thought to last about 15 years. BCG is an abbreviation for Bacille Calmette-Guérin.

When should a premature baby be immunised?

At the usual time *after birth*, i.e. 3 months (2 months in the USA and other countries) after birth irrespective of prematurity or weight. On the other hand, BCG should not be given until the child is at least 40 weeks from *conception*. For example, a baby born at 34 weeks should wait 6 weeks before BCG is given.

Should children with eczema or asthma be immunised?

The answer is very definitely *yes*. Many children with these conditions continue not to be immunised as a result of 'old wives' tales' and are thereby exposed to unnecessary risks.

What is Haemophilus influenza vaccine?

The recent recommendation that this vaccine be given routinely in the USA has led to much controversy. *Haemophilus influenza* is a germ normally found in the nose and throat. In certain young children it commonly causes otitis media (p. 213), meningitis (p. 293) and croup (p. 222). The current vaccine is not effective against all types of haemophilus but is highly effective against the type causing meningitis and croup, but the child's system will not fully respond to the vaccine before age 2. This is unfortunate; in the USA where there are about 10 000 cases of haemophilus meningitis annually as many as three-quarters occur before 2. The vaccine will, however, prevent the most serious form of croup (acute epiglottitis) which usually occurs after 2. The effect of the vaccine lasts only 18 months and at present there is no firm recommendation about whether the vaccine should be repeated. It is almost certain that within the next 3 years vaccines which protect children much longer than 2 will be licensed in the USA.

When should tetanus immunisations be repeated?

It would be advisable to repeat tetanus immunisations at 10-yearly intervals throughout life.

When does a child with a wound need a tetanus booster dose?

For a clean minor wound no booster is needed for a *fully immunised* child unless 10 years have elapsed since the last dose. For a contaminated wound a booster should be given if more than 5 years since the last dose. Needless to say, if immunisation is incomplete or if there is any uncertainty a booster dose should always be given.

There are 4 other vaccines which are used in children from time to time:

1. Influenza vaccine – this is indicated before each winter in children with chronic chest or heart disease. Egg allergy is a contra-indication. In the USA it may be given from 6 months, in Britain it is usually not given before age 4. The formulation of influenza vaccine varies from year to year. If there is no change from one year to another the child still requires revaccination because immunity declines after a year.
2. Hepatitis B vaccine – this is given to children who suffer from blood diseases which necessitate frequent blood transfusions or injections with blood components. It is also given to some babies immediately after birth when the mother has previously had hepatitis B and remains infectious.
3. Pneumococcal vaccine – this is a vaccine against infections caused by bacteria called pneumococci, which cause pneumonia, men-

ingitis and other serious infections in children. It is given to children over 2 who have had removal of the spleen. It is also given to children with sickle cell anaemia (a blood disease (p. 315)) and recurrent nephrotic syndrome (a kidney disease (p. 160)). The vaccine which has been used until very recently was effective against 14 types of pneumococcus. In 1983 a new vaccine effective against 23 types of pneumococcus was licensed in the USA. Children who have had the old vaccine need not have the new one: the increased benefit is marginal. At present revaccination with pneumococcal vaccine in adults is not recommended; in children the need for revaccination and the risk have not yet been clearly worked out.

4. Meningococcal vaccine – this vaccine is used in certain parts of the world where meningococcal meningitis is very common.

It is not recommended in Britain or North America for the following reasons:

(a) the risk of infection is low

(b) the vaccine is effective against types A and C. In Britain and North America more than half of the infections are caused by type B

(c) much of the disease occurs among infants too young to benefit.

Vaccines for going abroad

Children as well as adults travelling to certain parts of the world, particularly underdeveloped countries, may require vaccination against typhoid, infectious hepatitis, cholera or yellow fever.

Parents wishing to obtain up-to-date information about which countries require vaccination and also where there is a risk of malaria should contact:

UK

International Relations Division, DHSS, Alexander Fleming House, Elephant and Castle, London SE1 6BY. Telephone: 01–407 5522 ext. 6749/6711

Public Health Laboratory Service, Communicable Surveillance Centre, 61 Colindale Avenue, London NW9 5EQ. Telephone: 01–200 6868

USA

State Health Departments/Centres for Disease Control, Atlanta, Georgia 30333. Telephone: 404–329 3311

Chapter Four

Nutrition

INFANT FEEDING

Breast or bottle?

Breast feeding is the natural and best way of feeding a baby. Most mothers find this a very pleasurable experience. However, there are countless millions of infants dearly loved by their mothers, who have been reared on bottle feeds. While breast is undoubtedly best those mothers not wishing to breast feed, for whatever reason, should not feel guilty.

Is breast milk best for the premature infant?
It probably is but there is at present some controversy; some paediatricians believe that a premature infant formula may be more suitable. Milk from a mother of a premature infant is different from the mother of a term infant; it contains more protein. Most paediatricians would agree that pooled breast milk, as supplied by milk banks is inappropriate for the very premature infant, because the vast majority of mothers contributing milk have term infants.

How frequently should the infant be fed?
The first feed is usually given 4–6 hours after birth. Parents have a choice of waking the infant every 3–4 hours according to a schedule or feeding on demand, i.e. when the child cries. It should be borne in mind that infants cry for reasons other than hunger; he may be wet or just bored. Within a few weeks it may be more convenient to omit the night feed.

Is it necessary to warm bottle feeds?
Warming is not necessary as feeds at room temperature or straight from the refrigerator are just as well tolerated. If feeds are warmed,

always check the milk temperature before feeding, particularly when the feed has been warmed in a microwave oven.

How much should he get?

The infant should be put to one breast and when sucking slows be transferred to the other. Half the milk is consumed in 2 minutes and almost all by 4 minutes, but the infant can be left on the breast until he falls asleep, or as long as the mother desires. Contrary to the belief of many parents and midwives long periods on the breast do not cause sore nipples. True lactation failure does occur but is uncommon and a healthy child who is put to the breast at regular intervals will almost certainly get enough. The amount of milk produced bears no relation to breast size. Milk production is influenced by emotion so the excitement associated with discharge from hospital does often cause a temporary reduction in volume. Drinking extra fluids does not increase milk volume.

One advantage of bottle feeding is that the volume consumed can be measured. The average amount taken on the first day is 60ml/kg, increasing to 150ml/kg/day at the end of the first week. With the introduction of solids this volume should be gradually reduced.

Will the milk agree with him?

It is frequent for mothers to change the preparation for some trivial reason, often on the advice of grandparents or friends. There are differences between preparations, but these are negligible and for practical purposes should be ignored. If you have a problem take expert advice rather than change the milk.

Does breast feeding cause constipation?

A breast fed infant may pass 5 or 6 stools a day or 1 every 10 days, both are normal. Infrequency of stools is a very common cause for maternal concern, being attributed to 'constipation'. Unlike the stools of constipation these are soft and do not require treatment. The stool colour of a breast fed infant may be orange yellow or bright green, both being normal.

How should feeding bottles be sterilised?

They can be boiled for 10 minutes or soaked in water to which a chemical steriliser has been added, the duration being given in the instructions. Both methods are effective, so choose the most convenient.

How long should bottles be sterilised?

It is safe to stop sterilising bottles at about 6–9 months, but attention to hygiene while preparing feeds should continue well after this time.

Is it safe to take drugs while breast feeding?

Many drugs, including alcohol, are excreted in breast milk. The amounts are, however, so small that it would be most unlikely for any to affect the child.

When should solids be started?

It is the recommendation of the Department of Health in Britain, and the American Academy of Pediatrics that solids should be introduced between 4–6 months. It is best to start with cereals, then single fruits, then meat and vegetables.

How long should formula feeding continue?

Whole pasteurised milk can safely be introduced at any time after 6 months. It does not provide sufficient iron or vitamins which should be taken as supplements until the first birthday. In America most marketed milk is fortified with vitamin D so that there is a need for iron supplements only. Many parents find it more convenient and prefer to continue formula until the first birthday. It avoids the need to provide supplements.

What about skim milk?

Skim milk or half skim milk should not be used in the first year.

Cow's milk protein intolerance (CMPI)

Although large numbers of parents and doctors attribute all kinds of ailments to CMPI, it is in fact uncommon. The true incidence is difficult to establish because of a lack of objective evidence on which to base the diagnosis. It is, however, the most common cause of food intolerance. There are two types of CMPI; first a temporary variety which may occur in association with gastroenteritis, second a condition of unknown cause limited to the first 2–3 years of life, which need not be associated with a family history of allergy. Details follow about this latter type.

What are the signs and symptoms?

These usually develop in the first 6 months. Most children develop vomiting and bloody diarrhoea immediately after drinking milk, the presentation often being indistinguishable from gastroenteritis. Rarely the child may develop pallor, a fall in blood pressure (shock) and loss of consciousness. Swelling of the face and mouth, wheezing and an urticarial rash (p. 252) may accompany these symptoms.

A less common form presents after 24 hours, sometimes days later. It too presents with diarrhoea but may cause malabsorption and failure to thrive, showing a marked similarity to coeliac disease (p. 121). There are two other presentations with slow onset. The first occurs in older infants and is not associated with diarrhoea or vomiting. These children lose protein and blood in the stool so that they present with generalised swelling (oedema) or anaemia. The second is known as milk-induced colitis. These children present with a persistent bloody diarrhoea which may become apparent as early as the first week of life.

How is CMPI diagnosed?

The most practical and reliable but potentially dangerous way of diagnosing it is by challenging the child with milk and gauging the response. If there is a reaction it might not necessarily be due to CMPI, but could be caused by an intercurrent infection. The child should, however, be placed on a milk exclusion diet until he is challenged again. In the past it has been recommended that three challenges should be performed before the diagnosis is confirmed, but this seldom happens as most parents not surprisingly are extremely reluctant to challenge the child again when he is well and thriving on a milk exclusion diet. Children who do not react to a milk challenge should be started on a milk containing diet and carefully observed over the ensuing weeks to see if there is a recurrence of symptoms. A word of warning is necessary for parents wanting to attempt milk or any other food challenge in the home because there is some risk involved. It would be preferable for this to be done in hospital, where if the child collapsed appropriate facilities and expert help would be to hand. Parents wanting to start the child on a milk exclusion diet are advised to consult a dietitian, who will make sure that the diet is nutritionally adequate and that foods containing milk proteins are not inadvertently given in the diet.

Are there any other ways of diagnosing CMPI?

It has been well established that there are changes in the small intestine which are similar and at times identical to coeliac disease.

Another way of confirming the diagnosis is to perform an intestinal biopsy (p. 122). If abnormal, the child is started on a milk exclusion diet. At a later date a milk challenge will be given with a biopsy being performed before the challenge and after symptoms recur. A normal biopsy before, which becomes abnormal after challenge, establishes the diagnosis. This method has much to commend it in purely scientific terms, but most parents find it undesirable, seeing no need for further biopsies when the child is making good progress on a milk exclusion diet.

What about skin tests or a blood allergy test (RAST)?

In their present form these tests neither confirm nor refute the diagnosis and are of little use.

What is the treatment?

As outlined previously the treatment is a properly supervised milk exclusion diet. The child is given a milk formula containing a protein hydrosylate (Nutramigen or Pregestimil). The protein which has been broken down into its constituent amino acids is well tolerated. Many children with CMPI are also intolerant of cow's milk sugar (lactose). These milks do not contain any lactose.

What about a soya bean formula or goat's milk?

These are sometimes used but are not ideal. Many children who have CMPI will not tolerate soya protein or goat's milk protein.

Are there any drugs which may help?

There have been a few reports indicating the benefit of sodium cromoglycate, but others have not been so encouraging. There does, however, seem little place for drug treatment of food allergy.

What is the outlook?

As stated earlier CMPI is a temporary problem. About half the children have grown out of it by a year and all by 3 years.

IRON DEFICIENCY ANAEMIA

Iron is essential for the formation of haemoglobin, the part of the red cell which carries oxygen. After being absorbed in the diet it is normally stored in the body before use. When the stores become depleted haemoglobin cannot be formed in sufficient amounts, the resulting deficiency being known as iron deficiency anaemia.

How is anaemia defined?

After the first 6 months until 6 years a haemoglobin below 11g/dl is regarded as anaemia. After 6 years until puberty the lower limit of normal is 12g/dl. After puberty the haemoglobin of males is slightly higher (lower limit 13g/dl).

How is iron deficiency diagnosed?

It can be diagnosed by examining red cells under the microscope. Iron deficient cells are smaller (microcytic) and do not stain as well (hypochromic). Other types of anaemia do occasionally produce similar red cell changes. The diagnosis can be confirmed by measuring the amount of iron in the blood and by another blood test measuring ferritin which will indicate the amount present in the stores.

How common is it?

It is very common, usually among socially deprived communities. In Britain it is particularly common among Asian immigrant children, because cow's milk which contains little iron constitutes a high proportion of their calorie intake.

What causes iron deficiency?

Iron is needed for growth, the more rapid growth the more iron consumed. At birth only a quarter of the body's iron is in the stores, the remainder being in the blood haemoglobin. Iron deficiency arises when as a result of rapid growth or blood loss there is insufficient iron in the diet to make up the shortfall.

Why does iron deficiency matter?

There is now substantial evidence that iron deficiency has an adverse effect on brain function. Several studies have shown that iron deficiency with or without anaemia is associated with abnormal behaviour and mental performance, which improve with iron treatment. These findings have obvious implications for learning in the developing child. Other than pallor the signs of iron deficiency anaemia are more subtle. The child may be irritable, or apathetic showing little interest in his surroundings. He may be off his food and gaining weight slowly. Many have a craving (pica) for unnatural things as food. Reports from the USA suggest that eating excessive ice (pagophagia) is common.

Why is iron deficiency common in premature infants?

Iron is transferred from mother to fetus in the last third of pregnancy, the amount not being influenced by the mother's iron stores.

A premature infant is more likely to develop anaemia for two reasons: first he grows more rapidly, second he is born with very little iron. Both term and premature infants are born with a haemoglobin between 14–20g/dl. The haemoglobin then falls, reaching its lowest point (nadir) between 4–10 weeks. The fall which occurs earlier and to a greater extent in premature infants (lowest average haemoglobin 9g/dl is normal and is called physiologic anaemia). Giving iron to treat or prevent physiologic anaemia is of no use at all. Iron deficiency anaemia only becomes apparent at 4–6 months and can be prevented.

How can it be prevented?

The daily iron requirement is 1mg/kg/day (2mg for premature infants). Most formula milk is now fortified with iron so that consumption of the daily requirement is guaranteed. In the case of a premature infant milk alone will not meet the daily requirement. These infants are given iron supplements within a few weeks in Britain, while in the USA they tend to be given later at about 8 weeks.

The iron in breast milk is well absorbed, term breast fed infants do not require iron supplements. Most paediatricians, however, recommend iron supplements for premature breast fed infants.

What is the treatment?

The treatment is iron in a dose of 6mg/kg/day. This is the dose of elemental iron, which is the iron part of an iron salt. For example 100mg of ferrous sulphate contains 20mg of elemental iron and 80mg of sulphate. The iron is best absorbed when taken 2–3 times daily between meals. The iron may make the stools loose and gives them a black colour. Liquid preparations may cause a temporary discolouration of the teeth. This can be prevented by sucking up the iron with a straw or washing out the mouth with water after each dose. Treatment should be continued for 2 months until stores are replenished.

In addition to providing iron the diet should be modified so that there is no recurrence. In young children a reduction in the amount of cow's milk and replacement of the calories with an iron rich food may be all that is required. The advice of a dietitian may be very helpful.

RICKETS

Rickets is a bone condition usually caused by a deficiency of vitamin

D. In industrialised countries it is uncommon, occurring mostly in dark-skinned children who have a vegetarian diet, particularly when large quantities of unfortified cow's milk are consumed. In these countries rickets is more likely to be caused by kidney disease, malabsorption and other rare conditions rather than a deficiency of vitamin D.

Vitamin D occurs naturally in certain foods. Common sources of vitamin D are eggs, butter, fish and fish oils, the best known being cod liver oil. Exposure to sunlight also causes its manufacture in the skin. Whether skin pigmentation interferes with vitamin D formation is not known, but is suggested by the tendency for it to occur in dark-skinned children.

Vitamin D is essential for bone development; when in short supply the bones become soft, pliable and prone to deformities and fractures. One of the early signs is softening of the sides and back of the skull (craniotabes), which can also occur normally. Pressing on the skull will cause it to indent in a 'ping pong ball' like manner. Other signs are bossing on the front of the skull, beading on the sides of the rib cage, often with a deep groove (sulcus) below the lower end. There is widening of the ends of long bones and eventually bone deformities and poor growth occur. Rickets also affects muscles making them floppy, many children developing a pot belly from poor abdominal muscle tone.

The diagnosis can be confirmed by blood tests and x-rays which typically show thinning of the bone and concavity ('cupping') at the end. The treatment consists of appropriate dietary modification and big doses of vitamin D or smaller doses of the modified more potent form. Treatment is usually given for at least a month. An alternative is for the child to have a large dose of vitamin D by a single intramuscular injection. The outlook is excellent and most deformities, often quite severe, will correct spontaneously with treatment.

Rickets of very premature infants (usually weighing less than 1kg) is now a common problem, the cause and significance of which is not known for certain. Because of their rapid growth both breast fed and formula fed premature infants are usually given vitamin D supplements, which are continued until the feeding of solids is fully established.

OBESITY

What is obesity?

There are various definitions although ultimately it is defined by the eye of the beholder. If a child looks fat, he is obese. Where there is doubt it may be helpful to compare his weight with his height. Weight and height charts are shown in Figures 1/1, 1/2, 1/10, 1/11. Obese children are much fatter than they are tall.

Why do we want to help obese children?

There are two reasons: firstly, obesity is unhealthy and in adulthood is associated with a reduced life expectancy. Obese adults are at risk of developing heart disease, high blood pressure and diabetes. In children obesity has no medical risks although there seems to be a high incidence of chest infections, particularly in the pre-school child. The second reason is that fat, school age children are nearly always teased. This causes much unhappiness and may distort personality, education and family relationships.

What causes obesity?

There are many causes. Contrary to public belief simple overeating by itself is seldom the cause. Certainly most children with established obesity eat no more, and frequently less, than non-obese children. Whatever the cause, it is true to say that calorie intake is in excess of requirement, this being influenced by exercise and the efficiency with which calories are utilised for bodily functions. It is well known that lack of exercise may cause obesity. Whether obese children require less calories because they utilise them more efficiently is not known for certain. Obesity runs in families but whether genetic influences or common family environment are responsible for this readily observable fact has been difficult to identify. At present, on the basis of studies of identical twins living apart and families with natural and adopted children, it can be concluded that there is both a genetic and environmental component to obesity. In this context environment means type and amount of food eaten.

Many parents fear a medical cause for the child's obesity. I have often been asked 'Has he got something wrong with his glands, Doctor?' There are some genetic and hormone (gland) causes of obesity. These are characterised by short stature or mental retardation or both, so the child who is of 'normal' height and intelligence does not have one of these causes. Normal in this sense obviously depends on the parents' height and intelligence to a major extent.

Do fat children become fat adults?

The outlook for an obese child in the first year or two is much better than the older child; the majority will not become obese adults. The older the obese child the more likely the prospect of adult obesity. The obese 7-year-old is likely to become an obese adolescent and the obese adolescent is very likely to become an obese adult. As many as 75% of obese adolescents will eventually become obese adults.

How should obesity in childhood be managed?

The objectives of treatment are to produce, in the short term, slimming and, in the long term, a permanent change in eating habits. Best results are achieved by a programme of calorie restriction, exercise, nutritional education of the child or family and attempts at behaviour modification. The treatment of obesity will not succeed unless the child is motivated. When a child of school age is referred because of obesity my first step is to find out whether the child dislikes being overweight. A boy may volunteer that he hates being called 'fatty' or that he cannot move fast enough to be a good footballer. A girl may feel ugly or be unhappy that she cannot wear fashionable dresses. If the child is quite content to be fat, attempts to impose a low calorie diet are likely to cause arguments and unhappiness in the family with almost certain failure.

Most children will lose weight on an 800–1200 calorie diet. Diets should be composed of usual foods in proportions of a 'balanced' diet. Advice about diets can be obtained from a dietitian. There are on the market various reasonably priced books which parents may find very useful. Many provide recipes specially designed, or which can be adapted, for children who are slimming. It is important that the child should be given a rough guide about the calorie content of various foods so that certain foods can be avoided or reduced. Most parents have a good idea about which foods are 'fattening' and this information should be passed on to the child. In the event of uncertainty, a list of the calorie content of a variety of foods can be obtained from a dietitian. Fat has double the calories of protein and carbohydrate and fatty foods should be avoided. Fruit and vegetables, which have few calories, are satisfying and prevent constipation, should be encouraged. It goes without saying that 'junk foods' (chips, hamburgers, etc.) should be severely restricted. Simple commonsense measures include the use of skimmed milk and low-fat spread instead of butter. Drinks, especially fizzy drinks, should be of the low calorie variety. Chewing gum and sweets where possible should be 'sugar free'. It is always advisable to introduce these measures for the family as a whole rather than for an individual child. This is not only easier but it also prevents friction between children, and parents also derive some benefit.

Most studies have shown that dieting will enable children to shed a large amount of weight, but unless there is a permanent change in eating habits this weight will eventually be regained. Appetite suppressant drugs have been tried in children but are seldom used because their effect, like dieting, is only temporary. The need to eat is brought on by many factors other than hunger: social occasions, displays of food, feelings of unhappiness, being in the kitchen, watching television, boredom. Parents should attempt to define those situations in which the child snacks. Commonly these include times of stress or tiredness, occasions such as coming home from school or before going to bed, and periods of television viewing or studying. Having pinpointed the situations when snacking is most common a concerted effort should be made to avoid snacks.

Exercise is an important part of a slimming programme. It causes calories to be used up and should be encouraged. There are many ways activity may be increased. A simple measure may be walking to and from school each day. Those sports activities which the child likes most should be pursued. Where possible good behaviour should be rewarded with sports related items, e.g. ballet lessons or new football boots. Good behaviour should never be rewarded with sweets or food.

What about Weight Watchers?

Joining Weight Watchers is often very beneficial for older children and teenagers. They provide a well-run, sensible weight reducing programme, although some parents may find them expensive. They do, however, have a reduced price for children.

In conclusion, obesity is common and very difficult to treat, but with will power, a commonsense diet and exercise some improvement can usually be made.

ANOREXIA NERVOSA

Anorexia nervosa is one of the most perplexing medical conditions; the reason why someone would want to starve herself in the midst of plenty seems inconceivable. It is also one of the most frustrating conditions, for both parents and professionals. To be told by an emaciated teenager that she is not eating because 'it will make her fat' leads one to despair. The parental feeling of helplessness and bewilderment is soon followed by anxiety as the weight continues to fall. In the midst of all the parental concern the child appears totally oblivious, communication becoming impossible.

What is anorexia nervosa?

The literal meaning of the name is a nervous lack of appetite. There are many definitions of anorexia nervosa, none of which is perfect. The main features of the condition are listed below:

1. It affects mainly females – the female/male ratio being about 20:1.
2. The onset is usually from puberty to 25.
3. They have an intense concern about becoming obese which does not diminish as weight loss progresses.
4. They have a disturbance of body image, such as claiming to feel fat even when emaciated.
5. Their weight loss is greater than 15% of their original weight (25% if over 18). They do not have any known physical cause to account for the weight loss.
6. All females have amenorrhoea (no menstruation). When weight loss falls below a critical level menstruation ceases.
7. Their attitude and behaviour become distorted so that their whole life revolves round food and weight. They refuse to eat enough to maintain a 'reasonable' weight and are unmoved by feelings of hunger, threats or attempts to persuade them to eat. In their preoccupation with weight and their control over it they will avoid 'fattening' foods and may take plenty of exercise. They may even resort to additional methods such as self-induced vomiting or taking laxatives (opening medicines).

How common is anorexia nervosa?

It is difficult to get a very accurate incidence, as many instances may be mild and not come to medical attention. It seems, however, that of those severely affected the number in female teenagers may be as high as 1 in 100. In Britain it has been estimated that there are at least 10 000 affected at any one time and the numbers appear to be increasing.

What are the causes?

We do not know. It is very common for teenage girls (and boys) to diet and to be concerned about their weight and appearance. Why some develop anorexia nervosa is a complete mystery. There are two theories about the cause. The first theory proposes that the cause arises from a conflict and uncertainty about early womanhood. Loss of breast tissue, cessation of menstruation and a loss of any sexual feelings are commonly cited as the girl's way of retreating into childhood. This theory does not, however, explain why some women with children develop the condition or why it may develop for the first time during a pregnancy.

The second theory proposes that the girl's refusal to eat is a means by which she is striving for her independence, although somewhat misguidedly. It boils down to the question of who is really in control. Knowing a bit about the parents and families of anorexics helps put this theory in perspective. The parents are generally reasonably affluent in that they are mainly business or professional people. For many the relative affluence was recently acquired, they themselves not brought up with all the advantages and opportunities their children now have. The families are often excessively close with rather rigid attitudes. In a general way the parents could be described as overprotective, overconcerned and overambitious. While these qualities might generally be considered to be quite admirable it is thought that anorexia nervosa may occur as a culmination of the child's desperate fight against feeling enslaved and exploited, not permitted or competent to lead a life of her own. In this blind search for identity and selfhood she does not accept anything that her parents, or the world around her have to offer; she would rather starve than continue a life of accommodation. This theory has been widely expounded by Hilde Bruch and has much to commend it.

What type of personality does the girl have?

The type of personality is remarkably varied, there is no single personality type. Intellectually these girls are usually well above average and are academically quite advanced yet when it comes to dealing with their emotions and personal problems they are quite immature.

Could anorexia nervosa be a food phobia (unnatural fear)?

No, the central issue is about food control and not fear. Anorexics feel hunger but have learned to control it. People with unnatural fears (phobias) realise they get 'silly feelings' but cannot explain why; this is totally unlike the anorexic.

What are the physical effects of starvation?

There are various effects all of which are reversible when weight is gained. These are the main effects in order of their frequency:

1. Amenorrhoea (absent menstruation).
2. Sensitivity to cold – the limbs become bluish-mauve in colour and feel cold even when it is warm.
3. Weakness – it soon becomes evident that she is unable to undertake the same physical activity as previously. With increasing weakness she becomes accident prone.
4. Dry skin.
5. Constipation.
6. Hair changes – her hair will become brittle and dry. Fine hair (lanugo) appears on the face, arms, legs and back; at times it may be quite marked. As weight starts to increase the fine hair goes and this is accompanied by loss of scalp hair. The hair may become obviously sparse but there is no danger of the girl's going bald.
7. Puffy swelling of the legs (oedema). This is one of the last signs to develop and should be regarded as serious.

Anorexics do not get many infections, but when they do occur they are more severe as starvation lowers the body's resistance.

What are the psychological effects of starvation?

Like the physical effects these are also reversible. It is not generally appreciated that starvation changes the way people think, the more severe the starvation the more distorted thinking becomes.

1. Perceptual distortion – this means that the eyes see normally but what is seen is misinterpreted by the brain. Before weight loss occurs anorexics have the same ideas about fat and thin as anyone else. As weight loss occurs their judgement becomes impaired so what would previously have been regarded as 'thin' now becomes 'fat'. This explains why an emaciated teenager gives her reason for

not eating as 'it will make me fat'. What to us is a preposterous reply is quite genuine in the mind of the anorexic.

2. Inability to concentrate – her ability to concentrate on academic work will be diminished and she will notice this herself. The ability to think abstractly will be first affected, the deterioration most noticeable in subjects like mathematics.

3. Social isolation and increasing pre-occupation with food – they become selfish, withdrawn and lose all sexual interest. As weight loss continues they become pre-occupied with thoughts of food and the world round them gradually shrinks. Important things in their lives are valued in terms of food so that success is seen as control over food and loss of control as failure.

4. Attitude of mind – attitude of mind changes according to the degree of weight loss or weight gain after treatment. As weight is lost she will pass through a stage of depression, anxiety, low self-esteem and difficulty with even minor decisions. At the extreme end of weight loss she will feel very different; she will have peace of mind and a self-satisfied feeling of being in control. This is one reason why she may resist treatment; when she has peace of mind weight gain which is good is regarded by her as 'bad' because it makes her depressed and anxious.

5. Poor communication – there is a gradual worsening of communication as weight is lost.

6. Increasing restlessness (hyperactivity). As weight falls she will show increasing activity. She will be restless in her sleep, waking up frequently, particularly in the early hours of the morning.

What is the treatment?

The treatment is often prolonged, more often months or years rather than days or weeks. The aim is twofold:

1. To restore weight to normal.
2. To persuade the girl to change her attitude.

The top priority is weight restoration because trying to reason with her is of little value while her thinking remains distorted. In the beginning many parents develop a sense of impatience and anger as they feel not enough is being done. It is important to realise that there is a good reason for the lack of activity at this stage when the only effective treatment is food.

How is weight restored?

The usual approach is to arrange a 'contract' between child and doctor in which a 'target weight' is agreed. The girl is then closely observed as an outpatient over the following weeks to see if she gains weight. A suitable target weight is usually about the 25th centile for her age (see Fig. 1/11, p. 19).

If this regimen does not work or if she is extremely emaciated then hospital admission is necessary. While in hospital she is maintained on total bed rest until an agreed amount of weight has been regained, or until she can prove she is gaining weight steadily each day. As she gains weight so she is allowed privileges: she is allowed to go to the lavatory, have a bath, use the telephone, etc. At first she is permitted no visitors and this may include even keeping the parents away; visitors are a reward to be won later. It may be distressing but is regarded by many therapists as an important part of the management. Parents may feel isolated and ignored and may even feel that they are being blamed. As there is little to be said at this point parental attempts at discussion will often be met with a polite version of 'no comment'.

The hospital diet is carefully adjusted at first so as not to 'overload' the girl; her gut is not used to big meals so calories need to be increased very gradually until she is having about 4000–5000 calories a day at about a fortnight. Many are initially very difficult to persuade, but eventually they do give in and co-operate. Occasionally, however, it becomes necessary to force feed them and tube (gavage) feeds are given. Hospital discharge usually takes place after an agreed weight has been attained.

How can we get the child to change her attitudes?

This can be achieved over many months by winning her co-operation. The therapist will win her confidence by being flexible and not holding an entrenched attitude towards her which might be misconstrued as criticism. This part of the treatment is known as psychotherapy (treatment of the mind). The therapist will have regular meetings with her. He will explore her feelings and emotions and deal with underlying issues and conflicts that produced the anorexia. The aim of psychotherapy is to boost the child's confidence in herself and to instil a more mature mental attitude to her problems so that ultimately as she approaches adult life she is self-reliant and independent.

Anorexia is not just a problem of the child, but a family problem. Parents who believe otherwise are mistaken; they also need help. In many families the relationship between the parents is likely to be strained; they are depressed and demoralised, particularly the mother. The parents should also have regular meetings with a therapist. Ideally the therapist dealing with the parents should not be the one directly concerned with the child's treatment, although close communication between the two is important. The aim of the adult therapist is to support the parents and give them some insight into the problem so as to create the right family atmosphere for the child to develop a sense of independence and self-worth.

What about drugs?

Drugs are sometimes used. The drugs most commonly used are chlorpromazine and various types of antidepressants. Chlorpromazine reduces anxiety and restlessness and encourages eating. Antidepressants are particularly helpful in the depressive phase of the condition.

What is the outlook?

It is difficult to give a prognosis because cases vary so much. For some it is a brief and rapidly overcome snag in their development; for others it is a problem which arises from time to time throughout early adulthood with ups and downs, weight loss and amenorrhoea occurring and then being restored. Older age at onset, longer duration of illness and severity of weight loss are generally worse prognostic signs. A few (probably less than 5%) die from starvation.

What is bulimia?

It is the name given to the condition in which people (mainly women) of normal or near normal weight regularly gorge themselves and then vomit. This attitude to food control is not unlike that of an anorexic, but as a group bulimics tend to have rather different characteristics. They are generally women in their twenties and older rather than in their teens and are more likely to be sexually experienced. Many have 'chaotic' lifestyles, alcohol and drug abuse being common.

Are there any anorexia nervosa support groups?

Anorexia nervosa is one condition where families often wish there was some such support. Fortunately there are now several organisations in Britain, the USA and other parts of the world (see p. 351) which provide support and self-help for the anorexic and her family. Many of the organisations work through a network of local groups linked by occasional general meetings and a newsletter. There is no doubt that many anorexics and their families derive great benefit from these organisations.

Chapter Five
The Diabetic Child

On hearing their child has diabetes most parents are shocked and guilt feelings are common. At this emotional time much information given by medical and nursing staff is not remembered. The purpose of this chapter is to provide information which can be looked at from time to time in the weeks after diabetes has been diagnosed.

What is diabetes?

When we eat carbohydrate (sugar and starch) it is digested in the intestine to form glucose, which is absorbed into the blood. Glucose is used by the body as a source of energy. Behind the stomach lies a gland, the pancreas, one of whose functions is to produce the hormone insulin, which passes into the blood and plays an essential part in changing glucose into energy. Normally the supply of insulin is automatically regulated by the pancreas according to the amount of glucose present in the blood, the more glucose the more insulin is released. *The basic problem in diabetes is that the pancreas is damaged and is unable to muster sufficient insulin in response to a high blood glucose.* The net result is that glucose builds up in the blood and eventually passes through the kidneys into the urine. The glucose in the urine draws water from the rest of the body, producing frequent and excessive urination. This loss of body water creates an intense thirst. The glucose energy loss increases appetite and causes weight loss. Most newly diagnosed diabetics give a history of frequent urination, excessive thirst and weight loss despite a good appetite. The diagnosis is made by finding persistently high amounts of glucose in the blood or urine.

How common is diabetes in children?

Diabetes affects about 1 in 1500 children under 16. There are 30 000 diabetics under 16 in Great Britain. The most common ages at which it is first diagnosed are at 5 and 11.

What causes diabetes?

We do not know. What we do know is that certain groups of people have a tendency to develop diabetes. The cause of the pancreatic damage in these people remains a mystery. At the present time a viral cause seems most likely, but this does not in any way imply that diabetes is infectious.

Does diabetes run in families?

Yes, this often happens. It is not uncommon to find a clustering of diabetes in some families, through several generations.

What is the treatment?

Treatment consists of giving insulin. Because there is no glucose/insulin regulatory system as in the non-diabetic, diet needs to be modified so that the blood sugar remains as far as possible within the normal (non-diabetic) range.

What is the normal range?

The normal range of blood sugar is 4–7mmol/l before meals and less than 10mmol/l one hour after meals.

Why should a diabetic try to keep his blood sugar in the normal range?

There are two reasons:
1. He will feel better.
2. It may reduce the risk of complications.

What are the so-called diabetic complications?

These complications are first apparent after the child has had diabetes for 10–15 years. People with diabetes are:
(a) 25 times more prone to blindness.
(b) 17 times more prone to kidney disease.
(c) 5 times more prone to gangrene of limbs.
(d) 2 times more prone to heart disease, which is the main cause of death.

We do not know why some diabetics develop these complications while others do not. The reason would seem in part to be genetically determined. There is no proof that keeping the blood sugar in the normal range would prevent them, but there is strong evidence both in the animal and the human to suggest that it may help. Diabetic eye complications (retinopathy) can be stopped by special treatment given by an eye specialist, if picked up early. It is therefore most important for adult diabetics to have regular eye checks.

What are ketones?

Whenever the body cannot use glucose as a source of energy it starts to break down fats. This may happen during starvation and also in diabetes. During the conversion of fats to energy ketones are formed. Whereas a low blood sugar and ketones would indicate starvation, in diabetes there is a *high* blood sugar and ketones. In a diabetic ketones in the urine mean that, because of insufficient insulin, glucose cannot be used for energy. This leads to fat breakdown and, in turn, ketone formation giving a characteristic sweet smell to the breath.

Questions about insulin

Will he always need to take insulin?

Yes, insulin will need to be taken for the rest of his life because the pancreatic damage is permanent.

Can insulin be taken by mouth?

No, insulin only works when it is given by injection. When taken by mouth it is destroyed during the digestive process.

Are there any tablets which can be taken instead of insulin?

When diabetes is first diagnosed in *adulthood* tablets can sometimes be taken as an alternative. In childhood, however, the only effective treatment is insulin by injection.

Where does insulin come from?

Until recently insulin could only be obtained from cows and pigs. In the last few years a third source has become available, bacteria. Genetic engineering has led to the manufacture of insulin by bacteria. Because of the higher frequency of allergic reactions beef insulin is now seldom used.

What is 'human' insulin?

'Human' insulin is called human because the chemical composition is identical to that of the human. There are two types of human insulin; bacterial produced and pork insulin which has been modified so that it is chemically the same as the insulin of man.

What are the differences between insulins?

Although the source of insulins varies there is little to choose between pork and bacterial insulins. The main difference between insulins is their speed and duration of action. Two types of insulin (fast and slow acting) are commonly used in children, often in combination. Fast-acting insulins (clear solution) start working after 30–60 minutes and last about 8 hours. Slow-acting insulins (cloudy solution) start working after 1–2 hours and the length of action varies from 12–24 hours. A knowledge of the time of day when each insulin is having its maximal effect is essential for two reasons. First, it enables the parent or child to decide which insulin needs adjusting when the blood sugar is too high or low. Second, it helps with planning meals and snacks throughout the day. Your paediatrician will tell you all about your insulin if you ask him.

Where should insulin be injected?

Insulin should be injected into subcutaneous tissue, which is the tissue between the skin and muscles. Subcutaneous tissue is found in all parts of the body but the following parts are considered best because they are far away from joints, nerves and large blood vessels: the upper outer area of arms; front and sides of thighs; the abdomen and the top of buttocks (Fig. 5/1). The needles of diabetic syringes are designed so that if the syringe is angled at 75–90° to the skin and the needle pushed in full length to the hub, the injection will be in the subcutaneous tissue (Fig. 5/2). The injected insulin will then cause only minimal discomfort and will be absorbed into the blood at a steady rate.

It is wise to rotate the injection sites. If the injection is given into the 'favourite spot' each time it will become sore and lumpy and the insulin will not be well absorbed. At rest the speed of insulin absorption varies slightly from one site to another but this is of little practical importance.

Where should insulin be kept?

It is best stored in a refrigerator – *but not in the freezer part*. This will ensure that it lasts longer. The bottle in current use need not be kept in the fridge but should be kept away from heat and out of direct sunlight. Many children find that insulin straight from the fridge causes discomfort and prefer to keep the bottle in current use out of the fridge. Insulin stored in a fridge has a shelf life of about 2 years; the shelf life at room temperature (less than 25°C) is about 1 month.

Can fast and slow insulins be mixed?

Fortunately yes, but the following procedure should always be fol-

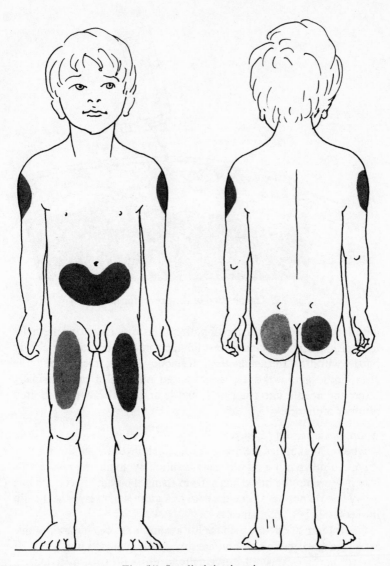

Fig. 5/1 Insulin injection sites

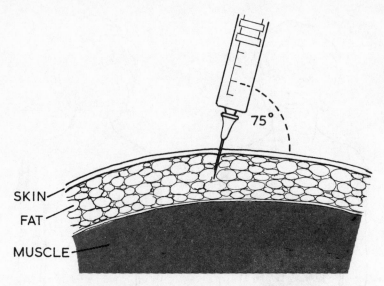

Fig. 5/2 The position of the needle for injection

lowed. After cleaning the top of both bottles with industrial methylated spirits, mix the cloudy insulin then inject air into the cloudy
bottle; withdraw the needle from the cloudy bottle; inject air into the
clear bottle and withdraw the required number of marks; finally
insert the needle into the cloudy bottle and withdraw the required
number of marks.

When should insulin be injected?

About 30 minutes before a meal. Carbohydrate in the meal is
absorbed much more rapidly than insulin. By giving the insulin this
way it prevents the blood sugar from rising too high. If you are in a
hurry and do not have time to spare it is quite safe to give the insulin
immediately before the meal.

It is the aim of doctors to make life as simple as possible and for this
reason most diabetic children are given only one injection a day. If
control becomes unstable, especially at puberty, then injections in
the morning and evening may be required.

Does insulin dose depend on age?

No, the dose of insulin has nothing to do with age. The total daily
dose is very variable but is usually between 0.5 and 1 unit per kg.

During the first weeks or months after the diabetes has been diagnosed the child goes through a 'honeymoon' phase during which the
insulin dose may be considerably less. Some children may even be
able to stop their injections temporarily.

Does it matter if the child forgets to inject himself?

It is quite safe to forget to give an injection, but forgetting to give a
few injections is very dangerous.

Must the skin be cleaned before an injection?

This is not necessary. If you wish to use something use cotton wool
and water.

Must the insulin bottle be shaken?

Never *shake* the bottle. Mix the insulin by rolling the bottle slowly
between your hands, or by inverting it several times.

Which insulin syringe is best?

There are two types of insulin syringe – glass and plastic. Until recently only glass were available free of charge in Britain. Plastic
syringes are very convenient and cheap (about £1.30 for 10 syringes
and needles). Each one can be used for a month before it is discarded.
No cleaning is required and after each injection the syringe and
needle should be placed in a refrigerator.

Glass syringes should be used with 26 gauge ⅝ inch stainless steel
needles which can be obtained on prescription and should be
replaced when they become blunt or painful to use. It is always advisable to have a spare syringe and needle ready for use in case of break-
age.

Glass syringes are dressed with a special chemical which makes the
plunger stick. It must be removed, by washing the syringe in warm,
soapy water, and then thoroughly dried before the first use – syringes
with needles attached should be kept in the container, needle down.
The container should always be kept three-quarters full of industrial
methylated spirits. It is not necessary to boil the syringe or needles at
all but the spirit should be changed once a week.

Before each use, all the spirit must be drained out of the syringe or
the injection may sting. The spirit can be removed by gently discon-
necting the plunger from the barrel of the syringe and giving them
both a good shake. When the spirit has evaporated the syringe is put
together again and, after working the plunger up and down the barrel
several times, is ready for use.

Disposable needles are also available on prescription. Each may be used many times if kept in a refrigerator between use.

When should the child inject himself?

The sooner the better. By age 9 most children should be injecting themselves. If a child is having difficulty in doing this it may be worth trying an injection aid. There are three which are worth considering. A 'Hypoguard' injector is a device which hides the needle from view. The 'Palmer' injector is a gun type device which mechanically inserts the needle into the skin when a trigger is pulled. The 'Auto Injector' not only hides the needle but inserts it and injects the insulin. Your paediatrician will be able to demonstrate these to you and will provide information about how they can be obtained.

What is the 'insulin pen'?

It is a sophisticated syringe and needle which looks like a fountain pen and can be worn like a pen. Insulin is provided in cartridge form.

The 'insulin pen' is a new concept in the management of diabetes which has been specifically designed to simulate artificially the natural response of the body to food. The child has about 40% of his daily insulin requirement in the evening as a long-acting (cloudy) insulin injection given by syringe and needle. This provides a low (basal) insulin level in his blood for a 24-hour period. During the day he carries a 'pen' which contains quick-acting (clear) insulin, which is given by the 'pen' needle before meals. The insulin dose is given according to the size of the meal and may even be omitted when a meal is missed. Unlike other insulin regimens the 'pen' concept allows for flexiblity in mealtimes and is particularly suited to the lifestyle of teenagers. There is, as yet, no proof that its use facilitates better control, but it would not be surprising if it did. The only disadvantage is the cost of the pen (about £30) and the need for as many as 4 injections daily.

Questions about diet

Why is a special diet necessary?

It helps to keep the blood sugar in the normal range.

In order to keep the blood sugar in the normal range should the diet or insulin dose be adjusted?

It is important *not* to adjust the diet more often than every 6–12 months, when all diabetic children should have their diet reviewed by a dietitian. Daily changes in blood sugar should be controlled by altering the dose of insulin.

Does a diabetic diet differ from a normal diet?

There is no difference between a diabetic diet and the normal diet recommended by the Department of Health in Britain. While in theory there may be no difference, in practice the difference is considerable. Several surveys have shown the majority of British children consume the wrong foods; eventually as a nation they are likely to pay the cost of consuming an unhealthy diet. In the case of diabetic children there is far more at stake, making it even more important that they should have a healthy diet. A healthy diet is one in which 50–55% of the calories are in the form of carbohydrates and 30–35% in the form of fat. Parents of diabetics should strive to maintain their children on such a diet.

Can a diabetic eat sugar?

A *small* quantity, e.g. on cereals at breakfast, is not harmful. However, in general we recommend that concentrated sugary foods such as sweets be omitted from the diet. The carbohydrate part of a diabetic diet is almost entirely starch, of which high fibre starch is especially recommended. Fibre is the name given to the cell walls of plants that we cannot digest or absorb. Like the straw in bricks or the gravel in concrete, fibre adds structure to carbohydrate foods. Foods with high fibre are wholemeal bread, bran, brown rice and beans. The presence of fibre slows down the rate at which food is turned into glucose and absorbed into the blood. For example, a whole orange is broken down by the body to glucose much more slowly than pure orange juice.

Can a diabetic go to children's parties?

Yes, of course. Diabetes does not prevent children from having a good time. Children will simply have to pay attention to what they are eating and drinking as they do for meals. A small 'indiscretion' here or there does little harm.

What is an 'exchange'?

An exchange is a 10-gram (g) portion of carbohydrate. Diabetic children, like all of us, like variety and the exchange system is used to give them a wide choice of foods. Carbohydrate foods are divided into 'exchanges' on the basis of the number of 10-gram portions. They are called exchanges so that different foods can be exchanged and, in this way, both total carbohydrate content and variety are maintained. Knowing how many daily exchanges the child requires will enable meals to be planned from a wide selection of food. An example of common foods which contain one exchange are a small banana, a large digestive biscuit, a small packet of crisps.

What about fat?

As mentioned earlier diabetics should eat less fat. A simple measure in the home would be the use of skimmed milk rather than full cream milk. The type of fat is also important; vegetable fats are much healthier than animal fats. For example, low fat spread should be eaten in preference to butter.

What about 'diabetic foods'?

These are seldom necessary but the sweets may be useful for children who want to eat sweets between meals. It is recommended that diabetics drink only low calorie fizzy drinks. Drinks such as tea or coffee should be sweetened with a sweetening agent such as saccharin. Teenagers should avoid 'diabetic' beer or lager. These drinks contain no carbohydrate but are more alcoholic.

Why should a diabetic always have regular meals?

The insulin injection is working throughout the day and if meals are missed the blood sugar will become very low and the child will feel unwell and may even pass into low sugar (hypoglycaemic) unconsciousness.

What information should the dietitian give me?

1. She will tell you how many calories and exchanges are required each day. Knowing the daily calories and exchanges will enable you to calculate the percentage of calories consumed as carbohydrate each day (1 exchange = 40 calories). Make sure that carbohydrates account for at least half the calories.
2. She will give you a list of foods showing the number of calories, exchanges, amount of fibre and type of fat.
3. She will show you how to spread the exchanges throughout the day.
4. She will give you a list of diabetic recipe books available. These will give you many ideas for meals and make cooking more enjoyable.

At first many parents have difficulty in gauging quantities of carbohydrate. You may find a cheap weighing scale useful until you 'get your eye in'. For example, a small potato which weighs 50g contains 10g carbohydrate. The word 'small' is open to misinterpretation and if you judge for yourself you may find your estimate of the weight way off the mark.

There are many outstanding and very comprehensive publications covering all these subjects which can be obtained at a small cost from the British Diabetic Association.

Questions about monitoring diabetic control

Why is it necessary to monitor diabetic control?

It enables each diabetic to know how well he is doing and helps him decide how much insulin to give.

What is 'good control'?

This is generally regarded as a blood sugar regularly within the normal range.

Which tests should be done – blood, urine or both?

Only regular blood tests need be done. Urine tests are not as accurate. Sugar appears in the urine only when the blood level is more than 10mmol/l; absence of sugar in the urine could indicate either a normal blood sugar or one that is too low. For children who do not want to do regular blood checks urine tests are acceptable, but occasional blood checks are advised to make sure the blood sugar is not too low or too high. There is no blood test for ketones and when blood or urine sugar is persistently high a urine test for ketone should be done. The presence of ketones would indicate an increase in insulin dose.

Which method of blood or urine testing is best?

There are several methods for estimating sugar in the blood and sugar and ketones in the urine. There is little to choose between them in terms of accuracy but some are more convenient and easier to use. Your paediatrician will advise you about this. Blood strips are expensive but the cost can be halved by dividing them in two; provided the coloured areas are not fingered the split strip is accurate. Urine testing strips are very convenient and accurate; there now seems little place for using tablets to test for sugar in the urine.

Should we buy a blood sugar meter?

This is usually not necessary as most children can get by with the strips only. There are, however, a few children or parents who find reading colours difficult and prefer to use a meter which gives a digital reading. A meter may also be necessary if the child or parents are colour blind. There are currently several meters on the market. In Britain a diabetic never need pay VAT on items of diabetic equipment.

Which 'pricking' device should be used?

There are several devices on the market and all cause a 'painless' prick. Probably the most widely used are the Autolet, the Glucolet and the Autoclix, the latter two having the advantage that the lancet cannot be seen entering the skin. Before the finger is pricked the hand should be washed in warm water and then dried.

At what time of the day should readings be made?

Ideally, for 'perfect' control, readings should be taken before and after meals as well as before going to bed. This is obviously impractical and a compromise is necessary. The tests should be done either before meals *or* one hour after meals and always at bedtime. A good scheme is to alternate before and after meals from one week to another. In practice, you will find that the times of testing are dictated very much by convenience. If the diabetic control is stable it is not necessary to do tests every day but tests should be made on at least 3 or 4 days a week. Your paediatrician will give you a diabetic diary in which you should record your insulin dose and test results. *Always* bring the diary to the clinic.

Can I make changes in the insulin dose?

Yes, you are expected to do that. Most diabetics do not visit the clinic more than 3 or 4 times a year. Between visits they are expected to make appropriate changes in their insulin dose. If you want some advice about changing the dose ask your family doctor or telephone the hospital.

Are there any other ways of checking control?

Yes, by measuring a part of the blood called glycosylated haemoglobin we are able to tell whether the blood sugar has been high in the previous two months; the higher the blood sugar the more the glycosylated haemoglobin. Normal levels of glycosylated haemoglobin are less than 9%. It is, however, not always a true reflection of average blood sugar; despite good control for most of the time a few episodes of very high blood sugar will register as an inappropriately high glycosylated haemoglobin. Ask your paediatrician for the result so that you know how it compares with the recordings in your diary.

Questions about hypoglycaemia

What is a 'hypo'?

It is an abbreviation for hypoglycaemia which means low blood sugar.

What are the symptoms when the blood sugar goes too low?

There are various symptoms, the most common are: weakness, sweating, poor concentration, irritability, excitement, pallor, palpitations, hunger, confusion, blurring of vision, tingling of lips, tongue or fingers, naughtiness, mood changes. Hypoglycaemia during sleep may lead to nightmares and a headache on wakening.

If these signs are not treated the child may become unconscious or have a fit.

What is the cause?

It could be any of the following:

1. A late meal.
2. Too little carbohydrate.
3. Extra exercise.
4. Too much insulin.

What is the treatment?

The treatment is to take sugar or a sugary drink as soon as possible. Two large sugar lumps, glucose, 3 Dextrosol tablets, Ribena, Lucozade, Coca-Cola or milk are all suitable. The symptoms should go within 10 minutes and, if not, take more sugar. *Because of the risk of hypoglycaemia a diabetic should always carry sugar, sweets or Dextrosol tablets with him.* The risk of hypoglycaemia necessitates that a diabetic carry something on him indicating that he is a diabetic. School teachers should always be told. There are commercially available information systems which are rather nicer than 'doggy discs'. The two most commonly used are Medic Alert and SOS talisman. See pages 350–1 for addresses. Information about these can also be obtained from your paediatrician or the British Diabetic Association.

What is glucagon?

Your paediatrician may issue you with a glucagon kit and will then instruct you about its use. It is very helpful when a hypo causes unconsciousness and the child is unable to eat or drink. Glucagon causes a rise in blood sugar; 10–15 minutes after the injection the child wakes up and he should then be given sugar by mouth. I routinely issue glucagon to parents of diabetic children but they seldom need to use it.

Questions about illness

What happens when a diabetic becomes ill?

The blood sugar may rise and both sugar and ketones appear in the urine. The child may be flushed, feel thirsty, drink more and pass a lot of urine. Loss of appetite and refusal to eat are common.

How should the diabetes be managed during illness?

The five most important principles of management are as follows:

1. Regular blood and/or urine tests should be made.
2. Even if he is not eating *never* stop the insulin.
3. Give him extra insulin. It is best to give fast-acting insulin, a supply of which should always be kept at home to be used on such occasions. With experience you will be able to judge how much extra insulin to give. In the beginning, if you are unsure, ask your paediatrician or family doctor to advise you.
4. If he does not eat give him his carbohydrate in liquid form. Most children will drink Lucozade, Ribena, cold 'flat' Coca-Cola or milk.
5. If the child vomits and is unable to retain liquids contact your doctor immediately.

What about exercise?

Exercise and sport are part of growing up and are to be encouraged in diabetic children. They promote fitness and help prevent obesity. During exercise glucose is used for extra energy and a 'hypo' may occur. The following measures are recommended to prevent the fall in blood sugar:

1. Before exercise take an extra 10 or 20g carbohydrate. This may need to be increased to 40g before vigorous or prolonged exercise. Dextrosols or mini Mars bars are ideal for this.

2. Alternatively, reduce the insulin dose slightly before planned exercise.
3. Before running exercise inject insulin into a site other than the thighs. Injection of insulin into the legs before running causes rapid absorption of insulin and a consequent quick fall in blood sugar.

Is there any advice about holidays?
Yes, the following points should be noted:

1. Depending on where you go you may need to adjust the diet accordingly. Take your exchange and calorie book/pamphlets with you.
2. Take plenty of insulin, syringes and needles as well as any other equipment you may require.
3. In case of delays or lost baggage *always* carry the insulin kit in your hand luggage. Insulin can pass through the x-ray machine at the airport without any harmful effect.
4. In temperatures below 30°C insulin need not be kept in a fridge but should always be kept out of direct sunlight and away from heat. In temperatures above 30° insulin should be stored in a refrigerator or wrapped in cotton wool or wet tissues in a wide-mouthed vacuum flask. If this is not done the shelf-life (expiry date) will be dramatially reduced.
5. Children who suffer from motion sickness should take tablets. In case of vomiting make sure you have some sweet drinks with you.
6. During travel, especially when crossing time zones, the times of meals may need to be altered. Ask your paediatrician for advice about this.
7. During camping holidays, where refrigerators are not available, plastic syringes and needles may be used for a week before being discarded.

What should the school be told?
The school should be told that diabetics require regular meals and from time to time carbohydrate (biscuits or sweets) may need to be taken in the classroom or on the playing field when the child has a hypo. With regard to meals, a packed lunch is obviously easier. If your child eats the school meals it is worth while visiting the catering officer to discuss the meals with him. I have found that when dietary help is required kitchen staff at schools are usually very obliging.

Make sure that the catering manager orders low calorie drinks for the canteen or tuck shop.

What jobs can a diabetic do?

Few employers today refuse to employ someone on the grounds that they are diabetic, but the police, armed forces and fire brigade usually do not accept diabetics. Certain jobs are unsuitable because a severe hypo could endanger not only the diabetic but others as well. Jobs falling into this category are drivers of heavy goods or public service vehicles, working at heights or controlling moving machinery. All other jobs are open to diabetics.

Can a diabetic drive a car?

It is only under exceptional circumstances that diabetics are denied a driver's licence. In Britain licences are granted for 1, 2 or 3 years at a time, not until age 70 as for the non-diabetic. The licensing department and the insurance company must be informed of the diabetes. Diabetics are advised always to carry carbohydrate in the car in case of a hypo. Diabetics who are being stabilised on insulin should not drive until the control is satisfactory. Driving should also be avoided in the event of unrecognised hypos which can be extremely dangerous to both the diabetic and others. Licences for heavy goods and public service vehicles are not granted to diabetics.

What is the effect of diabetes on the family?

The answer is not simple for it depends very much on the individual child and his family. Diabetes does put a strain on family relationships and marital breakdown or behaviour problems do occur more frequently. These are a few hints which you may find helpful:

1. After the diagnosis of diabetes in a young child parents frequently go through phases of shock, denial, sadness, adaptation and reorganisation. Problems arise when parents fail to adapt and reorganise. Remember life is not going to be the same as before. You should accept this and adjust.
2. A diabetic child will require a lot of your time and attention. Other children also need you to make a fuss of them. Try to distribute your time and attention equally among all the children.
3. The best way to discipline a diabetic child is by 'educated persuasion'. Try to get him to see that you really do love him and are doing everything for his benefit. This is not easy; a 5-year-old with a few toffees in his pocket is not much concerned with com-

plications likely to develop 20 years hence. Nevertheless, it is worth pursuing this line, for eventually the child will be convinced that you have his interest at heart. If the child does eat the toffees or raid the biscuit tin reprimand him but do no more. By being too punitive you will encourage the child to rebel and he will become dishonest. It is much better for relationships and for control if these 'forbidden activities' are out in the open and not in secret. Good behaviour and attention to diet should be rewarded with lavish praise. Remember, there are many ways of rewarding a child other than by giving him sweets.

4. Never threaten him with complications. A threat such as 'if you eat toffees you may go blind' is indeed very harmful and never succeeds.

5. A diabetic child is in every other way a normal child. Do not overprotect him or make him feel different.

6. If you feel there are family or behaviour problems let your paediatrician or family doctor know. Expert psychological help can be obtained at an early stage and these problems can then be nipped in the bud.

Can diabetic girls have babies?

Yes, diabetes does not impair fertility. Diabetic girls do, however, have more problems in pregnancy and should book early. Strict control during the pregnancy is also important.

What are the risks of a diabetic parent passing diabetes on to a child?

The risk is about 1 in 100 if one parent is a diabetic and 2 in 100 if both parents are diabetic. These risks are indeed very small.

What are the risks for a brother or sister of a diabetic child?

The risk is about 1 in 100. If two children have diabetes the risk for subsequent children rises to 2 in 100.

Should we join the BDA?

The answer is a very definite *yes*. The British Diabetic Association (BDA) supplies a wide range of free advice and help for diabetics. They publish books and leaflets, organise conferences, sponsor research, run holidays for diabetic children and teenagers and campaign on behalf of diabetics.

Every two months you will receive *Balance*, an excellent newspaper with news, features and articles of interest to diabetics and their families. Almost every town has a local branch of the BDA. The local branches help with fund raising and run many social and educational activities. They provide useful advice and are always happy to welcome newcomers. See page 351 for BDA address.

What is the Novo Award Scheme?

In Britain, Novo Laboratories are currently running an award scheme whereby a child can progress from a bronze to gold award by answering a series of 3 questionnaires correctly. At each successful attempt the child is presented with a certificate and badge. This is an excellent service for the promotion of diabetic education and I strongly recommend that school age children take part. Ask your paediatrician for the forms.

Chapter 6

Alimentary Tract Problems

COELIAC DISEASE

What is coeliac disease?

It is the name given to a condition in which gluten, a substance in wheat and several other grains, causes damage to the lining of the small bowel. Consequently, normal food absorption cannot take place.

How common is coeliac disease?

The incidence differs markedly from one country to another. In England, where the incidence has recently fallen, it is uncommon, affecting about 1 in 3000 people. In the west of Ireland it is common, as many as 1 in 300 have coeliac disease.

What causes coeliac disease?

Neither the way gluten causes damage, nor the reason why it affects only certain individuals is known. It is not an allergy to gluten. The disease tends to run in families and is in part genetically determined.

What are the symptoms?

The extent of the symptoms is very variable so that there are often delays in making the diagnosis; many people go throughout life with the diagnosis never having been made. In England most children are diagnosed between 9 and 12 months. A typical story is that of a child who has been on gluten-containing foods for 3–4 months who presents with failure to thrive, diarrhoea, intermittent vomiting, lack of appetite and irritability. The abdomen may become distended, the child becomes thin with an obvious appearance of weight loss. Older infants and children may present with short stature and a wide range of symptoms usually related to anaemia, protein or vitamin deficiency.

How is coeliac disease diagnosed?

The only way to diagnose coeliac disease is by intestinal biopsy. After the child is sedated he swallows a small capsule attached to a thin feeding tube. The child is later examined under an x-ray screen. When the capsule is in the small bowel a small piece of the lining (mucosa) is sucked into the capsule, which is then removed. The bowel specimen is sent to the laboratory for microscopic examination.

Normally the mucosa has finger-like projections (villi) through which food is absorbed. In coeliac disease the villi are sheared off and the mucosa is flat. This is permanent as long as gluten is consumed, but when it is removed from the diet the villi regrow. A small number (less than 5%) have a temporary coeliac disease, the mucosa eventually being able to tolerate gluten. Other common causes of a flat mucosa are cow's milk protein allergy and infection by a bowel parasite called giardia.

For the diagnosis to be beyond doubt, a biopsy should be taken after gluten has been eliminated from the diet to show that the mucosa has returned to normal. The child should later be challenged with gluten and a further biopsy taken to show that gluten has damaged the mucosa again.

What is the treatment?

The treatment is the avoidance of all foods which contain wheat and rye. While it is not known for certain whether barley and oats should be excluded, most paediatricians recommend their exclusion.

Common foods which contain gluten are bread, rolls, buns, crispbread, biscuits, cakes, pastry, pasta, breadcrumbs, sausages, gravy, semolina, foods cooked in batter. Flour is often an ingredient in tinned and packeted foods.

As you see gluten forms a large part of our daily diet and its avoidance may be inconvenient, nevertheless in recent years gluten-free products have increased and are now widely available; their taste is very palatable. Many gluten-free products are specially labelled with a crossed sheaf of wheat, the symbol of the Coeliac Society. The hospital dietitian should provide you with a list of gluten-free foods and information about where they can be obtained in your area. She should also provide recipes and information about gluten-free cooking. Rather than single out the child with coeliac disease it is usually kinder and more convenient to switch the whole family to gluten-free household foods such as bread, biscuits and cakes, but some families may find this too costly.

At present in Britain, gluten-free biscuits, bread, flour, pasta and rusks are issued free of charge by prescription, and can be obtained through chemists' shops, but may have to be ordered specially. For children over 16 a 'season ticket' helps reduce the cost of prescriptions. To obtain a season ticket, Form FP95 (EC95–Scotland) should be obtained from any post office.

How long does the treatment take to work?

Within a few weeks of starting the gluten-free diet the symptoms will disappear and the child will start to gain weight. Often the first sign of improvement is a change of mood; the child will be much less irritable and generally more pleasant.

When the child is challenged with gluten will he go back on a normal diet?

Having got the child used to a gluten-free diet it would be more convenient to maintain the same diet but to add 10–20 grams of gluten to the diet each day. Your paediatrician or dietitian will arrange for you to obtain the gluten.

How long should he remain on the diet?

At present paediatricians are recommending a gluten-free diet for life; this is why it is so important that the diagnosis is correct. The reason for the lifelong diet is based on theory rather than fact. Malignancy in the bowel of middle-aged coeliacs although very uncommon does appear to be more frequent than among the normal population. At the moment it is not known whether a lifelong gluten-free diet will protect against malignancy, but, in view of the chance that it might, long-term gluten avoidance is recommended.

Besides obvious symptoms of a relapse, what other reasons are there for staying on the diet?

If the diet is not assiduously followed, children may not grow as well as they should and adults may become anaemic.

What is the risk of coeliac disease in a child of a coeliac parent?

The risk is the same as for a sibling of a coeliac, namely between 2–5%.

What is the Coeliac Society?

It is a society for coeliacs which was formed in 1968. The society provides information about coeliac disease and has done much good work on behalf of coeliacs. Local groups exist in many parts of the country and I would advise all coeliacs to join. You will receive their magazine *Crossed Grain* twice yearly; news and information about coeliac disease are regularly featured. A gluten-free food list which is updated every 18 months is available from the society. For the address see page 351.

CYSTIC FIBROSIS

Cystic fibrosis is the commonest inherited illness of white children: about 400 new cases occur each year in the UK. 1 in 20 white people carry the gene for cystic fibrosis and about 1 in every 400 marriages produce a child with cystic fibrosis. The population incidence in early childhood is generally given as 1 in 2000 children.

What is cystic fibrosis?

It is a condition in which the glands producing mucus and sweat are abnormal. The mucus glands, which are present in organs in many parts of the body, secrete mucus which is very sticky. It is sticky mucus which causes damage in these organs. Sweat glands produce salty sweat which is used to diagnose the condition.

Which organs are damaged by the sticky mucus?

The organs most affected are the lungs and pancreas (85%); lung involvement is the more serious.

In the lung thick sticky mucus blocks the small airways. Blockage not only causes lung damage through back pressure but predisposes the child to repeated chest infections which cause further lung damage.

The pancreas is a gland which lies behind the stomach in the abdomen. It has two functions; it makes insulin and produces digestive enzymes, which are secreted into the bowel so that food is digested. Sticky mucus in the pancreas causes blockage and back pressure so that the pancreas is damaged and malabsorption ensues.

The lining (mucosa) of the bowel contains mucus-producing glands. About 10% of newborns with cystic fibrosis present with bowel obstruction, which may require surgery to relieve it. The obstruction is caused by sticky mucus and is known as 'meconium ileus'.

When cystic fibrosis was discovered in the 1930s it was noted that the pancreas was fibrosed (scarred) and contained several cysts (cavities) hence its name. It is also known as 'mucoviscidosis' which is probably more accurate in that it reflects the basic problem, viscid mucus.

What symptoms do children have?

The severity of symptoms is very variable, even within the same family. At times symptoms may be so mild that the diagnosis is in question, at other times the diagnosis is very obvious. Children usually present with failure to thrive and/or chest infections. Most have a voracious appetite and parents may be puzzled that they are not gaining weight. Many have foul-smelling, greasy stools which, because of the fat, float in the toilet after it is flushed.

How is cystic fibrosis (CF) diagnosed?

The sweat of children with CF has about 4 times more salt than normal and the skin may have a salty taste. CF is diagnosed by a sweat test; sweating is induced and sweat is collected on paper placed on the skin. By carefully measuring the volume and the concentration of sodium and chloride an accurate diagnosis can be made.

In the first weeks of life it may be difficult to obtain sufficient sweat for an accurate test. A blood test (serum immunoreactive trypsin) can then be used. Trypsin is a pancreatic enzyme which is forced into the blood because the pancreatic ducts are blocked and it is unable to escape. The concentration in the blood is very high in the first weeks of life after which it falls as the pancreas becomes damaged. This test is thus unsuitable for the older child.

How is cystic fibrosis inherited?

A child with CF has 2 CF genes. His parents are normal but because each has one CF gene they are called carriers. When mother and father are both carriers the risk in each pregnancy of an offspring with CF is 1 in 4 (25%). The chance of a normal, non-carrier child is 1 in 4 (25%), while the chance of normal carriers (like the parents) is 2 in 4 (50%) (Fig. 6/1). Unfortunately as yet there is no simple way of detecting carriers. The situation is changing, however. A recently developed genetic technique (DNA probes) has made it possible to detect carrier status of siblings of a child with CF in certain families.

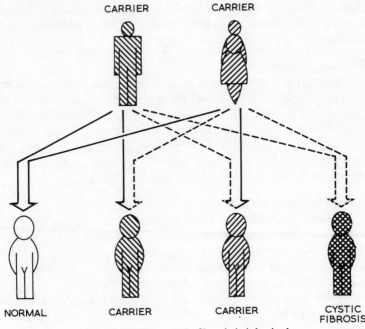

——— = Normal gene

– – – – – = Gene for cystic fibrosis

Fig. 6/1 How cystic fibrosis is inherited

This work is at the moment still being fully researched; families would be well advised to avail themselves of this facility should they have the opportunity.

Are there any antenatal screening tests?

Antenatal screening for cystic fibrosis has made rapid progress in the last 5 years, further progress will almost certainly be made in the next year or two. At present routine antenatal screening is not generally available for all pregnancies. Screening is limited to those families in which a child with CF has already been born. At present 2 tests are available, the DNA probe test and the alkaline phosphatase test.

The DNA probe test is done by taking blood from the parents and performing a chorion biopsy (p. 335) between 8–12 weeks. In two-thirds of pregnancies it will be possible to detect an affected fetus. The risk of abortion following chorion biopsy has not been accurately determined, but is probably no higher than 3–4%.

The alkaline phosphatase test is performed at 17–18 weeks by amniocentesis (p. 335). Alkalaine phosphatase is then measured in the amniotic fluid (fluid around the fetus); the amount is very low when the fetus has CF. The risk of abortion after amniocentesis is about 0.5–1%.

Both tests are currently being used; whether one or the other or both are eventually used as the preferred method for antenatal detection remains to be seen. In the meantime parents are advised to take expert advice about these tests and advances that are likely to occur.

How serious is cystic fibrosis?

Cystic fibrosis is a serious disease because there is as yet no cure and the risk of lung damage continues throughout childhood and adult life, but the outlook has improved dramatically over recent years. Untreated, a large number of CF children would still die in early childhood as was the case some years ago. Now, early diagnosis and effective treatment, which need not interfere with home or school life, is transforming the outlook. More and more are emerging into adult life with little lung damage.

What is the treatment?

Treatment has 2 parts; the chest and malabsorption.

Chest treatment: Physiotherapy is a very important part of the treatment. It should be carried out on a regular basis, particularly when the child is 'chesty'. Parents are instructed how to give physiotherapy; older children and adults are taught methods of carrying out physiotherapy for themselves.

There is controversy among paediatricians about the permanent need for antibiotics. All agree that when the chest becomes infected antibiotics should be given early and in a high dosage. Antibiotics may be given by mouth, injection or inhalation; the choice depends on the bacteria in the sputum. The two most common bacteria in young children are staphylococcus and haemophilus. As the child becomes older infection with pseudomonas is common. Unfortunately, it is virtually impossible to get rid of pseudomonas, but treatment does improve symptoms and makes the child feel much better.

Malabsorption treatment: The enzymes which are lacking because of pancreatic damage can be taken with meals as a powder, granules, capsules or tablets. The dose is variable and needs to be adjusted according to the appearance of the stools and the amount of weight gained. It is better to give too much than too little, but too much may cause soreness of the lips and bottom. Recently two new preparations have been introduced in Britain, Creon and Pancrease; unlike the older preparations these have a higher enzyme concentration. Because they can be taken in smaller doses they are preferred by many children.

Not all paediatricians are agreed on the best diet for children with CF. Most now recommend a normal high energy, high protein diet while the majority in the past favoured a high protein, low fat diet. All children with cystic fibrosis should regularly have vitamins, particularly vitamin E.

In Britain, prescription charges are free for children under 16. For those over 16 a 'season ticket' is available to reduce costs.

What about school?

This obviously depends on the child's disability; the vast majority attend normal schools. The child should partake in all school activities. Physical exercise is good for CF and sports should be encouraged within the child's capability. Teachers usually do not know much about CF. You should arrange to see the head teacher and the class teacher to explain what CF is.

What about employment?

For obvious reasons any job involving physical work is unsuitable. All other forms of employment are open to adults with cystic fibrosis.

Are adults with cystic fibrosis fertile?

Only females are fertile, males are sterile because the tube which carries sperm (vas deferens) becomes blocked in early life. The risk of a female producing an infant with CF is about 1 in 40, which is indeed small.

What about immunisations?

The child with CF should have all the childhood immunisations. Many paediatricians recommend annual influenza immunisations in older children and your doctor will advise you about this.

What is the Cystic Fibrosis Research Trust?

The Cystic Fibrosis Research Trust was founded in 1964 to finance research to find a complete cure and, in the meantime, to improve on current methods of treatment; to form regions, branches and groups throughout the United Kingdom for the purpose of helping and advising those with cystic fibrosis and their families with any problems that may arise; to educate the public about the disease and thereby, through increased knowledge, help to make earlier diagnosis possible.

The Trust is now supporting research by skilled doctors and scientists with modern apparatus at many universities and hospitals in the UK and progress is being made.

A network of regional, branch and group organisations has also been established, and help and advice is being given to those with problems caused by cystic fibrosis, while through publicity and education a wider awareness about the condition is being achieved. The address is given on page 351.

DIARRHOEA AND VOMITING (GASTROENTERITIS)

Other than the common cold, gastroenteritis is the most common illness affecting families in the UK. Most children experience between 1 and 3 episodes of severe diarrhoea in the first three years.

What is meant by gastroenteritis?
It means sudden onset of diarrhoea with or without vomiting caused by an infection of the bowel. The infected bowel is unable to function normally, water and salts are lost. This loss is due to active secretion into the bowel and not a failure of absorption.

What is diarrhoea?
Diarrhoea means an increase in stool volume. Many parents have difficulty in knowing what is 'diarrhoea', particularly in young children. It is quite common for healthy young children to have frequent watery stools of varying colour or smell, particularly when breast fed.

What causes gastroenteritis?
Gastroenteritis is caused by viruses, bacteria and parasites. Viruses are the most frequent cause.

How is it acquired?
Although laboratory studies sometimes may detect the source of infection, it is usually not possible or practical to do this. In the UK viral gastroenteritis is particularly common in winter and may spread

rapidly through the community. All gastroenteritis may spread by the oral faecal route (infected stools of one person spreading to the mouth of another). Bacteria may also be acquired from infected food, milk or water. On some occasions pets may be the source of infection.

What are the symptoms?

These depend to a large extent on the severity of the condition and the amount of fluid lost. Most children have mild gastroenteritis and present with a few vomits and disinclination to feed followed by diarrhoea for a day or two. In a more severe form vomiting and loss of appetite are more marked and the diarrhoea lasts much longer, often a week or more. The profuse fluid loss from the bowel may cause dehydration.

Are there any clinical differences between viral and bacterial gastroenteritis?

It is usually not possible to distinguish between a viral and a bacterial cause. Certain features may suggest one or the other. In young children (less than 2) a preceding or concurrent cough, runny nose, inflamed throat or ears are often associated with viral diarrhoea. A very high temperature, abdominal discomfort or blood in the stool are highly suggestive of a bacterial cause.

What are the signs of dehydration?

These are usually very evident but in fat babies may not always be so. Dehydration is categorised as mild, moderate or severe on the basis of definite clinical signs or the percentage of weight reduction as a result of fluid loss.

Mild dehydration – less than 5% weight loss. The face becomes pale and there are dark shadows under the eyes; the lips, by contrast, remain very pink. The child is miserable and sleep may be disturbed. He is irritable when handled and cries a lot.

Moderate dehydration – 5–10% weight loss. In addition to the signs and symptoms noted in mild dehydration the following are also apparent:

1. Sunken eyes.
2. In children under 18 months the dimple (fontanelle) on the front part of the skull becomes sunken and the skull bones become prominent.
3. Skin changes. These are most evident when a fold of skin on the

abdominal wall is pinched up between finger and thumb. Normally this should spring back instantly when released but in moderate dehydration the fold remains or springs back very slowly.

Severe dehydration – more than 10% weight loss. Because of the sudden loss of large amounts of fluid these children become shocked as well as dehydrated. They are pale, blue or mottled, look very ill and have cold, limp limbs and take very little interest in their surroundings.

What is the incubation period after exposure to infection?
Most gastroenteritis, whether bacterial or viral, develops between 1 and 3 days after exposure.

What investigations are necessary?
A mild gastroenteritis requires no tests. For the more severe form the only domiciliary test worth doing is a stool study to determine whether the cause is viral or bacterial. In the hospital, blood tests to measure the acidity and salt content (pH and electrolytes) may be done.

When should a child be admitted to hospital?
The vast majority of children with gastroenteritis can be treated satisfactorily in the home by the family doctor. A child with mild dehydration requires admission when oral feeds cannot be retained. Children with moderate and severe dehydration require admission for regular observation and probable intravenous therapy. A very common non-medical reason for admission is excess maternal (sometimes paternal) anxiety.

What is the treatment for gastroenteritis?
The mainstay of treatment is fluid replacement. It is most important to realise that fluid treatment is *not* a cure. Diarrhoea will continue, fluids only affect the state of hydration until the illness has run its course. Particular care in the choice of fluid is required. Many drinks and soups contain high concentrations of sugar or salt; their use will not only make the diarrhoea worse but may be dangerous. Trying a different milk does not make any difference. 'Doorstep' (pasteurised cow's milk) milk should never be used as a rehydration fluid because the salt concentration is unsuitable.

Water is the ideal fluid for the child with mild dehydration. It can be given as 'plain water' or be added to feeds (dilute feeds). 'Sugar water', which the child may find more palatable, is also suitable provided the sugar concentration is not too high. The concentration of white table sugar (sucrose) should not exceed 20g (approximately 4 teaspoons) in 200ml (approximately 7fl oz). If glucose is used the concentration should be half (approximately 2 teaspoons) that of sucrose.

A child with moderate to severe dehydration loses a large amount of salt in the stool. These children require extra salt in addition to water. It is unwise to add salt to drinking water, the amount required needs to be measured precisely, any inaccuracy may be harmful. The concentration of salts in the stool has been carefully measured and there are now commercially available sugar and salt solutions which have a similar salt concentration, making salt replacement more precise. In Britain preparations commonly used are Dioralyte (with or without flavour) and Rehidrat (flavoured) which come in sachets and are easily made up in the home. There is little to choose between the preparations, the flavour being the most important difference. A child who does not like the taste may refuse to drink despite his thirst. I usually advise parents to try more than one flavour to see which one the child prefers. Flavours available are cherry and pineapple (Dioralyte), and lime and lemon and orange (Rehidrat).

In the USA ready-to-use solutions (flavoured and unflavoured) are available in large cans in supermarkets. Coca-Cola is also widely used for mild gastroenteritis in the USA. While the use of Coca-Cola may be all right in an emergency it is not ideal and cannot be recommended for general use.

What about feeding?

If possible the child should continue to be fed *despite* the diarrhoea. As with fluids great care should be taken in the choice of food. A *bland* diet is recommended. Spiced or salty foods, together with sweet desserts, should most definitely be avoided. A suitable bland diet for a toddler would be fish and rice or chicken and boiled potato. In the very young child breast or bottle feeds should continue but the extra fluid should be given as water or sugar and salt solution. Extra fluids are generally required for 2–3 days but sometimes longer. It is common for mothers to be advised to give *only* salt and sugar solutions for 2 or 3 days. In my view this is inappropriate; sugar and salt solutions contain few calories and by the third day the 'starved' child will not only have lost weight but will be extremely hungry and miserable.

How much fluid does the child require?

Most children with diarrhoea become thirsty and should be allowed to drink as and when they like. The volume required depends on the weight (before illness) and the degree of dehydration. If the required volume cannot be met because the child is not drinking enough or there is persistent vomiting, intravenous fluids may be required.

The following table provides a rough guide for the calculation of the required volume:

Volume in ml/kg/24 hours

Weight	Less than 10kg	10–20kg	More than 20kg
No dehydration	150	100	50
Mild dehydration	175	125	75
Moderate dehydration	200	150	100
Severe dehydration	250	200	150

For example an 8kg baby who is moderately dehydrated will require 8 × 200ml (= 1600) in 24 hours.

The fluid volume should be calculated each day so that water or a sugar and salt solution can be increased or decreased according to the degree of dehydration. Eventually the dehydration will be corrected and the extra fluids (water or a sugar and salt solution) can be withdrawn.

What about antibiotics?

Antibiotics are seldom used to treat gastroenteritis even when the cause is bacterial. Although some bacterial infections are eradicated sooner with the use of antibiotics, the improvement in clinical symptoms is negligible. Indeed, there are some infections which persist longer when antibiotics have been used. There are, however, occasions when antibiotics are prescribed, in which case the doctor will be acting on the result of a stool culture and should be able to provide a reason for using an antibiotic.

Are there any 'constipating' drugs which slow the bowel or reduce bowel secretions?

Loperamide has both functions and has been shown to be effective. It is unlikely to be widely used because it is not a cure, the small reduction in stool volume hardly justifies the use of a drug in so benign a condition.

What about kaolin?

This is found in many over the counter diarrhoea preparations. There is no evidence to suggest that it is of any benefit.

When will the stools be back to 'normal'?

This usually takes a week or two but at times may take a few weeks though seldom more than a month. The common reason for the prolonged loose stools is the inability of the bowel to absorb milk sugar (lactose). It is not necessary to switch to a lactose-free milk but this may occasionally be necessary when the baby's bottom becomes very sore or there appears to be no let-up in the diarrhoea. Occasionally a transient cow's milk intolerance follows gastroenteritis and it may cause the diarrhoea to persist, switching to a lactose-free milk also helps this.

What is the outlook for children with gastroenteritis?

The outlook for children with gastroenteritis with mild to moderate dehydration is excellent. With severe dehydration the outlook is not as good. Fortunately this seldom occurs in the UK.

When can the child return to the nursery/school?

As soon as he is well. A child who has recovered from gastroenteritis may continue to harbour the virus or bacteria for a number of weeks afterwards. It would seem unreasonable to exclude these well children from school or nursery. There is, however, a risk that other children may be infected and there should be strict attention to hygiene by attendants at the nursery or by the child himself in the case of an older child. Gastroenteritis can spread very rapidly in children's nurseries. To prevent such spread it is wise to notify the staff that the child is recovering from gastroenteritis so that appropriate hygienic precautions can be taken. A commonsense measure would be to delegate the work in the nursery so that personnel handling food are different from those changing nappies (diapers).

TODDLERS' DIARRHOEA

Toddlers' diarrhoea is also known as chronic non-specific diarrhoea syndrome or the irritable colon of childhood. It is the commonest cause of prolonged diarrhoea in otherwise healthy children.

The onset may be slow or dramatic and is often preceded by a period of constipation. The age varies between 6 months and 2½ years, most children developing diarrhoea towards the end of the 1st year. Loose, watery stools with mucus and undigested vegetable matter (peas, carrots, etc.) occur. Three or four stools per day are usual and as many as ten may occur, most being passed in the early part of the day. With increasing frequency the child's bottom can become very sore. Diarrhoea can last a few days to many weeks with varying intervals (days or weeks) between episodes, when the child may even be constipated. Unlike other cases of diarrhoeal illness, these children have a normal appetite and do not lose weight. Episodes of diarrhoea are frequently brought on by viral infections and teething. In over 90% of children the diarrhoea ceases by the age of 3½ and does not persist beyond 5.

The cause of toddlers' diarrhoea is not known. What is known is that the time it takes for food to travel from the mouth, through the intestines and into the nappy is much faster than normal. Most foods cause slowing of intestinal movements (peristalsis) after meals, this slowing action being ineffective in children with toddlers' diarrhoea.

Many children have a parent with 'bowel problems'. In my experience there are few conditions that generate as much parental anxiety as toddler diarrhoea. Some imagine the child has something 'seriously wrong', others on seeing vegetable matter in the stool worry about malabsorption. Occasionally parents fear difficulty with toilet training and social embarrassment, particularly when placement in a nursery has just started or is being considered. Conflicting dietary advice given by various health care workers is a frequent and often major cause for parental distress.

There are no diagnostic tests for toddlers' diarrhoea, the diagnosis being made by the history. By the time most children see a paediatrician many stool cultures may have been done, all of which are normal. Because there is no treatment parents should always be reassured about the good outcome. A normal diet is recommended and there is *no* need to restrict milk, fruit or bran-containing foods. Chilled drinks may, however, make the diarrhoea worse and should be avoided. A drug, loperamide, is used by a few paediatricians with some success. In my view drug treatment for so benign a condition is not necessary; I do occasionally prescribe it on a *short-term* basis for the mother's convenience when the diarrhoea is severe.

NB: Loperamide, although widely used, is *not* licensed in Britain for children under 4. The dose usually used is 0.8–1.2mg/kg per day. This may be divided into 2–4 doses.

GASTRO-OESOPHAGEAL REFLUX

Gastro-oesophageal reflux means the upward movement of food (usually milk) from the stomach into the oesophagus. Vomiting of milk by babies is so common as almost to be normal. Small vomits are generally tolerated by most mothers but when large amounts are vomited after every feed or between feeds anxiety arises. The paediatrician is usually consulted because of this anxiety which is made worse by the ever-present smell of vomit and the constant soiling of the child's clothes. Vomiting seems to improve at about the same time as solids are introduced (between 4 and 6 months) and usually ceases by the end of the 1st year. It is indeed rare that vomiting continues beyond 18 months.

To understand the cause of reflux vomiting it is important to know some anatomy (Fig. 6/2). After swallowing, milk passes from the mouth through the oesophagus into the stomach. Normally, when the stomach is full the oesophageal valve tightens and very little milk can pass upwards. In young infants, for an unknown reason, this valve relaxes from time to time allowing milk to travel upwards and be vomited. Pressure on the stomach from tightening of the abdominal muscles, as in crying, may also cause vomiting by overcoming the resistance of the oesophageal valve. This resistance may be influenced by certain drugs and food. For example both fatty foods and chocolate lower the resistance and may make vomiting worse.

Despite a loss of large quantities of milk, the vast majority of vomiters gain weight normally and parental reassurance is all that is required. Rarely, complications do arise and these are of 3 main types which will be discussed briefly:

1. Failure to thrive. The child who is failing to thrive need not necessarily lose weight but weight gain may not be as good as expected. Charts showing the normal rates of weight gain can be obtained from your paediatrician (see Figs. 1/7, 1/8, pp. 13,14).
2. Milk inhalation. Refluxed milk may enter the lungs producing coughing and wheezing. The child may appear to have repeated chest infections or asthma.

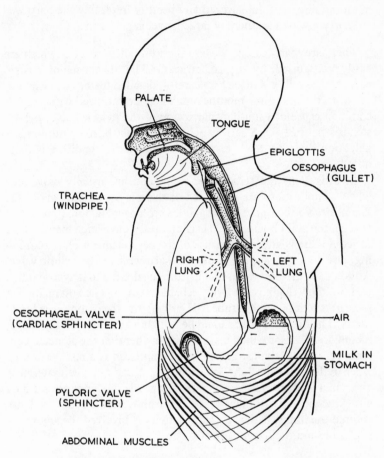

Fig. 6/2 Anatomy of the stomach and oesophagus

3. Acid effects. The stomach always contains acid which, when refluxed, may irritate the lower oesophagus causing loss of appetite, bloodstained vomit and blood loss (anaemia). The pain (heartburn) may cause the child to adopt abnormal positions of the head and neck, often leading to the mistaken diagnosis of a 'nervous problem'. Persistent acid irritation of the lower oesophagus may eventually destroy the lining and cause narrowing. This is a serious complication which may be corrected by repeatedly stretching the oesophagus with tubes of different widths. If

stretching does not succeed an operation replacing the narrowed portion with a segment of large bowel is performed.

There are many causes of vomiting in infancy, most of which are easily recognised by a paediatrician. The diagnosis of gastro-oesophageal reflux is made by a careful, detailed history and examination. In the first three months reflux may be confused with another common cause of vomiting, narrowing of the pyloric valve, pyloric stenosis (see p. 141). A narrow pyloric valve may be felt by abdominal palpation during a feed (test feed) whereby the condition is diagnosed.

Investigations are seldom necessary and are usually done only when complications are suspected or there is uncertainty about the diagnosis. The common investigations are a haemoglobin (blood) test to see if the child is anaemic, a barium meal x-ray which may be done to see if there is any abnormality of the oesophagus such as narrowing, also sometimes to see if there is narrowing of the pyloric valve. Although in the past we used a barium meal x-ray to diagnose reflux we now know that it is not a very reliable method. The best method at present is to insert a thin tube (pH probe) into the oesophagus for 24 hours. The tip of the tube should lie just above the oesophageal valve; it contains a sensor which measures acid whenever the stomach contents pass above the cardiac valve. A scintiscan is a test performed when reflux into the lung is suspected. A radio-active material is given in a feed and for some hours afterwards the lungs are scanned with a radio-activity detector to determine whether the feed has entered the lungs. Although radio-activity is involved the amount is negligible and the test is perfectly safe.

How should children with reflux be managed?

As mentioned before, the vast majority improve without any treatment, vomiting need be regarded only as a temporary inconvenience. Active management is only really necessary for the treatment of complications, but in practice when most children are actively managed it is because of parental anxiety created by persistent vomiting: explanation and reassurance alone may not have been sufficient to relieve this anxiety. The most effective measure for reducing reflux is lying the child on the front at an angle of 30° and maintaining this position for as many hours as reasonably possible both day and night. There are two methods of doing this:

1. Raise the head of the cot with bricks or alternatively elevate the mattress by placing pillows between it and the cot. Place the child in a harness and pin the harness securely to the mattress so that the child cannot slide down. The Mothercare 'Baby Carrier' is ideal for this purpose.

2. Obtain a 'reflux board', a specifically-designed elevated board which supports the child. Both board and harness are portable, and have the advantage of being able to be used anywhere. It is hoped that a light-weight 'reflux board' will become commercially available (see p. 141).

How does posture help?

This can best be demonstrated by a diagram which shows air fluid relationships in the stomach in different positions (Fig. 6/3). When the child lies on his back or is upright, fluid is trapped between air and the oesophageal opening, escaping air causes fluid displacement (reflux) into the oesophagus. In the front (prone) position there is no fluid displacement as the air lies between the fluid and the oesophageal opening.

Reflux can also be reduced by feeding more frequently with smaller volumes. It is not known why, but many children have a delay in stomach emptying. Large amounts of milk may accumulate and after a big feed the stomach may be very full. The risk of reflux can be considerably reduced by giving small amounts frequently so that the

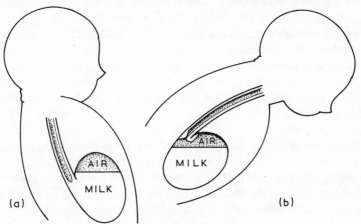

Fig. 6/3 To show the air/fluid relationship in the stomach in the sitting position (a) and lying on the front (prone position) (b)

stomach is not allowed to over-fill. For example, a child with reflux fed 80ml every 4 hours may be improved if 40ml were fed every 2 hours during the day at least.

The only drug which has been shown to be effective in reducing reflux in children is bethanechol, which seems to work by causing downward muscular contractions of the oesophagus so that milk or acid which enters the oesophagus is rapidly cleared back into the stomach. Side-effects may include sweating, increased saliva production and slowing of the heart beat. It can also cause colic and may even make vomiting worse. Although these side-effects are not common, bethanechol is seldom used because most children respond to the measures previously mentioned which should always be attempted first. Surgery is only performed when these methods, plus bethanechol, are unsuccessful. Indeed, the need for operation is now very rare. At operation a piece of stomach is wrapped around the oesophageal valve to tighten it and this produces a dramatic cure.

Children with reflux do not require a change in diet. Many parents try a variety of milks before discovering that each in turn is no better than the previous one. Traditionally parents have been told to thicken feeds. Nestargel, a seed flour, is widely used for this purpose. Although there is no proof of its value some parents do say it is helpful. Despite little scientific evidence of their value in an essentially self-limiting condition, a variety of medicines are widely prescribed for children with reflux. These include medicines which speed stomach emptying and tighten the oesophageal valve (metoclopramide), neutralise acid (antacids) or reduce acid production (H_2 antagonists – cimetidine and ranitidine). In Britain, the most commonly prescribed antacid is Infant Gaviscon which, in addition to neutralising the acid, also forms a gel in the stomach. I have often felt that these medicines are prescribed more for the parents' sake than the child's.

In conclusion, gastro-oesophageal reflux is a common, temporary inconvenience in the first year of life. An adequate understanding of the cause of the vomiting and knowing that it will soon stop helps relieve anxiety. Placing the child in the correct position and feeding frequent, small volumes will often produce a dramatic effect.

Equipment note: Information about the reflux board may be obtained from:

UK

Bio-Med Engineering Limited, 1 Headlands Road, Liversedge, West Yorkshire

USA

Cozcon, 24 Norwich Avenue, Colchester, Connecticut 06415

PYLORIC STENOSIS

Pyloric stenosis affects 2–3 children in every 1000 births. Male infants are 5 times more commonly affected, particularly first born.

What is pyloric stenosis?

The word stenosis means 'narrowing'. Food leaving the stomach for the duodenum normally passes through a valve called the pyloric sphincter. In pyloric stenosis muscle in the vicinity of the valve starts to increase in amount (hypertrophies) and bulges into the duodenum, eventually blocking the valve. Stomach contents (milk and acid secretions), prevented from leaving, are vomited. The reason for the muscle enlargement is not known.

Does pyloric stenosis run in families?

Yes, there is a familial tendency with about 7% incidence in children of affected parents. The incidence is highest in male infants of mothers who had pyloric stenosis.

What are the clinical signs?

The main sign is vomiting, which can occur at any time in the first 3 months, mostly between the 2nd and 6th weeks. Vomiting is never bile stained (yellow-green colour) and after a few days becomes projectile (shoots out). Generally, it occurs after feeding but can occur several hours later. At first the child appears well and will readily feed after vomiting. As nourishment and fluids are lost, weight loss and dehydration ensue. With increasing severity the infant becomes listless, limp and will not feed well. Depending on the amount of milk retained his stools may become small and infrequent.

How is pyloric stenosis diagnosed?

The doctor will do a 'test feed'. The infant will be placed on the knee of his mother or a nurse and his abdomen will be exposed while he is fed from a bottle. The doctor, who sits opposite the child, will observe the abdominal wall for movement (peristaltic waves). If the pylorous is narrowed the stomach muscle needs to work very hard to force feeds through the obstruction. The increased effort of the stomach muscle is seen as waves moving from left to right over the upper abdomen as the muscle contracts and relaxes.

The doctor will then place a hand on the abdomen in an attempt to feel the pyloric muscle enlargement. The enlarged muscle feels like an acorn or a large olive and is called a 'pyloric tumour'. Palpation of the tumour confirms the diagnosis. Very occasionally it may be difficult to feel the tumour: barium x-ray studies will show the narrowing and confirm the diagnosis. When the diagnosis is not confirmed the most likely cause for vomiting without diarrhoea is gastro-oesophageal reflux (p. 136).

What is the treatment?

The child will require a general anaesthetic and a small operation. There is no urgency about the operation. A delay of one or two days is sometimes necessary to prepare the child for surgery. During this time a check on blood chemistry will be made and dehydration will be corrected with intravenous fluids. Oral feeds will be stopped.

At operation (Ramstedt's pyloromyotomy) the muscle of the tumour is cut, but the lining (mucosa) of the duodenum is left intact. Feeding, breast or bottle, begins after 4–6 hours and is gradually increased. Most infants are feeding normally and ready for discharge after 2–3 days. At operation the mucosa is occasionally cut in which case the hospital stay may be a little longer. Of great concern to parents is the fact that about 15% continue vomiting postoperatively. This is caused by acid irritation of the stomach and lower oesophagus and seldom lasts more than a few days. The weight should rapidly increase in the weeks after operation. There are no long-term effects of pyloric stenosis or the operation.

In conclusion, pyloric stenosis is a life-threatening condition when untreated. It can usually be diagnosed with ease and responds well to surgical treatment.

CONSTIPATION AND ENCOPRESIS (SOILING)

What is constipation?

Constipation means hard stools. They are often infrequent and, because of the hardness, may be difficult to pass. When constipation is prolonged it is called chronic. Chronic constipation with soiling is a common childhood problem, affecting boys three times more often than girls. The average age is 7. Although most parents give a history of constipation starting in infancy or shortly thereafter, soiling is not apparent before age 3. The classic story is that of an early school age child who has an enormous stool every 2–3 weeks which may be large enough to cause blockage of the toilet. Between stools there may be soiling of underwear. Although large amounts of stool are retained and felt as masses in the abdomen, there is surprisingly little abdominal swelling, the reason being that gas which causes swelling can escape. Except for occasional bouts of abdominal pain or loss of appetite symptoms are infrequent.

By the time the child sees a paediatrician numerous laxatives, suppositories or enemas will have been tried as well as bribery or punishment. Few, rare medical conditions can cause chronic constipation. These can usually be excluded by the history and examination. Occasionally one such condition, Hirschsprung's disease, a congenital rectal narrowing, may need to be excluded by a barium enema x-ray. Constipated children have a tendency towards urine infections and some paediatricians routinely test the urine.

What is the cause?

This almost always dates back to an episode of constipation or deliberate attempts by the child to hold back defaecation. Constipation may occur during an illness, particularly if there is dehydration. Toddler dietary fads which avoid fibre produce constipation. Reasons for deliberate holding back include fissure in ano, a tear in the anus causing pain (see below) and not wanting to use school toilets which are often dirty and do not allow privacy. Some hold back as a protest against toilet training (see p. 26) particularly when attempted too early or in an obsessive and inflexible manner. Holding back may also be used as an attention seeking device when there is marital friction or sibling rivalry. Confusion arises when a young child goes red in the face and sits cross-legged after a meal. Such a child is presumed by the parents to be straining to pass a stool, but in fact the straining action may be an attempt to hold back the stool.

Stool retention causes water absorption and hardening, the longer the retention the harder the stool. The rectum contains pressure sensors which, when stretched, initiate a desire to defaecate. Unfortunately, when it is very full excessive stretch prevents the sensors from working and the desire to defaecate is lost. A vicious cycle is thus established: constipation produces excessive stretching which prevents the desire to defaecate and in turn causes further constipation. With further stretching voluntary control of the muscle (external anal sphincter) at the end of the rectum is no longer possible and soiling occurs. This may take the form of hard pellets of stool or a brown fluid, which can lead to the mistaken diagnosis of diarrhoea. Normally both bacteria and fluid are present in the lower bowel. Bacterial action around the edge of the stool causes small gaps through which fluid in the bowel above the rectum can escape.

Most children with chronic constipation have an emotional problem. They may be depressed and are typically timid and unwilling to talk about their problem. The cause of the emotional problem usually arises from attitudes of those around them. Punishment by parents or teasing by siblings or schoolchildren can cause immeasurable emotional damage. In my view the medical profession is not exempt either. A repeated number of, in most cases unnecessary, rectal examinations, suppositories and enemas could be expected to produce an emotional problem in any normal child.

The principles of treatment are the prevention of constipation and an encouraging, helpful attitude to the child's emotional needs. It is vital that parents realise at the outset that this problem will be cured but *not* in a week or two. It usually takes at least 4–6 months and on occasions much longer.

Many laxatives can be used for the prevention of constipation. I use Senokot, an old fashioned remedy which has stood the test of time. It acts by stimulating the bowel. Start with 2–3 teaspoons at night and increase by one teaspoon every day until there is a soft, regular motion. If the motion becomes very loose do *not* stop the Senokot but reduce the amount to the previous acceptable dose. The desired effect will usually be achieved with a dose between 4–15 teaspoons daily. Having established the correct amount it will need to be maintained for some months before making a very gradual reduction over a further few months. Many parents fear that the child will become dependent on the Senokot and will eventually be unable to cope without it. This does not happen; there need be no cause for concern. Children's schedules vary and the mother or child may find it more convenient to give the Senokot at differing times, depending on the time the child should be encouraged to sit on the toilet after the next meal. A full stomach initiates a reflex desire to defaecate (gastro-colic reflex) and it is worth while making use of this reflex at mealtimes. If Senokot is given at night, it is important to allow plenty of time for the child to go to the toilet between breakfast and going to school.

A constipated young child needs to increase intra-abdominal pressure to enable a firm, large stool to be passed. This is not possible unless the child is able to push with both feet. If a potty is not used make sure the feet rest on the floor or provide a foot step in front of the toilet.

Diet is important. A high fibre diet consisting of bran, cereals, fruit and vegetables is recommended. Many children like dried fruit which is sweet and reasonably cheap.

I have found this regimen of preventing constipation and emotional support very effective, indeed, it is seldom necessary to resort to suppositories or enemas. There are occasions, however, when such measures do not work. When this happens the problem is best dealt with by a child and family psychiatrist or clinical psychologist.

What is an anal fissure?

It is a small tear at the edge of the anus, where the skin on the outside joins the lining (mucosa) on the inside. It is a common problem which can occur at any age. The cause of the tear is usually not evident; it may arise from an episode of constipation in which there is stretching of the anus by a large hard stool. Explosive diarrhoea in which the anus is stretched by a sudden gush of gas and liquid may also be a contributing cause. Young children often have not just one tear, but several.

The child will scream with pain at defaecation, go red in the face and try to hold back his stools; constipation may result. Between episodes the child may be quite irritable. Bright red blood may be seen on the surface of the stool, bleeding sometimes following defaecation.

Anal fissures, especially in infants, should be treated promptly and vigorously to break the constipation-fissure-constipation cycle. The treatment consists of giving a stool softener or other type of laxative for a few weeks while the fissure heals. The consistency of the stool is very important: it should be kept soft, a hard stool or a runny stool both delay healing. The child's diet and medication will require careful adjustment in order to maintain a soft stool during this time. The stool should continue to be kept soft for a few weeks after the fissure has healed so as to avoid a recurrence. Many paediatricians recommend the application of a local anaesthetic jelly around the anal margin before the child defaecates. This is usually not very helpful because it is very difficult to predict when the child will need to defaecate, and to be fully effective the jelly needs to be applied about 30 minutes beforehand. Pain is best relieved by frequent hot baths, as many as four in a day for very severe pain.

On this regimen almost all fissures heal in 6–8 weeks; those that don't are usually treated by anal stretching and occasionally by other surgical procedures. Anal stretching is done under a short general anaesthetic after which the fissure usually heals, but occasionally recurs.

INFANTILE COLIC

Colic is one of the most frequent and distressing conditions affecting young babies. Mothers, advised by family, friends and various health professionals, become increasingly frustrated when nothing helps. They know that a baby cries when he is hungry, wet or bored; their inability to relieve the crying by feeding, changing or comforting him makes them very anxious.

What is colic?

Colic can best be described as bouts of painful screaming lasting from a few minutes to as long as half an hour. The attack ends suddenly with apparent pain-free crying (sobbing), only to be followed minutes later by a further screaming bout. During the attack the high-pitched screams, red face, clenched fists and flexed legs strongly suggest that the child is having pain. He is irritable, very active and may make sucking movements and appears to be searching for food. Colicky babies have an excess of wind, and 'tummy rumbling' is frequently heard. At times the painful screaming appears to be relieved by a motion or the passage of large amounts of wind.

What is normal crying and what is colic?

Studies of infants in the first 3 months have shown that crying increases during the first 3 weeks and reaches a crescendo of nearly 3 hours daily at 4–6 weeks. The amount then drops rapidly, stabilising at a reasonable level of less than 1 hour daily by 12 weeks. There is also a tendency for crying to be more in the evening, a trying time for parents. The definition of colic which is used by most doctors doing research on colic is as follows: 'Crying episodes occurring at least once every 24 hours, extending for at least 3 hours, and resistant to all attempts at soothing.'

How common is colic?

Colic appears to be a condition of industrialised societies, where it may affect as many as 1 in 4 babies. The incidence in underdeveloped societies is unknown.

At what age does colic occur?

Colic commonly occurs as early as the 1st or 2nd week after discharge from hospital and seldom persists beyond 5 months, most colic settling by the end of the 3rd month.

Is colic more common in the day or night?

Colic can occur at any time of the day or night. Studies, however, suggest that it is more common in the late afternoon and early evening.

Is there a sex difference?

No, it is equally common in males and females.

What is the cause of colic?

Although there are various theories, the truth is we do not know.

Does breast feeding help?

No, colic does not appear to be less frequent in breast fed infants.

Does constipation cause colic?

In an older child, perhaps, but *not* in the first months of life. The fact that passing a motion is often immediately followed by pain relief has led many parents to attribute the pain to constipation.

Why does he have so much wind?

We don't know. It does not appear to be connected with the way he is 'winded' after feeds.

Do colicky babies gain weight normally?

Yes, they are in every other way normal and may even gain weight faster than normal.

Does it help to try a different milk?

No, changing the milk does not help. Most mothers soon discover this.

What else may help?

Lying the child on his front over a covered hot water bottle placed on his mother's lap may help. An old-fashioned, frequently used method is to give 10–15 drops of an alcoholic drink in 60ml (2oz) of warm, slightly sweetened water.

Unfortunately, there are large numbers of infants who do not obtain relief from anything. Knowing that the child has been thoroughly examined and having been reassured about the diagnosis, most mothers are able to cope. However, there are times when even the most capable mother becomes worn out and unable to stand the child's relentless screaming. When this happens a short-term admission to hospital seems to provide relief for both mother and child. After she has had a rest a mother may be embarrassed by the fact that she was unable to cope and her 'healthy' child needed admission. She need not be embarrassed; hospitals are not only places for curing illness but are frequently used for relieving distress. After all, a happy mother and child is one of the fundamental aims of good child care.

Does colic have any long-term effects?

None that we are aware of. Sleep problems in early childhood seem to be more common in children who have had colic, the reason not being clear.

What is gripe water?

William Woodward, a pharmacist in Nottingham, first made gripe water in 1851 as a remedy for the watery gripes, as gastroenteritis was then known. It soon became well known as a medicine to be used for minor abdominal complaints in infants. The wives of British servicemen popularised its use throughout the British Empire, where to this day it still enjoys phenomenal sales. Readers in the USA will probably never have heard of it. In Britain there is surprisingly little gripe water advertising, its use is mainly spread by word of mouth. One of Woodward's original advertising slogans was 'Granny told mother and mother told me.'

There are many gripe waters on the British market, all containing alcohol, sugar and antacids; some contain ginger, caraway, dill, spearmint and peppermint. The latter ingredients are said to have carminative (flatus relieving) properties. Despite the consumption of millions of bottles of gripe water throughout the world each year there does not ever appear to have been a carefully controlled study to see if gripe water really does help. Judging by the numbers of children whom I see after gripe water has been tried I would say that it was no more effective than tap water! There are reports of dental caries in children where mothers have continued to use gripe water for various abdominal complaints throughout infancy.

What are colic drops?

Colic drops can be bought over the counter for colic, their main ingredient a substance called dimethicone. A recent study in Sweden has shown that dimethicone is of no benefit in colic.

THE PERIODIC SYNDROME

The periodic syndrome is a name given to bouts of abdominal pain and/or vomiting, occurring at periodic intervals (weeks or months) between which the child is perfectly well. It is also known as recurrent abdominal pain of childhood or abdominal migraine. When vomiting is the predominant symptom it is called cyclical vomiting. In most children the pain is around the umbilicus and this is often accompanied by nausea and sometimes vomiting. The child will not eat, will look pale and exhausted and often has the appearance of dark rings under the eyes. Fever, although uncommon, may cause flushing of the cheeks and when neck glands are enlarged the condition can be confused with tonsillitis. Occasionally children complain of limb pains or body aches. The length of these attacks varies from a few hours to several days. With bouts of cyclic vomiting the child may be irritable and off food, the vomiting lasting two or three days during which he may develop acetone (sweet breath) and 'hollow eyes' from dehydration. The smelly breath is often apparent a few feet from the child and may also occur in the child who does not vomit. Following attacks of pain or vomiting children are vigorous and surprisingly well.

The periodic syndrome is one of the most common conditions seen in paediatric practice in the UK affecting about 1 in 10 children. The problem can start at any time from infancy to early teens, although the majority present between 5 and 9 years. There is a slightly increased frequency in girls. The cause of this often very distressing condition is unknown. There is no firm evidence that diet, allergy or emotional problems are the cause, although in a few children attacks may be precipitated by emotional stress. Similar conditions in childhood for which we have no rational explanation or treatment are infantile colic and 'growing pains' of the limbs. Many children with recurrent abdominal pain suffer from constipation, but treating the constipation gives temporary relief only and the use of high fibre diet in this condition has not been shown to be of any value.

In over 90% of children investigations do not reveal any cause for the pain. When investigations are positive they usually indicate a urine infection and some paediatricians would routinely arrange urine tests in children presenting with the periodic syndrome. The decision about whether to investigate and which investigation is very much dependent on the individual paediatrician. His decision will be based on a very careful clinical history and a thorough physical examination. The history more than anything else assists me in deciding when to investigate. For example, if a child is repeatedly awakened from sleep by the pain I would arrange barium x-rays. The severity of the pain does not necessarily influence my decision, since many emotional children and anxious parents exaggerate, while the more easygoing minimise a complaint.

As a general rule investigations should be strongly resisted unless absolutely necessary. By the time most patients see a paediatrician the duration of the problem is many months and sometimes years, at which point the child and parents strongly believe that there is something 'seriously wrong'. A series of investigations, however well meaning, will often only perpetuate this notion and I have often seen a sudden deterioration in a child's symptoms following a battery of investigations.

Children with periodic syndrome do not have a specific personality type, but most paediatricians would agree that a large number have personality traits which could best be described as 'highly strung', 'worriers' or 'perfectionists'. They are often very sensitive, behave impeccably well and try hard to please. The vast majority of children I see are happy, from normal homes and have no educational problems. By the time they are seen by a paediatrician the parents will usually have explored a host of possible causes, but invariably draw a blank. Although the parents themselves are a mixed bag, I have often been impressed by the level of parental overanxiety. It is not uncommon to find parents very concerned about a child who, while complaining of abdominal pain, has a broad smile on his face. Some

parents also have 'bowel problems' and there is a high incidence of
migraine or headaches in the family. Interestingly, as in migraine,
children with periodic syndrome commonly suffer from motion sickness.

The mainstay of treatment is to convince the child and the parents
that there is nothing physically wrong. In some families it is more a
question of convincing the parents rather than the child. The explanation given by the paediatrician needs to be handled with some deli-
cacy and tact. It is difficult to resolve the dilemma of the child who is
experiencing severe bouts of pain yet is being told that there is nothing physically wrong. Most children and their parents accept the reassurance of the paediatrician and, for an ill understood reason,
symptoms somehow improve. Others are only reassured after a
gamut of investigations, while some are never reassured even after 3
or 4 'second opinions'. By the time most children see a paediatrician a
variety of analgesics (painkillers), antacids, sedatives or antibiotics
will have been prescribed and parents will volunteer the information
'that nothing seems to help'. Parents are astute observers of their children and their observations are correct, for no medication has ever
been shown to be of benefit in this condition. Although some paediatricians do prescribe sedatives, the use of drugs in this condition
can best be summed up as follows: doctors who treat the symptoms
give a prescription; doctors who treat the patient are more likely to
offer guidance. Hot water bottles placed on the abdomen during
attacks provide some relief. When vomiting is severe an anti-emetic
(drug to stop vomiting) is useful and can be given by injection or
rectal suppository if necessary. On rare occasions a child with cyclical
vomiting and dehydration will require a short hospital admission for
an intravenous infusion (a drip).

After the initial visit to a paediatrician, follow-up visits are seldom
required. The majority will have fewer and less intense symptoms;
others, having received some guidance, learn to accept the problem
and live with it. In the minority of families the child or parents have
difficulty in coming to terms with the condition and there is much
distress and anxiety, often with prolonged absence from school. It is
then very helpful to admit the child for a few days to a children's ward
equipped with a school. This has a dramatic effect in most children,
the reason not being entirely clear. It does, however, prove to every-
one that the child is educable even when unwell and school attend-
ance should then be firmly enforced by parents and teachers.

Although there is no demonstrable physical cause for the periodic syndrome the cause is not necessarily psychological and referral to a child psychiatrist or clinical psychologist is seldom required. When such a referral is made it is the family as a whole and not just the child that should be referred. I have dealt with a few families where psychological help was required to relieve parental anxiety rather than the child's abdominal pains.

'Will he grow out of it?' is a question every parent asks. The answer is that some children will, but, follow-up studies into adulthood indicate that this is not always the case. These studies show that many small belly-achers will grow into large belly-achers and in some migraine will develop. In an individual child it is impossible to predict the eventual outcome and no treatment has ever been shown to influence the outlook.

THREADWORMS

Threadworm, pinworm or seatworm are all names given to an infection with a worm called *Enterobius vermicularis*. This worm is found only in humans, is harmless and when it causes symptoms they are merely a social inconvenience. It is yellowish-white and lives in the lower part of the small bowel and upper part of the large bowel. Females are between 3 and 13mm long, males shorter. The child becomes infected by swallowing eggs which hatch in the upper small bowel eventually forming adults which then mate, the whole process taking 3–6 weeks. Shortly after mating the male dies. The pregnant female then moves down the large bowel and emerges at the anus, usually at night. She crawls several centimetres liberating thousands of eggs before dying. Figure 6/4 shows the life cycle of the threadworm.

Threadworms are found in both adults and children. It is the most common worm infection in British children, affecting as many as 20%. Girls are affected more than boys and the peak age is between 5 and 9 years. Many people, both adults and children, have no apparent symptoms and are unaware of the infection. The reason why some have symptoms and others none is unknown, but may be connected with allergy to the eggs. Those children with symptoms usually have an intense itch around the anus and genital area which is worse at night and may interfere with sleep. The scratched area

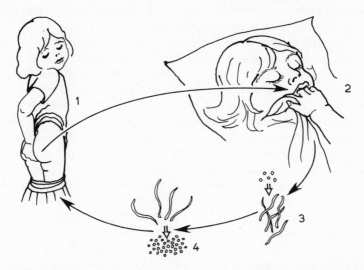

Fig. 6/4 Life cycle of the threadworm. 1. Scratching contaminates the hands and nails with eggs; 2. The eggs are transmitted to the mouth; 3. Eggs develop and hatch in the gut; 4. Adult worms emerge from the anus at night and lay their eggs

around the anus and genitals may become sore and infected and bleeding occur.

The eggs remain infective for several days. The child who scratches herself gets them on her hands and under her fingernails. She may self-infect herself by putting her fingers in her mouth or the infection may be spread by touching toys and other objects at home and at school. It is quite common for eggs to be found in dust in kindergartens and other areas where children congregate. It is often very difficult to prevent reinfection after treatment when the opportunities for ingestion and inhalation of eggs are so widespread.

Threadworms are diagnosed by seeing the worms around the anus or in the stools. When worms are not seen the 'Sellotape test' is done. As soon as the child is woken, before bathing or dressing, the adhesive side of Sellotape is repeatedly pressed against the skin around the anus. The Sellotape is then placed adhesive side down on a clean glass slide. Best results are obtained by repeating the test on three consecutive mornings. The slides can be stored in an envelope in the fridge until all three are ready to go to the laboratory, where they will be examined under a microscope to see if threadworm eggs are present. Remember to wash your hands after each Sellotape test.

Many paediatricians treat the whole family at the same time, but the benefit of such action is difficult to judge because eggs are to be found in so many places in the environment that reinfection is bound to occur sooner or later. In order to minimise the reinfection rate all treatment schedules require retreatment after 2–4 weeks. This should be accompanied by washing of underclothes, bed clothes and bedding, but more severe hygienic endeavours are unnecessary.

There are various effective treatments for threadworm: they can be divided into those that kill and others that paralyse the worms. With killing or paralysis of the worms their ability to adhere to the bowel wall is removed and they are then passed in large numbers in the stools. Piperazine, probably the most widely used treatment in Britain, acts by paralysing the worms. It may be given as a 7-day course followed by a further course after a 2-week, treatment free period. Pripsen is a combination of a large dose of piperazine and a laxative (Senokot). It is given as a single dose and repeated after 14 days. Side-effects of piperazine are minor but include nausea, vomiting, diarrhoea and skin rashes.

There are 3 other safe and equally effective de-worming preparations which are being used increasingly: mebendazole, thiabendazole, pyrantel pamoate. These are all given as a single dose which should be repeated after 2 and 4 weeks. Side-effects are uncommon.

It is not uncommon for children to get repeated threadworm infections. They are not harmful, only a minor irritation and treatment is necessary only when symptoms are present.

Chapter 7

Miscellaneous Abdominal Problems

APPENDICITIS

The appendix is a finger-like projection attached to the right side of the large bowel. When its opening becomes obstructed, bacteria in the appendix invade the wall causing it to become inflamed. If left untreated the wall will soon rupture into the abdomen, the bacteria then infecting the lining of the abdomen, a condition known as peritonitis. The most common cause of the obstruction is a lump of hardened faecal material known as a faecolith. Appendicitis can occur at any age, being most common in mid-teens and uncommon in the child under 3. The onset is *always* sudden: there is no such thing as a 'grumbling' appendix.

In the older child, the pain which is colicky at first then becomes constant, usually starts around the navel and moves to the lower abdomen on the right side. Vomiting, constipation and loss of appetite may initially accompany the pain, later diarrhoea and a high fever may develop. Any movement such as coughing will make the pain worse, particularly so when peritonitis has developed. The child with peritonitis lies very still and has an abdomen which feels rigid and very tender. Symptoms in the younger child are more vague; appendicitis is often difficult to diagnose. Most children are restless, irritable and unco-operative. It may be possible to feel tenderness on the right side of the abdomen.

The rapidity with which appendicitis progresses requires urgent treatment if a ruptured appendix is to be avoided. Removing the appendix is a small operation, after which the child should make a complete recovery. Immediately after the operation the child will have an intravenous drip and a suction tube in his mouth for a day or two. Analgesics (painkillers) will be given in the drip or by intramuscular injection. Most children are sent home after about a week. It is best to wait a few weeks after the operation before engaging in vigorous sporting activities.

What is mesenteric adenitis?

This condition may at times be very difficult to distinguish from appendicitis. The pain is caused by inflammation of the lymph glands in the abdomen. Children usually have a sore throat (p. 230), their temperature is higher and does not last as long as in appendicitis. The cause is usually a virus.

INTUSSUSCEPTION

When one part of the intestine telescopes into the adjacent portion so as to lie inside it an intussusception is said to have taken place. Although it is the most frequently encountered abdominal emergency of early childhood, it is not common. There are about 5 admissions a year to the average district hospital in Britain. The cause is usually a virus.

Most children are between 6–12 months. The characteristic features are colicky abdominal pain, vomiting, rectal bleeding (redcurrant jelly stools) and an abdominal mass. Although characteristic, these features need not always be present. In most children the intensity of the screams and pallor leave parents in no doubt about the child's pain. Screaming episodes last a few minutes, only to recur 15–30 minutes later. At first the child is well between attacks, but he later becomes pale, clammy and exhausted. When the child relaxes, a sausage-shaped mass may be felt on the right side of the abdomen. Diarrhoea may be present in the early stages when it is sometimes misdiagnosed as gastroenteritis. It can be differentiated from colic by its occurrence after three months and attacks of pain which come in waves.

Some surgeons arrange for the child to have a barium enema x-ray which will not only confirm the diagnosis but may cure the problem by pushing the bowel back into its correct position. Other surgeons perform a small operation immediately and the bowel is gently pulled back into its usual position. Hospital admission is seldom more than a week. A recurrence is unlikely to occur.

INGUINAL HERNIA

This is a common problem, affecting 1 in 50 boys and 1 in 500 girls. It is more common in premature infants. Hernias can occur at any age but most occur at either 2 months or 1 year.

What is a hernia?

It is a painless swelling in the groin or groin and scrotum. The lump may not be noticeable all the time, it may come and go, but is usually seen at the end of the day and often gone in the morning. At first it may be small but with time gradually enlarges. Crying or straining makes it larger. If it goes when the child stops crying or if it can be made to disappear by gentle massage it is said to be reducible. Hernias which are irreducible are particularly common in the first year of life. A hernia which is reducible causes only mild discomfort while one that is irreducible may cause pain.

What causes a hernia?

Before birth the testis is enclosed in the abdomen which is lined by a membrane called peritoneum. At the start of testicular descent (Fig. 7/1) it pushes against and stretches the peritoneum; the farther it descends the more peritoneum is pulled and stretched in its wake. Thus, a channel or sac of peritoneum linking the abdomen with the testis is created. This sac usually closes within a year of birth. Girls

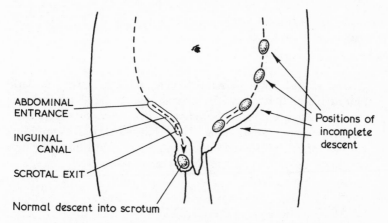

Fig. 7/1 Normal testicular descent showing positions of incomplete descent

also have a shorter but similar sac. When the sac does not close there are two common consequences; first a loop of bowel may move down the sac, when it is called a hernia; second, fluid from the abdominal cavity can pass down the sac into the scrotum, when it is called a hydrocele or fluid hernia.

Do hernias need treatment?

Yes, they do. There are two complications which may arise if they are not treated:

1. the bowel may become obstructed in which case the child will have pain, constipation and bile-stained vomit;
2. the blood supply to the bowel may be cut off; the hernia is then said to have strangulated. The lump over a strangulated hernia is inflamed, swollen and very tender; the child may be very ill.

What is the treatment?

The treatment is a small operation in which the piece of bowel is put back in the abdomen and the sac closed. If the hernia is reducible the operation should be performed sooner rather than later, particularly in the child under a year. If the hernia is irreducible the operation is performed straightaway, but the child may be held with his legs suspended in the air for some hours in an attempt to get the hernia to reduce before the operation. The child is usually perfectly well after operation, remaining in hospital for no more than a day or two.

UMBILICAL HERNIA

A bulge around a baby's navel is common, particularly in dark-skinned races. It is caused by a small gap in the abdominal wall through which a segment of bowel protrudes. It becomes bigger with crying, coughing and straining. An umbilical hernia does not cause any discomfort and there are no complications. Most disappear by a year, but some do take as long as 10 years.

DIVARICATION OF THE RECTI

A longitudinal bulge in the midline of the upper abdomen is quite common in the pre-school child and sometimes worries parents. It is caused by a laxity of the sinew which joins the two main abdominal muscles (recti). No treatment is required; the bulge disappears when the sinew tightens up.

HYDROCELE

As explained previously a hydrocele is a fluid hernia, the amount of fluid being to a certain extent dependent on gravity. A hydrocele is much more noticeable in a child who is sitting or standing than one who is lying down. Unlike a hernia a hydrocele transilluminates (lights up) when a flashlight is held against the scrotum. They are particularly common in the first year and require no treatment, eventually disappearing when the hernia sac closes. Only those that persist or develop after a year require treatment. They are treated because firm pressure of fluid against the testis may interfere with its function, the other reason being to avoid the embarrassment of an enlarged scrotum. The operation is similar to an inguinal hernia; the fluid is removed and the sac closed.

Chapter 8

Kidney and Genitalia Problems

THE NEPHROTIC SYNDROME

This condition affects 1 in 50 000 children each year in the USA. Most are between 2 and 7. Twice as many boys are affected.

Generalised swelling (oedema) develops slowly and is most evident on the face around the eyes and on the legs. In the abdomen fluid (ascites) may accumulate causing swelling. Despite the generalised swelling these children appear to be well. Urine output is reduced and on testing the urine there is a large quantity of protein.

Nephrotic syndrome is caused by a leak of protein from the kidneys. Why this leak occurs is a mystery. The high protein content of the blood normally prevents fluid in the circulation seeping into the tissues, the low blood protein in the nephrotic syndrome allows seepage to occur. The lower the protein, the more seepage, the more the tissues swell. More than 75% have a type of nephrotic syndrome called 'minimal change', which has an excellent outlook. It is called minimal change because changes are minimal when a segment of the kidney is examined under the electron microscope.

Steroids are used to treat nephrotic syndrome, the duration of treatment varying according to the treatment schedule the paediatrician normally uses. Most children respond within 2 weeks; they pass more urine which has diminishing amounts of protein. As the swelling subsides the weight falls. After steroid treatment is discontinued most children have at least 1 relapse in the following year, about 25% have frequent relapses. Again steroids are used and may at times be required for prolonged periods. Side-effects may be minimised by alternate-day dosage but do sometimes develop. When this happens steroid dosage is reduced and a group of drugs known as cytotoxics are used with good effect. Children with nephrotic syndrome have an increased risk of developing infections. If they are unwell or have a fever a doctor should be consulted. The child who picks up an infection may have a temporary relapse which improves spontaneously after a week or two. If there is an infection and a relapse there is no urgency about using steroids; a delay is not harmful. It does have the advantage of allowing time to see if the protein in the urine will clear so avoiding the need for steroids.

A very few children require a renal biopsy. This involves sedating the child and under local anaesthetic passing a fine needle through the loin into the kidney from which a sliver of tissue is removed. The tissue is then examined under a microscope. This procedure causes minimal discomfort. A renal biopsy is done for the following indications:

1. Failure to respond to steroid treatment.
2. A high blood pressure.
3. Visible blood in the urine.
4. Blood tests which suggest a type other than minimal change.

The most important point to remember about the nephrotic syndrome is that it is a temporary problem of early childhood. For the vast majority the outlook is excellent. No matter how many relapses the child may have his kidneys will eventually be perfectly normal.

URINARY INFECTIONS

Urine infections in children are common, the vast majority settling with a short course of treatment and no long-term complications. Although rare, kidney damage can occur and may present in later life as renal failure, high blood pressure or troublesome urinary infections. This damage may be minimised by early diagnosis, correct investigation and treatment.

How common are urinary infections in children?
About 5% of girls and 1–2% of boys are affected, except for the first 3 months when they are more common in boys, the reason not being known.

What are the symptoms of a urinary infection?
These are often non-specific and vary with age; in the first 5 years a urinary infection should be considered in any child who is unwell for

no apparent reason or has an unexplained temperature. In the child above 5 symptoms may be more specific. The child may have a temperature and complain of pain in the abdomen or side of back. 'Burning' when urine is passed, together with the need to empty the bladder frequently and inability to hold back urination are sometimes complained of by the older child. Urine infections may present as wetting (day or night) in a child who was previously toilet trained.

How is a urine infection diagnosed?

A urine infection can be diagnosed fairly accurately by examining urine under the microscope and looking for bacteria. The most accurate method is to use the specimen to grow bacteria in a laboratory or on a Dipslide (bacteria growing slide) and to count them. In the final analysis, the diagnosis will be based on both the count and the method of collection. Your doctor will be able to advise you on the accepted normal values of the bacterial count with each method of collection.

What causes urine infections?

Other than the newborn, when infection may come from the

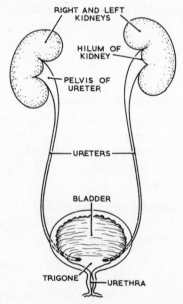

Fig. 8/1 Anatomy of the urinary system

blood, most arise when bacteria enter the urethra and infect the bladder (Fig. 8/1). These bacteria live in the bottom part of the bowel, the reason for the greater frequency in girls being the closeness of the urethral opening to the rectum and the shorter urethral length. Urine is warm and ideal for bacterial growth. Once bacteria enter the bladder they multiply rapidly if urine is present.

There are two main causes of urinary infection:

1. Causes that promote urine stagnation by preventing complete bladder emptying. Other than chronic constipation or a problem involving the nerves of the bladder, the cause for incomplete emptying is an abnormality of the urinary system, the commonest being reflux. This abnormality is found in about 35% of children with urinary infections, other abnormalities accounting for a further 15%.
2. Causes favouring the entry of bacteria into the urethra. Any irritation in the genital area favours the development of a urinary infection.

What is reflux?

On bladder contraction (urination) urine is normally forced into

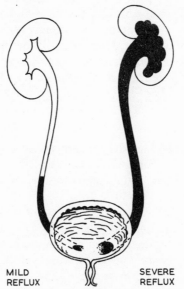

MILD
REFLUX

SEVERE
REFLUX

Fig. 8/2 Reflux of urine into the kidney

the urethra by opening the urethral valve (sphincter) and closing the openings of the ureters (Fig. 8/1). Reflux occurs when the openings of the ureters cannot close properly and urine is forced up the ureter; in a severe form it is forced up into the kidney (Fig. 8/2).

Is reflux harmful?

Yes, it may be. Besides preventing the bladder emptying completely severe reflux may cause kidney damage when the urine is infected. This mainly occurs in the first 7 years of life. After 7 years it does not cause damage but may cause further damage in kidneys already weakened.

Is reflux permanent?

No, in over 80% of children the ureteral valves eventually tighten up with age, and reflux ceases.

What tests should be done after a urine infection is diagnosed?

This will depend on the age of the child. The two common x-ray tests are an MCU (micturating cysto-urethrogram) and IVU (intravenous urogram).

1. MCU – a fine tube is passed into the bladder which is then filled with a dye. When the bladder empties x-rays are taken. Besides showing abnormalities of the lower urinary system an MCU shows whether reflux is present. After the MCU the child is given a short course of antibiotics if not already on treatment.
2. IVU – dye is injected into the blood and as it is excreted by the kidneys x-rays are taken. This outlines the urinary system and in this way we are able to detect any abnormalities, particularly those involving the kidneys.

For the child *under* 7 an MCU is normally done. If reflux is evident an IVU is then done. For the child *over* 7 an IVU is usually done first. If this shows scarring (kidney damage) the MCU is then done to detect reflux.

Two other tests which may be done and are now being used quite extensively are ultrasound and radio-isotope tests. Ultrasound is used to detect kidney abnormalities by passing sound waves through the abdomen. Radio-isotope tests are used for detecting kidney outline and reflux by injecting a radio-active substance into the blood and allowing it to accumulate in the bladder after excretion. On urination the direction of the radio-active material in the urine is measured by a radio-activity counter. Both ultrasound and radio-isotope tests are pain free and completely safe, ultrasound does not appear to be as accurate at detecting kidney scars as an IVU.

How should urine infections be treated?

Most urine infections are caused by a bacterium called *E. coli* and the antibiotic chosen will be one generally regarded as very effective against *E. coli*. Commonly used antibiotics are amoxycillin (Amoxil) and cotrimoxazole (Bactrim or Septrin). Treatment should be started immediately after a specimen has been obtained; a day later the laboratory may be able to confirm whether the bacterium is sensitive to the antibiotic.

Most paediatricians give antibiotic treatment for a week, although there is a strong case for continuing antibiotic treatment for some months. Within six months of discontinuing the antibiotic over two-thirds develop a reinfection with a fresh bowel bacterium. It has been shown that reinfection can be considerably reduced after antibiotic discontinuation if the antibiotic course is maintained at a lower dosage for 6–12 months.

Continuous low dose antibiotics (prophylaxis) are also used to prevent infections when a child has very frequent, painful urine infections. The main use of continuous antibiotics is to prevent kidney damage (kidney scarring). *Continuous treatment is necessary in the child under 7 with reflux and the child over 7 when both reflux and kidney damage are present*. In the younger child antibiotics may be discontinued after age 7 if the kidneys remain normal. In the older child antibiotics should be continued until the reflux ceases or until the kidneys are fully grown at about 14 years.

After a urine infection is diagnosed urine should be sent for bacterial growth (culture) monthly for 3 months and then 3-monthly. Children taking antibiotics continuously should *never* stop their treatment before the specimen is taken.

What other helpful measures should be taken?

1. The child should empty her bladder regularly. At bedtime in particular she should be instructed to try to pass as much urine as possible. A simple rule is to get her to pass urine before going to school, going out to play or watching television. The class teacher or nursery supervisory will often be willing to assist with this.
2. She should be encouraged to drink fluids. A regular drink with meals is advisable.

3. Make sure she does not become constipated.
4. She should wear cotton pants and avoid bath irritants. Do not add bubble bath or any detergents or antiseptics to the bath. If heavily chlorinated pool water causes irritation in the genital area apply petroleum jelly before swimming.

What about surgery?

Some children (less than 10%) have abnormalities which require surgery. The need for surgery for the most severe forms of reflux is controversial and is at present an unresolved issue.

Is it worth screening schoolchildren routinely for urine infection?

This does not appear to be worth while. The incidence of urinary infection without symptoms is about 0.03% for boys and 2% for girls. By school age most kidney damage will already have occurred, but in about 10% of children with damaged kidneys further damage will occur. The size of the problem is such that it would be impossible to investigate such large numbers of children to determine which may be at risk of further kidney damage. The alternative would be to keep them all on continuous antibiotics, which would be both morally and economically unwise.

In conclusion, although much has been written about kidney damage and its prevention, it should be emphasised again that the vast majority of urine infections in children settle with a short course of treatment and have no long-term complications.

UNDESCENDED TESTIS (TESTICLE)

The undescended testis is generally regarded as a testis which has not entered the scrotum (sac). The vast majority of so-called undescended testes are in fact retractile testes. A retractile testis is a normal testis, which by muscular action in response to anxiety, cold or fear, is drawn out of the scrotum. Most retractile testes are found in 5–6-year-olds. Testes can be coaxed into the scrotum by examining them with warm hands while the child is squatting. When doubtful, parents are asked to repeat the procedure at home with the child in a warm bath. Testes that cannot be induced to enter the scrotum are not retractile. Retractile testes do not require treatment; at puberty they remain permanently in the scrotum.

In early pregnancy testes are formed in the abdomen. Towards the end of pregnancy they gradually move along the inguinal canal situated in the groin, connecting the inner abdomen with the scrotum (see Fig. 7/1). By birth they should normally be in the scrotum; entry is usually some weeks later in the case of premature infants. Those which have not entered the scrotum by 1 year are destined to remain permanently undescended, by which time about 8 in 1000 boys are affected; one-third are incompletely descended testes and two-thirds maldescended or ectopic.

What is the difference between an incompletely descended and ectopic testis?

The incompletely descended testis is always abnormally small and lies anywhere along the normal pathway between the scrotum and abdomen. The inguinal canal remains patent allowing bowel to traverse it and produce a bulge (hernia) in the lower abdomen.

The ectopic testis is a normal testis which lies in an abnormal position (Fig. 8/3). It passes through the inguinal canal which then closes. Immediately before entering the scrotum it is deflected off course and moves sideways where it can usually be easily palpated. The reason why some testes do not come down properly and why others go to the wrong place is not known. Both types occur more often on the right and about 10% are bilateral. Ask your doctor which type your son has.

Why should the testes be brought down?
For these reasons:

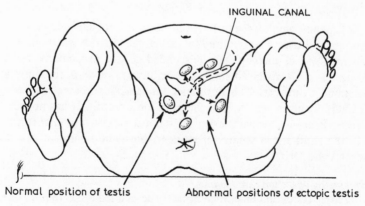

INGUINAL CANAL

Normal position of testis   Abnormal positions of ectopic testis

Fig. 8/3 Abnormal positions of the ectopic testis

1. There is an obvious psychological benefit in having both testes in the scrotum.
2. A testis in the wrong position at puberty will produce male hormones and secondary sexual development will occur quite normally. The effect on sperm production is, however, quite different; the sperm-producing cells will have been damaged and sperm production from the undescended testis is minimal, if at all.
3. Although the risk of malignancy is about 40 times that of a normally descended testis, it is extremely rare. Nevertheless, if such a malignancy were to develop it would be easier to detect by having the testis in the scrotum. Bringing down the testis does not lessen the risk but serves only to make early detection easier.
4. Undescended testes are more likely to be damaged by trauma.

At what age should the testes be brought down?

For many years testes were brought down shortly before school commencement at age 4–5. It was thought that damage to sperm cells occurred after age 5–6. From the psychological point of view it was thought that this was the best time for the operation.

There is now much firm evidence that sperm-producing cells become increasingly damaged after age 2 and for this reason most paediatric surgeons are recommending operation at that age. Before 2, when the anatomic structures are smaller, the operation is technically difficult and best delayed. The operation is mostly done at an earlier age when there is an accompanying hernia causing symptoms.

Is an operation always necessary?

It depends whether the testis is ectopic or incompletely descended. Surgery will always be required for an ectopic testis. A small number (about 10%) of incompletely descended testes, particularly when descent is at an advanced stage, can be brought down in response to hormone treatment. The hormone, luteinising releasing hormone (LHRH) is given by spray in the nose for a month. It has no side-effects. From 1–2, when the testis will not come down spontaneously and the child is too young for surgery, hormone treatment is well worth considering.

How many operations are required?

Ectopic testes and most incompletely descended testes require one operation known as orchidopexy. Two operations with about 6-month intervals may be required for some incompletely descended testes and when both testes are undescended.

Operations are done under general anaesthetic and hospital admission is seldom more than a night or two. Sutures are usually removed a week later.

What are the prospects for fertility?

The answer to this question has not been settled. Infertility is common when both testes are undescended, but the position with regard to one undescended testis is not clear. Early studies suggested that the prospects for potential fertility were good, but most recent studies have been more pessimistic. It is hoped that the earlier age of treatment nowadays will improve the prospect of fertility. As yet there have been no long-term studies comparing the effect on fertility of ectopic and incompletely descended testes.

TORSION (TWISTING) OF THE TESTIS

The testes, which dangle loosely in the scrotum, can easily become twisted causing interference with the blood supply. By the age of 25, 1 in 200 men have had a twisted testis. Testes can twist at any age but do so most commonly in the newborn and in adolescence. In the newborn the child presents with an enlarged, non-tender scrotal mass and remains surprisingly well. In the older boy there is a sudden onset of lower abdominal and scrotal pain, often associated with vomiting. The twisted testis is swollen and exquisitely tender.

A twisted testis is a medical emergency: unless the testis is untwisted within 4 hours it will be permanently damaged. There is a strong tendency for the other testis to twist so that, even if more than 4 hours have elapsed, an operation to stitch the other testis firmly in position should be performed.

HYPOSPADIAS

In hypospadias the opening of the penis is not at the end but along the undersurface of the shaft and in the most severe form at the base of the penis. Sometimes the shaft is relatively short and is bent in a downward fashion, this being known as chordee. Hypospadias occurs 2–3 times in every 1000 births. There is often a family history of hypospadias.

The hypospadias is corrected by surgery which is usually started at 3–4 so that it is complete by the time the child starts school. Some children have only one operation while others have 2 with about 6 months between. Occasionally an abnormal opening (fistula) appears soon after the operation, necessitating a further operation. The cosmetic effect of surgery is quite dramatic. Adults who have had a hypospadias repair in childhood have normal sexual intercourse and do not have any fertility problems.

Children who have a mild hypospadias where the opening is only slightly displaced do not require surgery. A child with hypospadias should never have a circumcision as the foreskin will be needed for the repair.

CIRCUMCISION

There is no medical reason for circumcision to be performed as a routine procedure and for this reason there are no neonatal circumcisions performed in the NHS in Britain. They are occasionally performed in older children when the foreskin opening is too tight, causing ballooning of the foreskin on urination or when the tip of the penis and foreskin become repeatedly infected. Despite the fact that the American Academy of Paediatrics and the American College of Obstetricians and Gynaecologists have repeatedly stated that there is no valid reason for neonatal circumcision, 1.25 million (75% of male births) circumcisions are performed each year in the USA. There are various spurious reasons for this, not least of which is the financial benefit to the medical profession. While there are no benefits there have been reports of serious complications directly attributable to circumcision, the most frequent being infection.

Because religious (Jews and Moslems) circumcisions are performed without pain relief it is wrongly believed by some that babies do not feel pain. Without wishing to become embroiled in a religious controversy I do feel that where circumcisions are deemed necessary for whatever reason, performing them under a short general anaesthetic would be the most humane way.

Should the foreskin retract?

At birth the foreskin is usually tightly stuck to the tip of the penis and cannot be pulled back. No attempt should be made to pull it back until the boy is 4, when almost all have foreskins which can be pulled back easily.

VAGINAL DISCHARGE

A vaginal discharge of mucus and some bleeding are quite normal in the newborn due to withdrawal of maternal hormones which were present in the blood before birth. Vaginal bleeding in the older child is commonly due to irritation from threadworm infection.

A frequent cause of intense parental concern, particularly maternal, is a yellowish-green, creamy vaginal discharge which stains the knickers. The discharge is usually not itchy, the only occasional symptom is a burning feeling on urination. The cause is probably a combination of irritation and bacterial infection. Most children I see have already had a few courses of antibiotics with little effect. The most effective treatment is a short course of twice daily applications of oestrogen (0.1% dienoestrol) cream. It thickens the vaginal lining making it more resistant to irritants and infection. The cream should not be used on a regular basis; feminising side-effects may occur from absorption. Irritants can be reduced by not adding anything to the bath water and wearing cotton pants which are well rinsed after washing.

On rare occasions a young child may push a bead or some other small object into the vagina. Suspicion of this may be aroused by the child's having a foul-smelling, bloodstained discharge. It may be necessary to examine her and remove the foreign body under general anaesthetic.

ADHERENT LABIA MINORA

When this happens the lips of the vagina seem fused so that there appears to be no vaginal opening, much to the consternation of the parents. If left the vast majority eventually separate. The level of parental anxiety frequently dictates that something be done. After applications of oestrogen cream (0.1% dienoestrol) for 10–14 days the lips can usually be parted easily. If this is not successful a small probe is used to separate them. Petroleum jelly should then be applied to the edges for a further fortnight to stop them adhering again.

Chapter 9
Enuresis

NOCTURNAL (BED-WETTING)

When writing about bed-wetting it is always worthwhile first to define the normal. Between 1½ and 4½ years about 30–40% of children become dry each year, thereafter about 14% a year. These figures can be expressed another way: at 5, 10% wet their beds; at 10, 5% and at 16, 2%. It is therefore important that both child and parents realise that with time there is a natural tendency for bed-wetting to cease and most paediatricians would not consider treatment before age 5. A number of children wet during the day as well, and the daytime wetting should be treated first. Treating both day and night wetting at the same time is not very effective.

It is rare to find a physical cause for bed-wetting. While most children referred to a paediatrician are examined, this is probably not necessary. A urine test to exclude infection and diabetes may be all that is required. The cause is unknown and is beyond voluntary control. Thus, it goes without saying that punishment has no effect and is indeed cruel. Boys are more commonly affected than girls and there is a strong genetic influence. It is frequent to find that one or both parents were bed-wetters as children. It is also more common in identical than non-identical twins. Although many parents attribute the wetting to deep sleep, scientific evidence shows that wetting is as common in light as in deep sleepers. The vast majority of bed-wetters are psychologically normal. When children have been dry at night for a few months or years before wetting starts again (secondary enuresis) parents invariably seek 'emotional factors' which may have been responsible. In most cases it is not possible to identify such factors.

The treatment of bed-wetting depends on age and frequency. Occasional wet beds, once or twice a month, require no action. After age

7 the treatment of choice is a bed-wetting alarm. Less mature children are not sufficiently motivated and poor co-operation seldom guarantees success.

Between 5–7 best results are achieved by parents' having an encouraging attitude and rewarding success. This is frequently done with star charts. A star is awarded for each dry night and a succession of stars is followed by further reward. Fluid restriction is not necessary and the child should not be put in nappies or plastic pants as they inhibit motivation. The mattress can be protected by a plastic cover and the blankets by a layer of plastic between the top sheet and blankets. Before school the child should be bathed or showered to remove the urine odour and so avoid teasing. 'Lifting' is sometimes very helpful for a child on the verge of becoming dry. This technique consists of making sure that the child empties the bladder before going to bed and lifting him on to a potty or toilet a few hours later. Although not very successful, these methods are worth trying because there is no effective alternative at this age.

After age 7 the enuretic alarm produces a permanent cure in about 70%. This figure can be improved even further by 'overlearning'. The principle of overlearning is that, after dryness has been achieved, the child is encouraged to drink considerable quantities of fluid at bedtime.

The mechanism of all alarms is that the triggering of the alarm when wetting completes a circuit between 2 electrodes. They are all battery operated and perfectly safe and although they are very effective we are not sure why they work. It is probable that the repeated sequential association of full bladder, noise, then awakening eventually means a full bladder will produce awakening without noise. When the alarm rings the child should immediately switch it off and then pass the remaining urine in the toilet or into a potty. Having a night light in the bedroom or corridor is very helpful. With continued use the amount of urine passed before the child wakes becomes progressively smaller and most children are cured in 2–3 months.

There are 3 commonly-used alarms: the double bed mat, single bed mat and 'in pants' detector alarm. The single bed mat is shown in Figure 9/1 and the 'in pants' system is shown in Figure 9/2. The traditional method has been to have the sensors (electrodes) in bed mats, but nowadays many families prefer the sensor in the pants and the 'in pants' detector alarms are very popular, particularly in the United States. To ensure success the correct use of the alarm is vital. Discuss

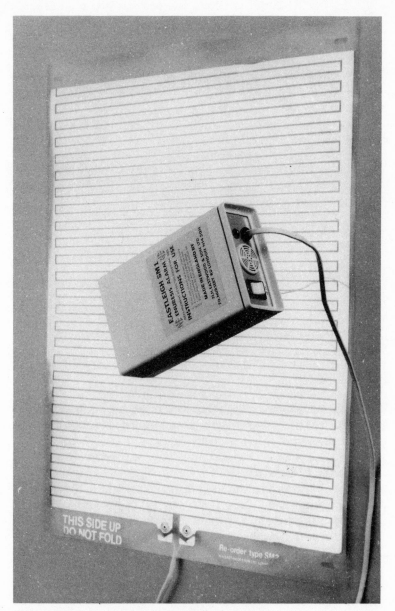

Fig. 9/1 Single mat enuretic alarm. The mat is placed under the top sheet.
The child should sleep without pyjama bottoms

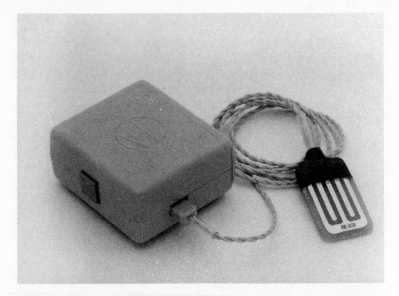

Fig. 9/2 'In pants alarm' available as audible or vibrator version. The alarm is attached to the child's pyjama top and the sensor pad is located in a disposable 'panty liner' in the pants. Immediately the child starts to wet, the alarm emits a pulsating audible tone waking the child. The sensor can be easily dried and re-used, reducing the necessity to make the child's bed every time he wets

the three types with your paediatrician and choose one best suited to your child. When you receive the alarm it should be taken to a clinic so that the paediatrician personally can show you and your child how it should be used. I have seen many failures arise because not enough attention was paid to detail.

At first most parents will need to get up at night to supervise the child when the alarm rings. If the parents' bedroom is far away, a commercially available extension alarm can be plugged into the child's alarm. This will ensure that both mother and child are awakened when the bed is wet. When a child shares a bedroom or is deaf a 'silent awakener' can be used. This device plugs into the alarm and is placed under the pillow. When the alarm is triggered there is no noise but instead the pillow shakes and causes the child to be awakened. An address list of manufacturers/suppliers of enuretic alarms in Britain is shown at the end of this section.

So far very little has been said about drugs. The two most commonly used drugs are imipramine (Tofranil) and amitriptyline (Trypti-
zol). These drugs cause a reduction in the number of wet nights or
complete dryness in about 40% of children. The way they work is uncertain, though it is commonly believed that they reduce bladder sensitivity. The bladder may be less sensitive to stretch so that more
urine can be held before there is emptying. Unfortunately the main
drawback of drug treatment is that when the drug is stopped there is
invariably a relapse. Another serious disadvantage is that the pleasant
tasting medicine has caused severe side-effects and even death
through children taking overdoses. It is for these reasons that many
paediatricians do not prescribe drugs, but they do have a place in the
short-term treatment of bed-wetting. Their effect is immediate,
making them ideal for situations where dryness is required for a week
or two, such as family holidays or school camps. They can also be
used to provide quick proof to the child that it is possible to become
dry.

Recently drug treatment by nasal spray has become established as
an effective and safe alternative to oral treatment (drugs by mouth).
The drug, desmopressin (DDAVP) is sprayed in the nose at bedtime
and has an immediate effect. It is thought that it works by causing the
kidney to secrete a smaller volume of urine. Like other drug treatment it is not a cure: when the treatment stops the child wets the bed
again. It is very much more expensive than oral treatment, but unlike
oral drugs has the major advantage of eliminating the serious risk of
accidental ingestion by younger children.

In conclusion, when we look at bed-wetting closely there is nothing
really bad about it. It is just a temporary inconvenience. Patience and
understanding can keep it from become anything more serious. Even
without treatment all children eventually grow out of it.

Manufacturers/suppliers of enuretic alarms in the UK include:

Astric Products Limited
Astric House, Lewes Road, Brighton BN2 3LG   0273 608319

Connevans Limited, 1 Norbury Road
Reigate, Surrey RH2 9BY   07372 47571

Downs Surgical Limited, Church Path
Mitcham, Surrey CR4 3UE   01–640 3422

N. H. Eastwood & Son Limited
70 Nursery Road, London N14 5QH   01–886 5458

Headingley Scientific Services
45 Westcombe Avenue, Leeds LS8 2BS   0532 664222

Medax Electronics, Derien House
Mount Bovers Lane, Hawkwell
Southend, Essex SS5 4JA   0702 202053

Nottingham Medical Aids Limited
17 Ludlow Hill Road, West Bridgford
Nottingham NG2 6HD   0602 234251

Wessex Medical Equipment Co Limited
Budds Lane, Romsey, Hants SO5 0AH   0794 518246

DIURNAL (DAYTIME WETTING)

Between 3–4 most children have bladder control during the day, but
about 1 in 100 children over 4 wet themselves during the day. Many
children have occasional 'accidents' in the years following toilet training and this is normal, as is the passing of a few drops of urine into the
pants throughout childhood. In general I only recommend treatment
of daytime wetting after age 4 in children who pass large volumes at
frequent intervals. About half the children with daytime wetting also
have night-time wetting (nocturnal enuresis). As part of normal development bladder control during the day is usually established first.
Thus, it seems logical to exploit this natural tendency by treating daytime wetting first. Treating day and night wetting at the same time
seldom gives good results.
    Almost all cases have a non-physical cause. A paediatrician will be
able to exclude a physical cause by the history and examination. No
investigations are required other than perhaps a urine test to rule out
infection. About half the children I see have been dry during the day
for some months or years before wetting starts again. In some there is
an obvious precipitating event such as a change of school, a new
brother or sister, divorce or bereavement. Most parents look for a
cause and may become very agitated when there is nothing obvious,
as often happens.
    In general there are three main causes for daytime wetting; stress,
bladder sensitivity and difficulty associated with toilet training. In

the young child (4–7) the commonest cause is stress. This affects boys and girls equally and in many a precipitating event can be found. These children are often timid and lacking in self-confidence, some having been dry for many months before wetting starts. The commonest cause in the older child (after 7) is bladder sensitivity. This group have very sensitive bladders and the slightest stretch, even with a small amount of urine, causes the muscle to contract and the bladder to empty. The majority are girls and most will never have been dry. In those who have been dry, wetting is frequently precipitated by a urinary infection. Children may need to pass urine frequently and when they get the urge are unable to hold the urine for any length of time. Because these symptoms are also caused by urine infections diagnostic confusion may arise. Persistent daytime wetting following a urine infection is frequently thought to be due to treatment failure or reinfection. By the time these children see a paediatrician, many will have been on repeated courses of antibiotics to no avail.

A third cause of daytime wetting is difficulty with toilet training. Most are boys and parents are often rigid and obsessive. In some there is an abnormal relationship between mother and child. Difficulty with toilet training leads to an emotionally punitive attitude. It is not uncommon to find that children have been physically punished. The child who is constantly reminded of the toilet, punished or has fluids restricted becomes angry and rebellious and deliberately wets himself. Unlike children with other causes of daytime wetting, this group also soil themselves frequently.

When the cause is stress or bladder sensitivity the outlook is very good, most responding to treatment within a few months. Wetting arising from difficulty with toilet training usually takes much longer to resolve. Children and their parents require a lot of time and expert psychological help. Most paediatricians refer this group of children to a child and family psychiatrist or a clinical psychologist. Best results are achieved by giving the child more responsibility and allowing him to decide when he needs to go. Parental attitude needs to be changed. The child should be encouraged but should not be constantly reminded to go or asked if he needs to go.

The principles of management for stress wetting and bladder sensitivity are as follows:

1. Increase fluid intake. The child with daytime wetting needs

plenty of practice at controlling his urine. This requires a large urine output. This is best accomplished by encouraging, but not forcing, your child to drink lots of extra fluids while he is home.

2. Encourage your child to go to the toilet whenever he feels the urge to urinate. He should not try to postpone this urge. If in doubt, he should go earlier rather than later, but he should not be reminded to go excessively or made to sit on the toilet against his will because these actions will foster a negative attitude about the whole process.

3. Practice stream interruption exercises. Your child needs better control over his bladder sphincter (the valve that holds the urine in and lets the urine out of the bladder). Once sitting safely on the toilet, help your child to relax and count slowly to 10. Then have him urinate but stop his urine flow when his bladder is only half-emptied. After counting to 10 again he can proceed to empty it completely. This should be done every time your child urinates, and gradually increase the interval by counting to a higher number. This simple exercise will help your child learn to suppress bladder contractions and is essential in overcoming this problem.

4. Reward child for being dry. If your child is dry, he needs to be rewarded. This includes plenty of praise, smiles, hugs and kisses. For the child who is wet several times a day, he should be rewarded every time he successfully urinates into the toilet. For the child who wets on some days but not others, this recognition and celebration should occur whenever he is dry for a complete day.

6. Respond gently to accidents by:
   a. Changing his clothes. Do not ignore wet clothes. As soon as your child is noted to be wet by odour or appearance, remind him to change himself immediately into dry clothing. The main role you have in this programme is to enforce the rule, 'You cannot walk around wet'. Encourage your child to change himself before anyone else notices the wetness, but do not expect your child to confess to being wet.
   b. Establishing a routine for handling wet clothes. Rinse these out in the sink until the odour is gone, hang them somewhere to dry, then store them until the next washday. Get your child to do this, but he will need supervision until he is 7 or 8.
   c. Avoiding punishment. Your child should not be blamed, criticised or punished. In addition, brothers and sisters should not

be allowed to tease him. Your child should never be put back into nappies.

6. Ask for the school's co-operation (only for children who wet in school). These children need ready access to the toilet, especially if they are shy and new at school. If the problem is significant, you might also temporarily supply the school with an extra set of dry clothing. If there is teasing at school, you may wish to discuss this problem with your child's teacher.

7. Help with record keeping. The paediatrician will give your child a record book to keep. Bring this to all clinic visits. This record should be kept until your child has gone two weeks without any accidents.

Do drugs which are used for bed-wetting help daytime wetting?
There is no evidence that drugs are of any use in daytime wetting.

Chapter 10
Heart and Chest Problems

COMMON HEART MURMURS

There are three heart murmurs commonly heard in children. These
are the 'innocent' murmur, the murmur of ventricular septal defect
(VSD) and the murmur of a patent ductus. On learning their child
has a murmur many parents become very anxious and immediately
think about heart surgery. Most children with these common murmurs do not have symptoms and grow normally; surgery is indeed
unusual.

The innocent heart murmur

What is a heart murmur?
   It is a noise heard with a stethoscope in that part of the chest over
the heart.

When is a heart murmur innocent?
   When a noise is heard in a *normal* heart the murmur is said to be
innocent. Other commonly used names for an innocent murmur are
'functional', 'physiologic', or 'insignificant'.

How common are innocent murmurs?
   They are very common, affecting at least 30–40% of school children.

What causes the noise?
   The noise is probably caused by a variety of mechanical factors.
The rapid flow of blood through the heart produces a noise in the
same way as rapidly flowing water in a stream.

182

How does the paediatrician know the heart is normal?

This can be established by carefully examining the child. Innocent murmurs have certain common features: they are soft, short noises which are heard only in a small area of the chest. They may become very loud when the heart speeds up, as during fever, exercise and nervousness. Their loudness is also affected by the position of the child (standing or lying).

Are any investigations required?

Innocent murmurs are diagnosed by listening to the heart and it is seldom that a heart trace (ECG) or chest x-ray are required.

Will the murmur go?

With time the chest wall thickens and they are no longer heard, however, some do persist into adult life. The fact that some persist does not signify any heart abnormality.

What action should be taken?

None, the child has a *normal* heart and can take part in all physical activities and no special precautions are required during dental extractions.

Should the heart murmur be checked again?

No. Very occasionally a paediatrician may have difficulty in deciding whether a murmur is innocent, in which case follow up visits are required until the situation is resolved.

Ventricular septal defect (VSD)

The two main pumping chambers of the heart are called ventricles. The ventricles are separated from each other by a common wall known as a septum. When there is a hole in the wall the child is said to have a ventricular septal defect.

It is the commonest heart abnormality, accounting for 30–50% of all heart abnormalities. About 3–5/1000 children are born with a VSD; 50–75% eventually close, most closing within a year or two. Generally the smallest holes have the best chance of closure but many large holes also close.

Some murmurs may be heard immediately after birth, most are heard between 2–6 weeks. Whether the child has symptoms depends on the age of the child and the size of the hole. *At all ages* the child with a *small hole* has no symptoms and grows normally. Most of these murmurs are detected at a post-natal examination or incidentally during some other illness or at a routine examination such as a school medical.

In those with a *big hole* who develop symptoms *before 2* most occur between 2–6 months. The following are the most frequent symptoms: (1) slow feeding, (2) poor weight gain, (3) breathing difficulty, (4) profuse sweating, (5) swelling of hands and feet. *After 2* there are few symptoms although repeated chest infections may occur.

What causes the hole?
We do not know, it is something that just happens. It does *not* seem to be caused by drugs or infections during the pregnancy.

Why does it matter if the heart has a hole?
There are 3 main reasons:

1. The hole causes the pumping chambers to function less efficiently, placing a greater strain on them.
2. Blood is pumped through the hole into the lung. The extra blood in the lung causes a high pressure which may result in lung damage.
3. Bacteria may enter the blood and settle around the edge of the hole and then spread to the rest of the body making the child very ill.

What investigations may be done?
1. Chest x-ray – this may show whether the heart is being strained and gives a rough idea of how much extra blood is going through the lungs.
2. Electrocardiograph (ECG) – this is a heart trace which not only shows heart strain but also shows which pumping chamber is having most difficulty.

Which children should be referred to a specialist paediatric heart centre?
Despite initial improvement a *few* children with *large* holes develop lung damage which is permanent if the hole is not closed before age 2. It is usually very difficult to know which children are at risk of permanent lung damage without performing highly specialised tests. For this reason it is most important that *all children with symptoms* in the first 2 years should be referred to a paediatric cardiologist, a children's doctor specialising in heart disease. Similarly, children over 2 with symptoms or when the diagnosis is uncertain should also be referred.

What tests are done at the paediatric cardiology (heart) centre?
The common tests are:

1. Echocardiogram – by passing sound waves through the chest a picture of the heart is formed. This not only confirms the diagnosis but may also show the size of the hole.
2. Cardiac catheterisation – the child is anaesthetised and a fine tube (catheter) is passed along a big blood vessel into the heart and lung where pressures are measured. Measurement of pressure in the lung is the best method of assessing the risk of lung damage. Some children require cardiac catheterisation to be performed on more than one occasion.

How should a child with a VSD be managed?
The child *with no symptoms* requires no treatment and should continue to be reviewed at 1–2 yearly intervals. Antibiotic cover should be given before surgical procedures such as dental extraction and tonsillectomy.

The child *with symptoms* may require drug treatment. The two commonly used drugs are digoxin and frusemide. Digoxin strengthens the heart beat and frusemide takes strain off the heart by removing body fluid. Antibiotics should be used before surgical procedures listed above and chest infections should be treated vigorously. Follow-up visits are more frequent (3–6 monthly). If the symptoms are very severe or if there is a risk of lung damage the hole is closed surgically with a patch. Should an operation be required the time varies from one child to another and this information can be obtained from the paediatric cardiologist.

Why should the child with a small hole continue to be followed?
There are 2 reasons:

1. If and when the hole closes the child or parents should be told so that antibiotic cover before dental extractions need not be taken.
2. Very rarely blood flowing through the hole will interfere with the function of a heart valve (aortic valve) and this will be detected.

How long before dental extractions should antibiotics be given?
A letter or card will be given to you by the paediatrician. This should be given to the child's dentist who will advise you. A cardboard advice sheet entitled 'Dental advice for children with heart problems' which I use in my hospital is shown in Figure 10/1. Insert-

DISTRICT HEALTH AUTHORITY

Dental advice for children with heart problems

1. Keep your child's teeth free from decay.

a) FLUORIDE

It is now well known that dental decay can be much reduced by the use of fluoride. Cleaning the teeth well using fluoride toothpaste will help, but dental decay can be further reduced by giving fluoride tablets or drops regularly. You can get these on the NHS from your family doctor – or buy them from the chemist. Make sure you give the correct dose. This depends on the age of your child, and whether there is fluoride in the tap water. *In areas where there is no fluoride in the water,* we suggest the dose as follows:-

Children from birth to 2 years	0.25 mg fluoride ion per day
Children from 2-4 years	0.5 mg fluoride ion per day
Children from 4-13 years	1.0 mg fluoride ion per day

(2.2 mg of sodium fluoride = 1 mg fluoride ion)

Your doctor, dentist or chemist will give further advice on this if needed.

The dentist can also reduce decay by painting the teeth with fluoride twice a year, and by putting a plastic coating onto the back teeth. These forms of treatment can be arranged free of charge through the Community Dental Service.

b) SUGAR IN THE DIET

Do please restrict sweet snacks and fruit cordials to meal times only. Give your child savoury snacks, if necessary, between meals, e.g. cheese, fruit, milk. Use a low calorie fruit drink. Clean teeth well after syrupy medicine.

TO WHOM IT MAY CONCERN

Your patient

This child has a heart problem. It is essential that he/she has antibiotic cover to prevent infective endocarditis before dental treatment involving breach of the gingiva, removal of tonsils or adenoids, and any procedure involving the upper respiratory tract.

When general anaesthesia is NOT required

Give amoxycillin 3g orally one hour before treatment. The dose is halved for children under 10 years.

If general anaesthetic is required

The patient should be referred to hospital and amoxycillin given by INTRAVENOUS injection immediately after the anaesthetic has been given.

IMPORTANT: Please see overleaf

2. In the event of dental treatment or tonsillectomy please show the special card above to the practitioner giving the treatment.

Produced by the Colgate Professional Dental Service in the service of preventive dentistry.
Colgate-Palmolive Limited. Colgate-Palmolive House, 76 Oxford Street, London W1A 1EN

Fig. 10/1 Dental health advice for children with heart problems (courtesy Colgate-Palmolive Ltd)

ed into the cardboard is a plastic 'credit card' which parents are advised to show the child's dentist. The fluoride supplementation schedule in the USA is different and is shown in Table 10/1.

Table 10/1   Fluoride supplementation schedule for children in the USA. Values are milligrams (mg) of fluoride supplement per day

Age (yr)	Fluoride concentration in local water supply (ppm)		
	<0.3	0.3–0.7	>0.7
0–2	0.25	0	0
2–3	0.50	0.25	0
3–16	1.00	0.50	0

Should activity be restricted?

A child who has no symptoms and is growing normally should partake in *all* childhood activities. Children with symptoms, by the nature of their symptoms, may need to restrict their activity.

What about school?

Almost all children with heart disease are able to attend normal schools.

What is the risk of a VSD in the next child?

The risk in the next child is very small, about 1 in 25. If two children have a VSD the risk rises to 1 in 12.

What about the future?

The outlook is excellent for children with small holes even if they fail to close. They can all expect to have a normal life expectancy. The outlook for children with large holes varies considerably and should be discussed with the paediatric cardiologist who performed the child's tests.

Patent ductus

What is a patent duct?

Before birth fetal lungs are collapsed, the fetus obtaining its oxygen from the placenta (afterbirth). Blood that is pumped from the heart to the lungs is normally diverted away from the lungs to the rest of the body by a vessel called the ductus arteriosus. After birth when the lungs expand the increased oxygen in the blood acts as a signal to the ductus to close so that blood from the heart passes to the lung for oxygenation. In some full-term babies (about 1 in 2500–5000) the duct is abnormal and fails to close, hence the terms patent ductus or persistent ductus. When the duct remains open the direction of blood flow reverses so that instead of being diverted away from the lungs as before birth the blood now enters the lung. If the flow is large, the lung may become congested. The fact that the duct normally closes at 40 weeks (full term) means that large numbers of premature infants have patent ducts, these ducts being open due to immaturity rather than defects. Unlike the full-term infant where the duct remains open permanently, the duct of the premature infant may close at any time in the first 2–3 months.

How does the patent duct present?

This depends on how much blood passes through the duct and the age of the child. When the flow is small the child is usually perfectly well, the duct is detected incidentally by hearing a murmur below the left collar bone (clavicle). When there is a large flow in infancy the extra blood in the lung may make the child breathless. He may have difficulty with feeding, a rapid heart rate, enlarged liver and swelling of the limbs. These children may fail to thrive and the lung congestion predisposes them to repeated chest infections. In sick premature infants with respiratory distress, particularly those given a lot of fluid, the size of the flow through the duct may be considerable so that they are very ill; their patent ducts need prompt attention.

Why is it necessary to treat a patent duct?

If symptoms are present the need for treatment is obvious. In the premature infant with no symptoms treatment is not required as spontaneous closure is likely to occur. Treatment for the symptomless older child is required for the following reasons:

1. Bacteria may become lodged in the duct forming small infected clots which then spread to the rest of the body. This is a serious complication.
2. In the third or fourth decade breathlessness and other symptoms which were not present in infancy may develop.
3. Rarely lung damage will occur so that blood flow to the lung will

be severely impaired causing a blue colour (cyanosis) from lack of oxygen.

What tests are needed?

Few tests are required, the diagnosis and need for surgery are usually decided on the basis of the clinical findings and history. Tests that may be done are a chest x-ray, ECG and echocardiogram. Cardiac catheterisation is seldom required.

What is the treatment?

A small operation is performed; the chest is opened and the vessel tied. With the exception of premature infants the operation is usually done shortly after the diagnosis is made. In premature infants fluid restriction and giving a drug, indomethacin, in the first days after birth may cause the duct to close, so avoiding an operation.

What is the outlook?

The effect of ductal closure on symptoms is usually dramatic, the child's condition often improves within hours. The long-term outlook is excellent, these children should be perfectly normal in every way and have a normal life expectancy. Antibiotic treatment with dental extractions is not necessary after ductal closure.

ASTHMA

Asthma affects about 1 in 10 children at some time. It is a condition affecting the airways of the lung (Fig. 10/2). The air tubes of the lung (bronchi) are over-sensitive and react readily to various provoking factors by going into spasm (narrowing), and secreting excessive amounts of mucus causing obstruction. (Fig. 10/3). The impaired movements of air through the lung gives rise to the most obvious sign of asthma, wheezing. Because the airways are narrower when breathing out than breathing in, the wheeze is most obvious on breathing out.

Children with asthma have repeated attacks of wheezing, cough or difficulty in breathing out. When there is severe spasm the difficulty may be so great that it is hard to move air, so no wheeze is heard but the chest feels very 'tight'. Between attacks the chest may be quite normal or there may be a persistent cough which is usually worse at night.

Childhood asthma has a wide range of severity, ranging from oc-

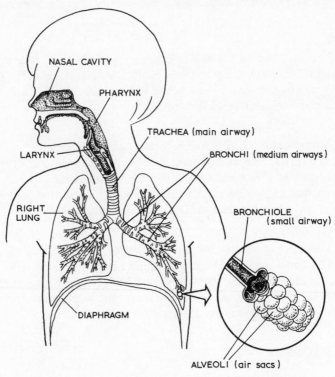

Fig. 10/2 Anatomy of the lungs and airways (bronchi)

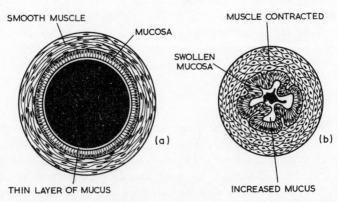

Fig. 10/3 Cross-section of a bronchial tube showing what happens in an asthmatic attack

casional mild attacks of wheezing that do not require treatment to the uncommon severe form, when attacks are frequent and the child does not grow as well as he should. Treatment will depend on the severity and your family doctor or paediatrician will make sure your child receives the appropriate treatment. Early, effective treatment results in normal growth and the small chance of a chest deformity is very unlikely. The very effective treatment now available has made interference with school or other activities a thing of the past.

What causes asthma?

There are many causes of asthma. The vast majority of asthmatic children have demonstrable allergies and there is no doubt that these allergies play the major role in producing symptoms. Allergy to the excreta of house dust mite is the most common. These mites are so small you cannot see them without a microscope and they live everywhere in the house but are most common in the bedroom. They feed on shed skin scales of the human and thrive in damp surroundings.

Other substances producing an allergic reaction are house dust, feathers, animal dandruff or fur. Like house dust mite these commonly produce symptoms all year round. Seasonal asthma is most commonly caused by pollen and moulds. Moulds are members of the fungus family. Unlike mushrooms and toadstools they grow on a relatively small scale producing colonies of growth, often just a few millimetres across, on decaying vegetation and damp walls. They spread by producing spores which are released into the atmosphere and when inhaled cause asthma.

Pollen is transferred from one plant to another in a variety of ways, by birds, bees, insects, sometimes by water and by wind. Flowers which are highly coloured and have a strong smell are insect pollinated. Their pollen is not windborne, so it does not usually cause problems. However, if you sniff a bunch of flowers it may bring on an attack.

It is the lighter pollen of grasses, trees and weeds blown by the wind which more commonly cause symptoms. Mould spores too are blown about by the wind. These different plants all produce pollen at different times of the year. So, if you are allergic to tree pollens, your symptoms could start as early as March. If you are allergic to moulds it may not end until October. Grass pollen, the main cause of seasonal asthma, is in the air during June and July but the date of its highest concentration varies throughout the country. In London the peak is usually during the third week in June, in Liverpool and Glasgow a week or two later.

Heavy, prolonged rainfall before the pollen season starts encourages lush plant growth and the production of pollen. And, as pollen is distributed by the wind, high winds during the pollen season can lead to a higher incidence of asthma especially if there are long dry spells. On the other hand, heavy rainfall during the season helps prevent the release of pollen and washes it from the air. For these reasons, symptoms can be worse on some days than on others. Generally asthma will be at its worst on hot, dry, windy days and better on cloudy or rainy days. Pollen released in the morning is carried high in the air around the middle of the day, only to descend again late in the afternoon. Consequently the highest pollen counts occur around mid-morning and late afternoon, although, in large towns where it stays hotter longer, the pollen count can stay high well into the evening.

Most children with asthma are allergic to a variety of substances rather than one. When exposed to these substances the tendency to an attack of asthma varies from time to time, depending on whether 'non-allergic factors' are also present, the greater the number the more likely the attack. The common non-allergic factors are:

virus infections (colds, coughs, sore throats)
emotion (excitement or upset)
cold air or atmosphere pollution
exercise.

For example a child who is allergic to cat fur may start to wheeze when he is upset and yet when he is not upset he can meet the same cat and have no wheezing.

Food allergy in asthma is very uncommon and when it does occur there is usually a rash or some other allergic symptom. Asthma is much more likely to be due to something inhaled into the lungs rather than something swallowed. From the above description of the causes of asthma it should be evident that the environment, whether it be stress, a particular house or climate, all have a profound effect on the number of attacks.

Is asthma hereditary?

The tendency to asthma seems to be inherited to a large extent. Children with asthma frequently have a parent or sibling who have had asthma, hay fever or eczema.

How early in life can asthma be diagnosed?

It is often possible to diagnose asthma within the first months of life. Most children with asthma have their first attack by the age of 5 years. In the past the diagnosis was frequently delayed because it was not widely appreciated by family doctors that the predominant symptom in young children may often be coughing and not wheezing.

How is asthma diagnosed?

The diagnosis is based almost entirely on the history. The diagnosis can sometimes be confirmed by breathing tests. These involve getting the child to blow hard into a meter called a peak flow meter (Fig. 10/4). The force of the blow is then compared with the values obtained from the normal child population. Children with asthma, particularly when severe, may not be able to blow as hard as normal children. A chest x-ray is seldom of help in the diagnosis of asthma.

What about allergy tests?

Allergy tests do not diagnose asthma. There are two types of allergy test – of skin and blood. Although slightly less accurate and expensive, blood tests are more convenient. About 80% of asthmatic children are allergic to one or more of the substances previously

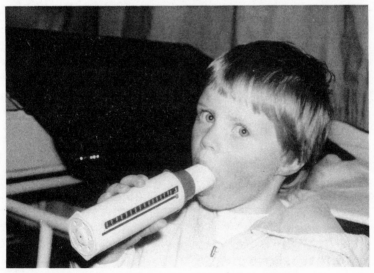

Fig. 10/4 Blowing into a peak flow meter

listed. About 20% of the normal population also give positive results (false positives). The information gained from allergy tests is of little benefit in the practical management of asthma and these tests are seldom necessary.

Do children grow out of asthma?

About half the children with asthma grow out of it. There is no magic age at which this happens and it is not possible to predict which children will grow out of it. Of the half that do not grow out of it a large proportion will be free of attacks during adolescence and early adult life before the asthma comes back.

How is asthma treated?

The most effective way of relieving symptoms or preventing attacks is by treatment with drugs. Treatment taken only when there are symptoms is referred to as 'symptomatic treatment' and treatment taken regularly (even if the child is well) is called 'preventive treatment'. Both treatments are frequently used in the same patient and this way even the most severe asthmatic can lead a normal life. The need for preventive treatment is best assessed by the parents or child after a discussion with the doctor. Remember, the doctor can advise on treatment but you know the child far better than he does.

The drugs commonly used for asthma treatment are listed below:

SYMPTOMATIC TREATMENT

Except for ipratropium these drugs are all similar and can be given by inhalation. Salbutamol or terbutaline can also be given by sugar-free syrup, tablets or slow-release tablets. Ipratropium is free of side-effects while the other drugs very rarely cause a rise in heart rate or muscle tremors. Both effects are harmless and cease with a reduction in dose.

Approved Name	*Trade Name*
salbutamol (albuterol, USA)	Ventolin; Salbulin
terbutaline	Bricanyl
fenoterol	Berotec
ipratropium	Atrovent

PREVENTIVE TREATMENT

These drugs have different actions and it is quite common to take more than one at a time. They are usually grouped in 3 categories: 1. theophyllines; 2. sodium cromoglycate; 3. steroids.

1. Theophyllines – there are many available, all given by mouth. The slow-release tablets or beads are best. Not only are they more convenient but are more effective and have fewer side-effects than the liquid preparations. When the beads are given with a 'bribe' such as ice cream, jam or fruit yoghurt, most young children will take them. Slow-release preparations should not be chewed. To determine the correct dose a blood test may be required. Do not alter the dose without medical advice. Some children experience a feeling of nausea when starting this treatment, this usually goes after a few days and may be helped by taking the treatment with meals. Side-effects such as headache, nausea, vomiting and bed-wetting are uncommon if the dose is carefully adjusted.

Approved Name	Trade Name
aminophylline	Phyllocontin
theophylline	Slophyllin

2. Sodium cromoglycate – this drug can only be given by inhalation, as a powder or aerosol. To be effective it must be given *at least* 3 or 4 times daily. It has been used for many years and has no side-effects.

Approved Name	Trade Name
sodium cromoglycate	Intal

3. Steroids – these may be taken by inhalation or mouth. Inhaled steroids are now widely used because it has been shown that they are very effective and have no serious side-effects. Oral steroids have side-effects when taken for a long time, the most serious being slowing of growth. Side-effects can be minimised by taking the tablets first thing in the morning on alternate days. Children taking oral steroids should follow the doctor's advice accurately and these tablets should never be stopped suddenly without medical advice. Oral steroids are prescribed as prednisolone or prednisone. There are two commonly used inhaled steroids:

Approved Name	Trade Name
beclomethasone dipropionate	Becotide
budesonide	Pulmicort

Minor side-effects of inhaled steroids are rare and include thrush (a fungal infection) at the back of the throat, and hoarseness.

How do asthma drugs work?

A simplified scheme is shown in Figure 10/5. The bronchial muscle has muscle cells and nerve cells. Present in these cells are chemical substances which cause the muscle to constrict or dilate thereby opening and closing the airway. During health these chemicals are formed and broken down at a similar rate to maintain balance and keep the airway open. The main dilator chemical in muscle cells is cyclic AMP, the main constrictor chemical in nerve cells being cyclic GMP.

Drugs which cause bronchodilation by stimulating an enzyme (adenyl cyclase) to produce an increased amount of cyclic AMP are known as sympathomimetic drugs or B_2 agonist. Examples of this type of drug are salbutamol, terbutaline, fenoterol and rimiterol. Drugs which cause a rise in the amount of cyclic AMP by inhibiting the enzyme (phosphodiesterase) which normally breaks it down are called xanthines. Examples of xanthines are aminophylline and theophylline.

Drugs which cause bronchodilation by inhibiting an enzyme (guanyl cyclase) to cause a reduction in the cyclic GMP are known as anticholinergics. An example is ipratropium.

Throughout the lining (mucosa) of the lungs, nose and eyes there are cells called mast cells. In the lung whenever an allergic substance such as pollen comes in contact with the mucosa the mast cells release histamine and other substances which cause the bronchial muscle to constrict. Sodium cromoglycate is a mast cell stabiliser, this means that it prevents mast cell release of these substances and in turn prevents airway narrowing. Interestingly, antihistamine drugs do not help asthma, but are of considerable benefit for allergy of the nose and eye; the reason is not clear.

Steroids take longer to work than other asthma drugs and the way they act is not known for certain. It is thought that by reducing inflammation in the bronchi they diminish mucus production and the chance of airway obstruction. By facilitating the production of cyclic AMP they seem to improve the response of the bronchial muscle to sympathomimetic drugs.

How should drugs be given – by mouth or inhalation?

If it is possible for the drug to be inhaled then this is the method of choice. It works quicker, has fewer side-effects and is more effective at only a fraction of the oral dose.

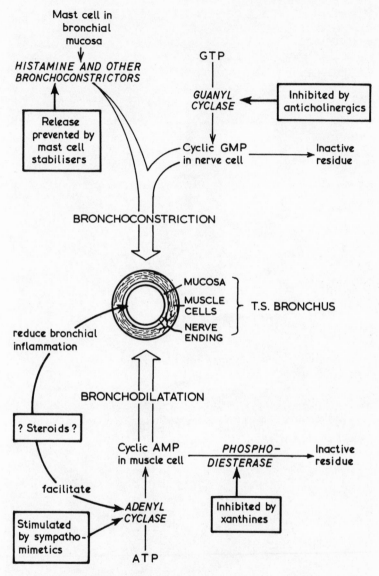

Fig. 10/5 Scheme showing how asthma drugs work. TS = transverse section (cut); GTP = guanosine triphosphate; GMP = guanosine monophosphate; ATP = adenosine triphosphate; AMP = adenosine monophosphate

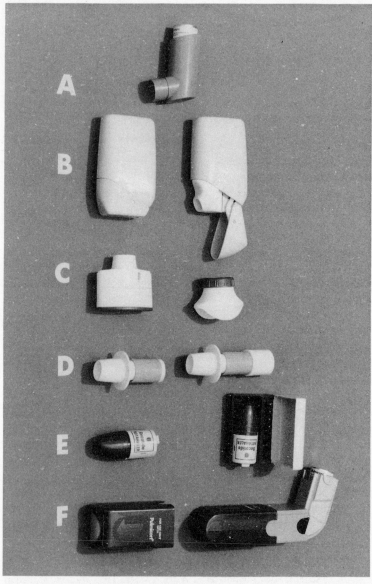

Fig. 10/6 Types of inhalers. A. Aerosol inhaler; B. Breath-actuated inhaler (Autohaler); C. Halermatic; D. Spinhaler and Spinhaler with whistle; E. Rotahaler; F. Spacer

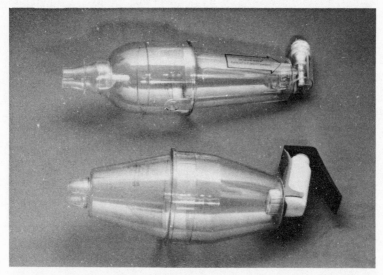

Fig. 10/7 *Upper*: Nebuhaler. *Lower*: Volumatic with a Haleraid attachment

Most children under 7 are unable to use the conventional aerosol (spray) properly and alternative methods of giving drugs by inhalation have been developed. The choice of device is dictated by the preference of the child and his ability to use it. Unfortunately, all the drugs cannot be given with the same device. Your doctor should be able to demonstrate each device and he will tell you which drugs can be used in each.

The inhalation devices currently available, together with the manufacturer, are shown below. Figures 10/6 and 10/7 illustrate some of the devices.

Rotahaler, Volumatic	– Allen and Hanburys Limited
Spinhaler, Halermatic	– Fisons Limited
Spacer, Nebuhaler	– Astra Pharmaceuticals Limited
Autohaler	– Riker Laboratores Limited (a new breath-actuated inhaler is due for licence in Britain in 1987)

Most children by age 3 can be trained to use any of these devices. Below 3 the most effective way of administering asthmatic drugs is by nebuliser. Nebulisers are small chambers which convert a liquid into a fine mist. They need a supply of air under pressure which usually comes from an electric compressor pump (Fig. 10/8) or can be mechanically operated by a foot pump. Unfortunately, nebuliser/compressor units are not available on the NHS and the alternative oral treatment is suitable only for mild, infrequent attacks.

How should inhalers be used?

Space does not permit me to give a detailed explanation of how the various inhalers should be used. There are many thousands of children whose asthma is not helped despite the use of very effective and expensive drugs, the reason being faulty inhaler technique. My advice would be not only to read the package inserts very carefully but also ask your doctor or a physiotherapist to observe your child using the inhaler.

Can the dose of symptomatic treatment be increased if necessary?

Advice about doing this should be obtained from the child's

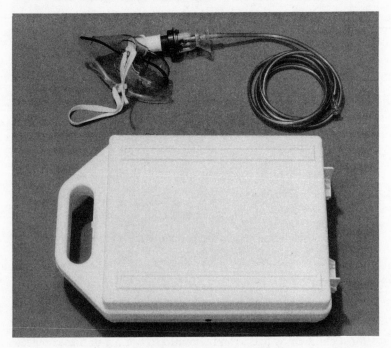

Fig. 10/8 Portable electric nebuliser unit

doctor. In general the worse the symptoms the poorer the response to treatment and the shorter its effect. Most doctors would recommend bigger inhaled doses and more frequently when the symptoms are very distressing. A gap of a few minutes between inhalations is also more effective than the usual regimen of inhalations in quick succession. The important point about increasing inhaled symptomatic treatment is: should there be no response or if the child is worse after 30 minutes then *urgent* medical advice should be sought.

During an attack when should the doctor be called?

If your child has not responded to the medication that has been prescribed then your doctor should be consulted. After you have helped your child through several attacks you will become a good judge of his condition and will know when to summon help.

How is asthma treated in hospital?

The only treatment given to the vast majority is 'symptomatic' treatment by nebuliser. Occasionally other drugs such as intravenous aminophylline and steroids (intravenous or oral) are also used.

Is it necessary to keep a record of the child's symptoms?

This is not always necessary but can at times be very helpful to the doctor in deciding the most appropriate treatment. Many parents like to keep a record as it enables them to make an objective assessment of the child's condition from time to time. In order to monitor the child's asthma carefully your doctor may give you a peak flow meter and a symptom diary card (Fig. 10/9).

What about trying to avoid allergic substances?

As mentioned earlier the mainstay of asthma treatment is with drugs. Measures to reduce exposure to allergic substances, even when assiduously carried out, are in the main ineffective. Nevertheless, simple measures may be worth trying provided they do not become an obsession and are inexpensive. Here is some simple advice which can be carried out in the home:

1. The bed – the mattress probably has thousands of mites in it at present! Make a cover from building grade polythene secured with plastic carpet tape obtainable from any large hardware store. Leave an end open to allow the mattress to ventilate. Vacuum the mattress before you fit the cover and remove about once a month and repeat. Damp dust the mattress cover weekly in between. This removes

Date this card was started:			1	2	3	4	5	6	7	8	9	10	11	12	13	14	15	16	17	18	19	20	21	22	23	24	25	26	27	28	29	30	31
1. WHEEZE LAST NIGHT	Good night	0																															
	Slept well but slightly wheezy	1																															
	Woke x 2-3 because of wheeze	2																															
	Bad night, awake most of time	3																															
2. COUGH LAST NIGHT	None	0																															
	Little	1																															
	Moderately bad	2																															
	Severe	3																															
3. WHEEZE TODAY	None	0																															
	Little	1																															
	Moderately bad	2																															
	Severe	3																															
4. ACTIVITY TODAY	Quite normal	0																															
	Can only run short distance	1																															
	Limited to walking because of chest	2																															
	Too breathless to walk	3																															
5. NASAL SYMPTOMS	None	0																															
	Mild	1																															
	Moderate	2																															
	Severe	3																															
6. METER Best of 3 blows	Before breakfast Medicines																																
	Before bedtime Medicines																																
7. DRUGS	Name of Drug	Dose Prescribed																															
Number of doses actually taken during the past 24 hours.																																	
8. COMMENTS	Note if you see a Doctor (D) or stay away from school (S) or work (W) because of your chest and anything else important such as an infection (I).																																

Fig. 10/9 A symptom diary card

mites and the skin scales which provide their food. Get rid of feather pillows and replace with a foam type.

Old-fashioned eiderdowns and duvets filled with feathers can cause problems and should be disposed of. Duvets filled with synthetic materials are satisfactory. Do not use nylon sheets – they carry a static electric charge and attract dust to them. Cotton cellular blankets are best, although difficult to obtain, all blankets should be washed and aired frequently. If a child is sharing a bedroom all other beds should have similar treatment. An asthmatic child should not sleep in the bottom bunk of a bunk bed.

2. The bedroom – children with asthma usually improve in hospital as wards are designed to minimise dust traps. Arrange the bedroom to be without dust traps as far as possible. Keep furnishings as light and simple as you can. Soft toys such as teddy bears contain numerous mites and should be removed from the bedroom. During the summer keep bedroom windows closed during the day and early evening so that pollen is not blown into the bedroom.

3. The rest of the house – damp dust and vacuum clean. Make sure the child is not around when you brush carpets and furniture. Empty the vacuum-cleaner bag frequently and check that the cleaner is working properly.

What about exercise?

Asthmatic children should take as much exercise as they can. Different exercises bring on varying amounts of wheeze or coughing; steady running brings on a lot and swimming much less. Help your child find a sport he enjoys and then give him encouragement. If you find exercise makes his asthma much worse and he is constantly needing to stop for a 'breather' then he should be given 'symptomatic' treatment a few minutes *before* exercise. If wheezing with exercise is severe and the child's activities are constantly restricted then, in addition, theophyllines or Intal should also be given on a *regular* basis to prevent symptoms.

What about pets?

While there are a few children who benefit from removal of a pet, the majority do not. Unless it is very obvious that the child is allergic to the animal there is no certain way of knowing whether removal will make any difference. A trial removal from the home would need to be for a few months if it were to yield any useful information. This is not desirable because of the emotional effect on the child. Having pets is part of growing up and in general I would not recommend removal of a pet unless the allergy was obvious or tests showed animal allergy only. For example, if within minutes of stroking a cat the child started to wheeze, and this happened repeatedly, then removal of the cat would be advised. In most asthmatics animal allergy is only one of many allergies and any decision to remove a pet should first be discussed with your doctor.

Can repeated severe asthma attacks or prolonged coughing cause heart or lung damage?

Heart 'strain' or lung damage never occur. Occasionally young children, particularly those with frequent and troublesome attacks, may develop some chest deformity. This often takes the form of a prominence of the upper part of the chest and broad grooves over the sides of the chest with flaring of the rib ends, which tend to stick out. The chest deformity usually becomes less obvious as the child gets older and the bones strengthen. Even severe abnormalities will improve or disappear if the asthma subsides or becomes less severe.

Do children die of asthma?

Yes, but it is very rare. The risk of dying from an asthmatic attack is considerably less than from road accidents.

What should the school be told?

Because asthma is a common condition most teachers are familiar with it and can be very helpful. The school should be informed of the problem and should be told that the child is able to take part in sport and all other school activities. Medication should be left at school and you should explain to the staff exactly how the treatment should be taken in the event of an attack or before physical education, if treatment is necessary.

Does physiotherapy help?

Physiotherapy does not help, but a visit to a physiotherapist may be useful. During an attack parents need to remain calm and confident. The physiotherapist will help you with this. She will teach your child breathing exercises that help him relax during the attack). She will also show you the best position in which he should sit or lie (Fig. 10/10). Checking or teaching inhaler technique is also part of the physiotherapist's job. Most asthma treatment does not work during the first year of life. During this difficult period a physiotherapist may play an important supportive role to the family.

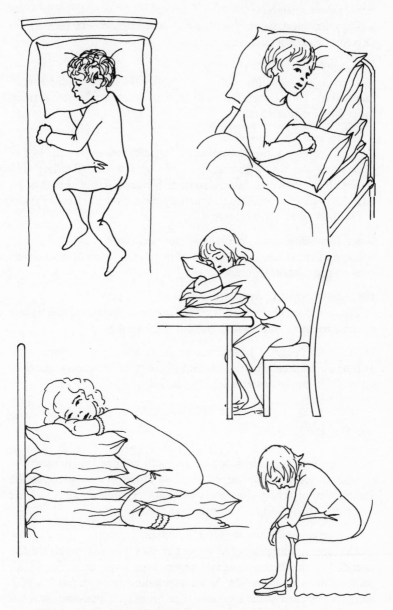

Fig. 10/10 Suitable positions into which to place a breathless child. The position should be selected to suit the individual child

Are antibiotics helpful?

They are *not*. Attacks of asthma are caused by viruses which are not affected by antibiotics.

Do cough mixtures help?

There is no place for the use of cough mixtures in asthma treatment. If the child coughs he needs 'proper' treatment, which is treatment with asthma drugs.

What about desensitisation?

Small, repeated injections of the allergic substance is a method of preventing attacks by getting the body used to the offending substance. It is known as desensitisation. Because most asthmatics are allergic to many substances this method is relatively ineffective and is not without risks. It is seldom used.

What about humidifiers, ionisers and dust extractors?

None of these has any proven use in asthma. In fact, humidifiers may do more harm than good.

What about hypnosis, acupuncture or homoeopathy?

These methods have been tried but are not effective. If you try any of these methods you should let your doctor know.

In these few pages I have listed most of the salient points about asthma in children. Should you require more information this can be obtained from the Asthma Society (p. 351).

BRONCHIOLITIS

In Britain bronchiolitis is one of the main reasons for admission of children to hospital during winter. The illness is widespread in the community affecting thousands of children; only a small number (probably about 5%) are admitted to hospital.

What happens to the lung during bronchiolitis?

The lung is comprised of tubes and air sacs (alveoli), which are surrounded by fine blood vessels. During inspiration (breathing in) air passes down the tubes into the air sacs where gas is exchanged with blood in the surrounding vessels. The bronchioles are narrow tubes which connect the wide tubes (bronchi) with air sacs (Fig. 10/2).

In bronchiolitis the lining (mucosa) of the bronchioles becomes inflamed and swollen and produces thick mucus. The obstruction caused by the swelling and mucus has two effects:

1. The diameter of the airways is normally reduced on expiration (breathing out). In bronchiolitis expiratory narrowing together with airway obstruction has the effect of producing a 'ball valve'; air entering the lung cannot be expelled, consequently trapped air causes the lung to be inflated like a balloon.
2. When the obstruction is severe enough no air can pass through the bronchioles, the air remaining in the air sacs is absorbed and the air sacs collapse.

The net effect of these changes is impairment of normal gas exchange. This causes a relative lack of oxygen which is compensated for by the lungs working harder by breathing faster.

What causes bronchiolitis?
It is a viral illness. A few viruses can cause bronchiolitis but by far the most common (about 90%) is respiratory syncitial virus (RSV). In Britain each year RSV infections start gradually in October to reach a peak in the middle of January and then disappear by the end of April. Although people of all ages are infected, bronchiolitis seems to develop only in children between 1 month and 2 years (peak incidence 2–6 months). In general boys seem to be more severely affected than girls.
The reason why bronchiolitis does not occur in the newborn, older child and adult is not known. RSV infection in the newborn causes feeding difficulty and episodes of arrested breathing (apnoea). After age 2 the symptoms are those of a 'cold' (runny nose and cough).

How does the child get infected?
Studies have revealed that most children with bronchiolitis acquire the virus from another member of the family, usually in the preceding week. It has also been shown that at the height of the bronchiolitis season admission to hospital for some other reason frequently leads to the child's being infected with RSV.

What are the signs and symptoms of bronchiolitis?
These are very variable ranging from the child with a cough who is off his food to a child who is desperately ill. The typical story is that of a child with a mild respiratory infection, runny nose, sneezing, coughing and a temperature. These symptoms last a few days during

which he feels poorly. He then gradually breathes more rapidly as he becomes progressively short of breath. The breathlessness is accompanied by wheezing and/or repeated spasms of coughing during which he is irritable and may vomit or be unable to feed. The illness is at its most severe 2–3 days after the onset of breathlessness when the child may appear very ill and may have episodes of apnoea (arrested breathing).

On examining the chest, wheezing and/or fine crackles are heard. The breathing rate is usually in excess of 50–60 per minute and the heart rate is also raised. Lung distension causes the liver and spleen to be pushed downwards making abdominal palpation of these organs easy.

Recovery from mild illness occurs within a few days from the height of the illness, but in those severely affected it may take as long as 2 weeks.

How is bronchiolitis diagnosed?

The diagnosis is usually made by the history and examination. A chest *x*-ray may be normal or it may show signs of air trapping and small areas of air sac collapse (atelectasis). The diagnosis can be confirmed by sending sputum or nasal secretions to the laboratory where a special technique (immunofluorescence) can be used to identify RSV and provide a result on the same day. The confirmation of the diagnosis by immunofluorescence is mainly academic in that it seldom influences the way the child is managed.

What is the treatment?

There is no treatment. Most children can be nursed at home under the supervision of their family doctor. Despite no evidence of their benefit, antibiotics and asthma treatment continue to be inappropriately used.

Besides parental anxiety hospital admission is mainly for vomiting, poor feeding and severe symptoms. In the hospital the child may be given tube feeds or intravenous fluids (a 'drip'). If symptoms are severe warm humidified oxygen may be required and regular checks of blood gases will be made to monitor progress. Very rarely (less than 3% of admissions) a child will become so exhausted from the increased effort of breathing that he needs to be placed on a respirator. A respirator is a 'breathing machine' which will breathe for the child for two or three days while he is most ill.

What is the outlook?

With the very rare exception of bronchiolitis caused by adeno-virus, virtually all children make a complete recovery.

Among the most severely affected infants who have been hospita-lised there does appear to be an increased tendency to develop further episodes of wheezing which may be indistinguishable from asthma. However, this tendency does not seem to be apparent in the majority who are mildly affected.

Is bronchiolitis infectious?

RSV, like all viral infections, is spread by tiny droplets in the air when the child coughs or sneezes. Although the infection is harb-oured for a number of days (average 9) after recovery there seems little point in isolating the child from other young children who will probably have been exposed to RSV from some other source. Most urban children have acquired RSV infection by age 2.

In conclusion, bronchiolitis is a common winter illness of wide-ranging severity affecting young children. Although there is no specific treatment, all children make a complete recovery in 1–2 weeks.

PNEUMONIA

What is pneumonia?

It is inflammation of the lung in which air sacs (alveoli (Fig. 10/2)) become filled with liquid (exudate) interfering with normal lung function. The inflammation may involve one or both lungs, 'double pneumonia'.

What causes pneumonia?

More than 90% of pneumonias are caused by viruses and, like all virus infections, pneumonia is more common in winter. The first month of life is the only time that bacterial infection is more frequent. In older children bacterial pneumonia is usually preceded by a viral infection. The lung is normally sterile, any bacteria entering are rapidly cleared. The preceding viral infection predisposes the child to bacterial pneumonia by causing impairment of the clearing mechan-ism. Both viral and bacterial pneumonias can occur at any age but are most common in the pre-school child.

There are two common causes of pneumonia which are neither viral nor bacterial. One affects infants in the first three months after birth. The organism, chlamydia is acquired from the mother's genital tract and very often also causes 'sticky eyes' in the first weeks of life. Chlamydia is common in the USA and probably in Britain but is not as well recognised. The other common non-viral/bacterial pneumonia is caused by an organism called mycoplasma and affects mainly the school-age child.

The bacteria most likely to cause pneumonia show some geographical variation. In Britain, the most common bacteria are called pneumococcus and staphylococcus, the latter almost always affecting children under 2. Infection with tuberculosis is uncommon but does occur, especially in the immigrant community.

What are the signs and symptoms?

There is a wide variation in the severity, ranging from the child with a few symptoms to another who is desperately ill. It is usually not possible to differentiate the various types of pneumonia according to the signs and symptoms. Children may have fever, cough, rapid breathing, loss of appetite and feeding difficulty. The child may experience discomfort such as headache, chest or abdominal pain. Involvement of the upper part of the lung may cause neck stiffness. A striking feature of mycoplasma pneumonia is the slowly progressive cough which may be confused with an allergic cough (asthma). Young children with pneumonia usually swallow their lung secretions while older ones, especially when the cause is bacterial, may cough up green or rusty coloured mucus.

How is pneumonia diagnosed?

For the most part the diagnosis can be made by examining the chest, but very young children and a few older children, especially those with mycoplasma pneumonia do require x-rays. The diagnosis may be missed by relying on the clinical examination alone.

Should the child be admitted to hospital?

Most are mild and can be treated at home by the family doctor. Only the most severe require hospital admission.

What happens in hospital?

Depending on the severity, oxygen, intravenous fluids and antibiotics may be required. Paracetamol (acetominophen (USA)) may be given for discomfort.

Investigations such as x-rays and blood tests will be done. In about half the bacterial pneumonias bacteria can be grown from the blood. When sputum can be obtained it will be sent for culture (bacterial growth). Swabs from the throat and mouth are of no value; the bacteria at these sites are not necessarily the same as in the lung. It is difficult to grow mycoplasma in the laboratory. The diagnosis can only be confirmed by blood tests, the results of which may take as long as a fortnight.

When tuberculosis is suspected in young children who swallow their secretions, a thin feeding tube is passed into the stomach first thing in the morning; the secretions are then removed and sent for culture. A skin test for tuberculosis will also be done.

Physiotherapy plays a major part in the treatment of pneumonia in hospital. The sooner the infected secretions can be cleared from the lung, the better. The physiotherapist will percuss the chest and get the child to lie in positions likely to facilitate drainage.

Which antibiotics are used?

The difficulty in distinguishing viral from bacterial pneumonia has necessitated the widespread use of antibiotics for what is in the main a viral illness. In Britain, pneumococcus is very sensitive to penicillin which is the drug of choice. In very ill young children, particularly when the response to penicillin is poor, flucloxacillin, an antibiotic effective against staphylococcus should be added. In practice the choice of antibiotic varies widely, paediatricians may use a single antibiotic or combinations all of which are effective against these bacteria. The antibiotic of choice for the treatment of mycoplasma and chlamydia pneumonia is erythromycin. Tuberculous pneumonia is now treated for 6 months, 4 drugs being used simultaneously in the first 2 months.

Is pneumonia infectious?

Neither tuberculous nor any other pneumonia in children is infectious. When the child is well enough, there is no reason why he should not attend school.

What is the outlook?

Although it is common for children to develop fluid on the lung (pleural effusion), it soon goes. Most children make a complete recovery within a few weeks, recovery being most rapid in the case of pneumococcal pneumonia. The mortality from pneumonia has fallen dramatically in the last 50 years. This owes more to improved social conditions (housing, nutrition, etc.) than the advent of highly effective antibiotics; 80% of deaths from pneumonia occur in the first year when it is still an important cause of infant mortality. A large number of these deaths are due to wrong or or too late diagnosis.

Pneumonia seldom recurs. Children with recurrent pneumonias should be tested for cystic fibrosis (p. 124) or immune deficiency (an inability to fight infections). Inhalation of a foreign body (usually a peanut or small toy part) may cause recurrent episodes of pneumonia. If this is suspected it may be necessary to pass a thin tube (bronchoscope) down the airways while the child is under a general anaesthetic. The doctor looks down the bronchoscope while a thorough search is made for the foreign body; if detected it is immediately removed.

Can pneumonia be prevented?

For children above age 2 there is now an effective vaccine against pneumococcus (see p. 82). In view of the infrequency of bacterial pneumonia it is not recommended that all children have the vaccine. Despite recent evidence that children predisposed to pneumococcal infection may not be fully protected by the vaccine, most paediatricians would still recommend it for them. Children with sickle cell anaemia and those who have had their spleens removed are at particular risk.

Chapter 11

Ear, Nose, Throat and Eye Problems

EAR PROBLEMS

There are two common ear conditions in childhood, acute otitis media and chronic otitis media (glue ear). Both affect the middle part of the ear.

Acute otitis media

This means inflammation of the middle ear. It is the diagnosis most frequently made by paediatricians. Occurring mostly in winter and spring it affects as many as 20% of children, the majority below school age.

What is the cause of otitis media?

To understand the cause it is necessary to know the anatomy of the ear (Fig. 11/1). The middle ear is a membrane-lined cavity which communicates with the back of the nose by the auditory tube. This tube has 3 functions: (1) to maintain gas pressure in the cavity, (2) to drain secretions formed in the cavity, (3) to prevent secretions from the throat and nose from entering the cavity. Infection (virus or bacteria) from the throat or back of the nose may enter the tube opening and travel to the middle ear where it causes inflammation (acute otitis media). Swimming under water or diving increases air pressure at the back of the nose facilitating movement up the auditory tube and may cause otitis media in a child with a respiratory infection. Some children (those with cleft palate or Down's syndrome) are unable to shut the opening of the auditory tube, and in consequence suffer from recurrent attacks of otitis media.

213

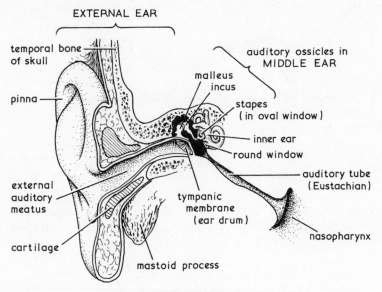

Fig. 11/1 The anatomy of the ear

How is acute otitis media diagnosed?

The child with otitis media has a temperature, is frequently irritable and may scream with severe pain. Deafness, although usually not noticeable, soon occurs. Examination of the ear by a doctor will show red ear drums. The ear drums are easy to visualise because on most occasions the warmth of the inflamed drum has caused the wax to melt.

What is the treatment for otitis media?

Treatment is directed at the infection and relieving pain. The need for an antibiotic and the type prescribed varies from one doctor to another. Ampicillin or amoxycillin are the most widely prescribed antibiotics for ear infections. It is most important that the antibiotic should be given for *at least 7 days*; any shorter course may eventually lead to chronic otitis media. Pain relief can be obtained by taking regular doses of paracetamol.

Nowadays complications of acute otitis media are rare. Occasionally pus in the middle ear cavity causes bulging and perforation of the ear drum or infiltrates the surrounding bone (mastoiditis). In the vast majority of cases the pus clears completely in 3 months, when the ear drums should be normal in appearance.

Chronic (serous) otitis media (glue ear)

Glue ear is the descriptive name given to this condition in which fluid, often of glue-like consistency, fills the middle ear cavity. It is the commonest cause of deafness in children and occurs in as many as 20% in their first 7 years. In most cases both ears are affected.

What causes glue ear?

The precise cause is unknown but it may be caused by any one or a combination of the following: (1) incomplete treatment of acute otitis media. It is common for parents to stop antibiotics after 2 or 3 days when the pain and temperature have subsided, particularly when there is difficulty in administering the treatment; (2) auditory tube blockage, the commonest cause being adenoid enlargement. This has two harmful effects. First, blockage prevents drainage of secretions from the cavity and, second, air is absorbed and pressure in the cavity is reduced. This reduction in pressure stimulates the lining (mucous membrane) of the cavity so that even more secretions are produced; (3) allergy – as many as 50% of children with glue ear have allergy (asthma, eczema or hay fever). It would appear that the allergic substance is able to enter the nose and gain entry to the middle ear cavity where it causes an outpouring of secretions by the lining.

How does the child present?

Unlike acute otitis media, pain is not usually a complaint, however, some children do experience a short, niggly pain which is most prevalent at night. There may be a feeling of fullness in the ear which is described as 'an ear that feels blocked'. Rarely buzzing noises may be described. Recurrent attacks of acute otitis media are common.

Deafness is the main symptom, though not always readily apparent. Most cases of glue ear are detected by screening procedures or routine examination of ear drums by paediatricians or other physicians. The difficulty in hearing may cause behaviour, educational, speech and communication problems. Common remarks by parents are: 'He only seems to hear when he wants to', 'he is always shouting', 'he wants the telly on loud'.

How is glue ear diagnosed?

Examination of the drum with a bright light by a doctor may show a dull appearance and fluid behind the drum. This is the method most commonly used but is not as accurate as a tympanogram, a graph which demonstrates the mobility of the drum. Performing a tympanogram is pain free and takes seconds and is suitable even for an unco-operative child. A small ear plug (probe) is placed in the ear and the presence of middle ear fluid is immediately apparent from the extent of ear drum movement which is shown by the graph. Wax in the ear interferes with the accuracy of a tympanogram and should be removed by placing five drops of warm olive oil or 'Cerumol' in each ear three times a day on the three days before the test.

Can glue ear be diagnosed by a hearing test (audiogram)?

This is *not* a reliable screening test. While most children with glue ear will have some hearing impairment and a hearing test may be helpful in making the diagnosis, others, even with a substantial amount of glue will have fairly normal hearing. It is because of the possibility of subsequent hearing impairment in these children that screening at school entry should include both a hearing test and a tympanogram.

Do children grow out of glue ears?

Yes, most glue ears resolve spontaneously over 3–4 months and often earlier. Resolution seems to be more common during the summer. It would therefore seem unreasonable to undertake any treatment of glue ears until a period of *at least* 4 months has elapsed.

Why is it necessary to treat glue ears?

For some children, a minority, glue persists for months or years and the temporary partial deafness at an important time in the child's development may be harmful. Removal of the glue restores hearing in almost all, sometimes producing dramatic changes in learning or behaviour. Another reason for treatment is that persistent glue ears predispose to recurrent attacks of acute otitis media and on very rare occasions cause complications which can lead to permanent deafness.

How may clearing of the glue be speeded up or delayed?

There is little evidence that any medication is of value in facilitating the clearance of the glue. However, in those cases which follow acute otitis media a 1–2 week course of antibiotics may help, some doctors may extend the time of antibiotic treatment for as long as 3 months.

In the presence of glue ears many paediatricians advise against swimming in chlorinated water which is very irritating to the lining of the nose and middle ear cavity. Others feel that swimming can be permitted provided there is no underwater swimming or diving. It is particularly harmful for the child to jump feet first into the water, thus forcing water through the nose into the auditory tube opening.

Air travel is harmful when a child has glue ears. Not only does it make the ear worse but it can be extremely painful. If it is necessary to fly, then immediately the aircraft *descends* the child should be encouraged to swallow as much as possible by providing a drink for an infant or chewy toffees for an older child.

What operation is performed for glue ear?

The operation is called 'myringotomy', a small cut is made in the ear drum and the glue is sucked out. Many surgeons remove the adenoids at the same time and if there have been frequent throat infections the tonsils may also be removed. The operation is done under a general anaesthetic and hospital admission is seldom more than a day or two.

About 75% respond to this treatment and nothing further need be done. In the remainder fluid recurs and another operation is required to insert a grommet in the ear drum (Fig. 11/2). A grommet is a plastic ventilation tube which prevents fluid formation by creating a normal pressure in the middle ear cavity. Some surgeons do not do a myringotomy as the first procedure but insert grommets instead. Grommets do not require removal but usually fall out spontaneously between 3 and 18 months; unfortunately it is not possible to predict how long they will stay in for an individual child. On occasions grommet re-insertion may be required two or three times. Most surgeons follow up children every 3–4 months to check whether the grommet is in place or if it has blocked. Re-insertion of a grommet which has come out is only required when the original symptoms are still present.

Must children with grommets avoid swimming?

No, provided underwater swimming and diving are avoided and

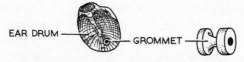

EAR DRUM —————— GROMMET

Fig. 11/2 A grommet and its fixation in the ear drum

ear plugs are worn. Ear plugs, while not watertight, prevent total flooding of the external ear canal and provide sufficient protection to allow swimming. Almost any plugs will do; special fitted plugs can be obtained from hearing aid dispensing firms, but may be expensive. A large cotton wool plug coated with petroleum jelly is effective and is commonly used. Contrary to common belief cotton wool by itself does allow water through. 'Silly putty' which is inexpensive and available in most toy shops is an effective alternative. It should be removed immediately after swimming. If not removed, on a hot day, it can melt and later harden in the external canal. Should an ear plug come out in the water most children will not develop an infection, but if pain or discharge develop then a doctor should be consulted.

The answer to the above question is controversial and the view expressed is a personal opinion. Should your child require grommets it is most important that you raise this question with the surgeon who performed the operation.

Does glue ear run in families?

Both glue ear and acute otitis media seem to occur more commonly in certain families; the reason is not clear.

In conclusion, glue ear is a common condition which produces temporary deafness in a young child. Treatment is initially conservative, at least 4–6 months' observation. Failure of resolution over this period may require surgery, usually producing a dramatic improvement in hearing.

NOSE PROBLEMS

Nosebleeds (epistaxis)

Nosebleeds are common in children and are sometimes recurrent. Usually the nose starts bleeding without any obvious cause, but it may follow a sneeze or a hard blow. Occasional nosebleeds may be inconvenient and messy but are of no significance. Frequent or prolonged nosebleeds may cause the child to become anaemic and medical advice should be obtained. Most nosebleeds are caused by rupture of one or more vessels on the nasal septum (part that separates nostrils). When nosebleeds are frequent it is usually possible to identify the source of the bleed. The bleeds can be stopped by spraying the nose with a local anaesthetic and then cauterising the vessel or vessels responsible.

First aid management of nosebleeds:

1. Sit the child up.
2. Pinch the nostril between a finger and thumb for a few minutes.
3. Apply an ice pack to the bridge of nose.
4. Allow the nose to drip freely over a basin or bowl. Swallowing may cause clot displacement. Swallowing can be prevented by placing a cork between the teeth.
5. Insert a pledget of cotton wool up the bleeding nostril.

These steps should be followed in sequence until the bleeding stops.

Snuffles

Snuffles are common in young children and usually form part of the 'common cold', a viral infection for which there is no treatment. A mucous nasal discharge occurs normally in the first months of life in many babies and is of concern to parents. The cause is not known and it does not require any treatment.

What about nose drops?

Nose drops are seldom given properly and even when given properly probably have little effect. The runny nose usually gets worse after the treatment has stopped and, if used for long, nose drops irritate the lining (mucosa) of the nose. The constituents of nose drops are absorbed and serious side-effects have occasionally been reported. Other than saline nose drops there seems little place for their use in children; if they are used it should not be for longer than 2–3 days. Saline drops are helpful for moistening thick dry secretions.

Sinusitis

The skull has membrane-lined cavities known as sinuses: when they become infected the condition is called sinusitis. The two sinuses most commonly infected in children are the maxillary and frontal, both connecting directly with the nose. The maxillary which lies behind the cheek is usually not formed until about 4 years, the frontal which lies in the forehead is not formed until 7–8.

A mild form of sinusitis is common when a child gets a 'cold'. He may have pain in the cheek or forehead and tenderness is elicited over these areas when pressure is applied. The pain may become worse when the child bends forward or lies down. There may be an accompanying yellow/green nasal discharge and fever. The symptoms usually resolve in 2–3 days, antibiotics may be helpful if symptoms do not appear to be improving.

Chronic sinusitis was at one time a fashionable complaint, large numbers of children being subjected to sinus 'washouts'. There is seldom a need for such procedures nowadays.

THROAT PROBLEMS

Sore throat (pharyngitis)

The treatment of a sore throat is one of the paediatric controversies. Most doctors, rightly or wrongly, have their own fixed views.

Most (85%) throat infections are viral. The remainder, except during epidemics when the incidence rises, are caused by a bacterium known as streptococcus. Clinically it is usually not possible to distinguish a viral from a bacterial sore throat. In general bacterial infections tend to be more severe and last longer while viral infections are usually associated with a runny nose and eyes, cough and hoarseness.

The child with a sore throat is usually feverish and unwell. If old enough he will complain of a sore throat, or he will just refuse to eat or drink. Neck glands may become painful and swollen. The throat appears red and follicles (pus) may be seen on the tonsils. Abdominal pain and vomiting (mesenteric adenitis) may occur with both bacterial and viral sore throats.

What investigations are done?

Some doctors take a throat swab to see if streptococci can be cultured (grown) in the laboratory. The need to wait 2–3 days for the result is a major disadvantage. Recently some paediatricians in the USA have started using 'office kits' to detect the streptococci while the patient waits. The test is designed to detect a protein (antigen) in the wall of the bacteria. Because the test is expensive, time consuming, has a high yield of false negatives and does not detect all throat infecting streptococci, it is unlikely to become widely used.

Does the growth of streptococcus indicate that the cause is bacterial?

No, as many as 40% of 'positive' (bacteria grown) cultures are from children who have a viral infection, but who normally carry the streptococcus in the throat (carriers).

Are antibiotics necessary?

Since the vast majority are viral, antibiotics are probably not necessary, but most doctors do prescribe antibiotics for sore throats on the chance that the cause may be bacterial.

What is the purpose of treatment?

The main reason for treatment is the belief that the severity or duration of symptoms will be reduced by early effective treatment. At present there is some support for this, but the evidence so far is by no means convincing.

The other reason for treatment is that the streptococcus also causes rheumatic fever and glomerulonephritis. In the past it was hoped that early treatment would prevent them. In Britain and the USA these illnesses have all but disappeared and this argument is no longer tenable.

Which antibiotic should be used?

There are many antibiotics which are suitable, but penicillin remains the one of choice. For those allergic to penicillin, erythromycin is a safe alternative.

What should he have for the fever?

Many parents have a misguided belief that fever is harmful. In a well-hydrated child there is absolutely no harm in having a temperature and no fever treatment is required. For a child with a sore throat or headache it would be reasonable to give a pain reliever, paracetamol (acetaminophen (USA)), which also causes a lowering of the temperature.

What about tonsillectomy?

Removal of tonsils is the most common operation of childhood and probably the most unnecessary operation at any time of life. Before subjecting a child to tonsillectomy a parent or doctor should balance the potential benefit of the operation against the fact that 200–300 children die each year in the USA (about 10 in Britain) as a result of the procedure. I have found that some parents have most unrealistic expectations about the benefits of tonsillectomy, and are often disappointed. These expectations may be quite irrational ranging from increasing appetite to curing bed-wetting.

There seems to be only one firm indication for tonsillectomy about which most doctors agree. Very rarely, large tonsil size interferes with the flow of air through the throat producing changes in the heart and lungs. Children with this problem are usually under 4. They snore loudly and have episodes of interrupted breathing (apnoea) during sleep, and, because of the disturbed sleep, may appear sleepy during the day.

Among doctors the main reason for recommending tonsillectomy has been the belief that the operation would reduce the number of throat infections. At present there is no evidence that operation will significantly reduce the number of days with a sore throat or the amount of school absence.

At tonsillectomy most surgeons remove the adenoids as well. The operation is performed under general anaesthetic and should never be done while the child has a sort throat. At most, 2–3 days in hospital are required during which it would be emotionally beneficial for the mother to room in with the child. Eating and drinking should be encouraged as soon as possible after the operation. Discomfort, which is usually mild, is treated with paracetamol.

In conclusion, the treatment of the sore throat and the need for tonsillectomy are controversial. Most medical practice is based more on custom than reason.

Croup

Croup can best be defined as a throat condition of children characterised by a hoarse cough and laboured breathing resulting from partial obstruction of the larynx (back of throat). The obstruction causes a characteristic inspiratory crowing noise called 'stridor'.

Boys are affected more often than girls and it occurs most often in the winter when respiratory infections are most common. Although primarily a throat condition the ears and lungs may also be affected. Croup can be categorised as 3 types, viral, bacterial and spasmodic.

Viral croup, the most common affects children between 3 months and 3 years. The virus usually responsible is called parainfluenza. Why some children just develop a mild respiratory infection and others croup is not known. Viral croup frequently develops in a family where the child and other family members may have a respiratory infection. After a 'cold' and mild fever for 2–3 days he develops a 'barking' cough, laboured breathing and stridor. The croup usually lasts several days during which the severity will wax and wane, but is usually worse at night during which the child may be restless and frightened. Crying makes it worse. The child will not eat but generally drinks normally.

The vast majority are mild and can be managed at home without any treatment. The use of humidity (steam) is controversial; despite little evidence of its benefit it continues to be widely used. Recurrences of viral croup do occur but there are no long-term effects.

Bacterial croup (acute epiglottitis) is usually caused by bacteria called haemophilus. It is a very serious form of croup with a high mortality if left untreated. Fortunately it accounts for less than 10%. The age range is usually between 2 and 12. A previously well child suddenly develops a swinging temperature, stridor and breathing difficulty. He looks ill, is anxious and restless and may complain of a sore throat. Refusal to eat and drink is common. Most children sit upright with an open mouth from which there is excessive drooling of saliva.

The seriousness of this form of croup lies in the fact that there is a very rapid progression of the illness. It is common for complete airway obstruction to develop within hours of onset. At times it may be difficult to decide which form of croup a child has. The gravity of this condition necessitates this general advice:

1. All children with croup should be seen by a doctor.
2. Any marked deterioration after the doctor has seen the child should not be ignored. Croup commonly occurs at night, a delay until the morning could be dangerous. If the child is getting worse after the doctor has been, call again, or take the child to the accident and emergency department of your nearest hospital.

When bacterial croup is suspected children are always admitted to hospital. At the hospital blood tests are done to confirm that bacterial infection is the cause. Intravenous fluids (a drip) are given and antibiotics started. Humidity may be given. The child is then very carefully observed and, depending on his condition, no further action may be required. He will usually be well enough for discharge after a few days.

A further deterioration in hospital may require the passage of a thin plastic tube (endotracheal tube) through the nose and down the throat so that the airway is kept open. The tube is kept in place for 2–

3 days during which the child is sedated. When the tube is removed the throat swelling will have subsided and only slight hoarseness remains. After a further 2 or 3 days he will be fit for discharge.

Very rarely, a small incision on the front of the neck (tracheostomy) is required for insertion of the tube. The operation is performed under general anaesthetic by a throat surgeon. The rest of the management is similar.

With preservation of the airway there is virtually 100% recovery from acute epiglottitis. There are no long-term effects and there is no chance of a recurrence. Recently a vaccine against haemophilus has been licensed for use in the USA. It is very effective in children over 2. With widespread use of the vaccine it can only be hoped that acute epiglottitis will become a thing of the past (p. 81).

Spasmodic croup usually affects children from 1–3 years. The symptoms are similar to viral croup but unlike viral croup the child and his family usually do not appear to have a respiratory infection. The cause is not known for certain but like asthma could be primarily allergic, with recurrent bouts of croup precipitated by viruses or emotion. A family history of recurrent croup and allergy is common. Like asthma and other forms of croup it is always worse at night.

The typical story is that of a child who suddenly wakes at night, has a few episodes of coughing followed by stridor. He become progressively breathless, frightened and anxious. Usually there is no temperature. Symptoms start to improve within hours so that by the morning he is well except for slight hoarseness and a cough. Similar but less severe attacks may occur over the next night or two. Not having seen the attack one often finds it hard to imagine the severity when the child is so well the following morning. Parents sometimes become annoyed when the doctor regards their story with total disbelief.

Although spasmodic croup can be very frightening for both the child and the parents it is a harmless condition. The main danger is that it should not be confused with acute epiglottitis which is a serious condition. Hospital admission is seldom necessary but may be required for relief of parental anxiety. Parents are advised to seek medical advice, following which symptoms will gradually go irrespective of treatment. There is no proof that the treatments currently recommended are of any value. These include exposure to humidity (steam) or cold air and vomiting induced by syrup of ipecacuanha – the dosage being one drop per month up to age 2, thereafter 1ml per year of age. The syrup should be given with an orange drink rather than milk and the dose should be repeated after 15 minutes if the child has not vomited and symptoms are still present.

In conclusion, croup is a common childhood problem. It is usually worse at night and can be extremely frightening for both child and parents. In a small number the illness is rapidly progressive and may have a fatal outcome if diagnosis and treatment are delayed. The vast majority of children have a mild illness which can be safely managed at home. Children with croup should always be seen by a doctor as soon as possible.

What is congenital laryngeal stridor?

Also called laryngomalacia, it is the commonest cause of stridor in newborn babies. The cartilage of the larynx (back of throat) is soft so that when the baby breathes in the negative pressures causes the walls to collapse inwards, narrowing the airway. The stridor is usually noticed at birth or shortly afterwards. Parents may be very concerned as the noise may be quite alarming. Characteristically it is worse on crying and feeding and quietest or absent at rest. The loudness also varies with the position of the child; it sometimes increases with upper respiratory infections when occasional children become breathless and may require admission to hospital. By 2 the cartilage of the walls of the larynx will have firmed up sufficiently to prevent the walls' collapsing and the noise will disappear.

EYE PROBLEMS

Squint (strabismus)

Squint is the most common eye problem of childhood affecting 3–4% of the pre-school population. It takes its name from the Greek word *strabismos* meaning to look obliquely. The direction of the squinting eye may be convergent (turning inwards), divergent (turning outwards) or vertical when one eye appears higher than the other. Most children have convergent squints.

When should a child with a squint be referred to an eye specialist (ophthalmologist)?

It is quite normal for a child to have an *intermittent* squint in the first months of life. Any persistence beyond 6 months is abnormal necessitating referral. A *constant* squint is always abnormal and the child should be referred as soon as it is noticed.

What is a false squint or 'pseudosquint'?
It is the false impression of a squint when the eyes are normal (Fig. 11/3). It is caused by a fold of skin (epicanthus) at the inner angle of the eye in a young child who has either a very wide or narrow base of the nose. These facial features cause the observer to see less white on the nasal side of the eye than would be expected, giving the impression that the eye is turned inwards. This is particularly obvious when the child is gazing from side to side or when the eyes are half closed when tired.

The pseudosquint requires no treatment: as the face grows it will disappear. At times when there is an epicanthus it may be very difficult to distinguish a false squint from a genuine one. Children never 'grow out' of a genuine squint and if there is any doubt you should seek medical advice. If the doctor is not sure, the eyes will be assessed by an orthoptist (optometrist in the USA), a specialist at evaluating squints.

Can the child with a squint see normally?
Yes, the brain switches off the image from the squinting eye. The effect is the same as looking down a microscope or sighting a rifle. The brain quickly learns to concentrate on the eye that is being used even though the other eye is open and seeing.

What happens if a squint is not treated?
There is an obvious cosmetic benefit in treating a squint. The other reason for treatment is to prevent the development of a 'lazy eye' (amblyopia). The chance of a lazy eye is the same whether the squint is mild or severe.

What is a 'lazy eye' (amblyopia)?
Over many months of switching off the image from the squinting eye it will become permanently switched off. This happens after 7 when the function of the eye is lost for ever. Although this does not in any way interfere with vision, future loss of the good eye would

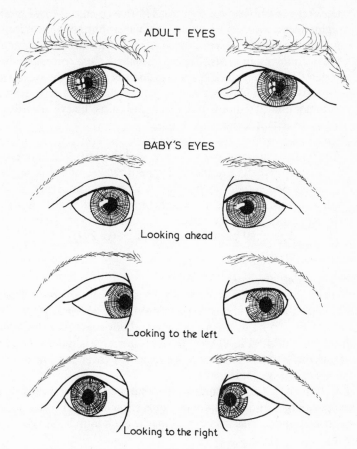

Fig. 11/3 Pseudo-squint. A false impression of squint when gazing from side to side caused by a wide nasal bridge and epicanthic folds. *Note* the difference in appearance between the eyes of infants and adults

render the child blind. This is obviously cause for concern: a 'lazy eye' is therefore more a psychological than a visual handicap.

What causes squint?

Squints frequently run in families. The causes can be divided into those causing an abnormality of eye function and causes affecting eye muscles.

(a) Abnormality of eye function – function may be abnormal because of blurring of the lens (cataracts), far-sightedness or abnormalities of the retina (back of the eye). The most common cause is far-sightedness: the eyes are able to see distant but not near objects. Normally, in order to see near objects the lens needs to refocus, the eye moving inwards. There is usually a close correlation between the amount the lens focuses and the amount the eye turns inwards. When children are very far-sighted this relationship does not hold; the brain over-reacts and turns the eye inwards to a greater extent, producing a squint.

(b) Abnormal eye muscles – muscles move the eyes up, down, and from side to side and any weakness in the eye muscles causes an imbalance and the eye moves in the direction of the strongest muscles. Some children are born with muscle imbalance while others acquire it. Conditions sometimes associated with muscular imbalance are hydrocephalus (excessive fluid in the brain (p. 318)) and cerebral palsy (spastic children (p. 297)).

How are squints diagnosed?

Usually the diagnosis is obvious from simple observation. When the eyes look straight ahead and a bright light is shone at them, the reflection should be at the same spot on both eyes. Any deviation indicates a squint (Fig. 11/4). In a co-operative child alternately covering the eyes and noting eye movements ('cover test') facilitates the diagnosis (Fig. 11/5).

Children with vertical squints sometimes hold their heads in a tilted position. The diagnosis of squint is often delayed because most parents and their physicians think that the neck muscles are causing the tilt.

How is squint treated?

Spectacles – these will correct the far-sightedness and may be all that is required.

Patching – in children under 7 who are developing a 'lazy eye', the good eye may be patched so that the squinting eye is used and a 'lazy eye' prevented.

Eye exercises – the orthoptist may give the child eye exercises to

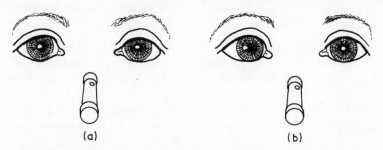

Fig. 11/4 The light reflex test for squint. The light is held about 30cm in front of the eyes. (a) Light reflex should be on the same spot on each eyeball. (b) Light reflex on different spots indicates squint

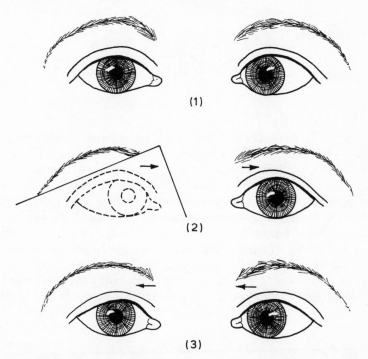

Fig. 11/5 The cover test showing: 1. left convergent squint; 2. covering the right eye causes the non-functioning left eye to move outwards as it takes over vision. The covered eye moves inwards; 3. uncovering the right eye causes it to move outwards and the left eye inwards as both eyes revert to their former position in 1

improve eye muscle function. Eye exercises are used to complement other forms of treatment.

Surgery – about two-thirds eventually require surgery, a small number (about 1 in 3) requiring more than one operation. The purpose of surgery is to straighten the eyes by altering the position of the muscles.

The operation is done under general anaesthetic. Admission to hospital is seldom for more than 2–3 days. The operated eye will be padded. Redness and mild discomfort may last as long as a month.

In conclusion: squint is common in children. It does not interfere with normal vision and the benefit of treatment is in the main cosmetic. For most success, early diagnosis and treatment are required.

Absent tears

Tears are normally absent in the newborn. In most infants they are apparent by 2–4 months, but sometimes appear later.

The watery eye

A tube (nasolacrimal duct) connects the inner aspect of the eye with the nose. Tears, which are formed by the lacrimal gland below the upper eyelid, drain through this tube into the nose. In the first months of life the tube is commonly blocked giving a persistently watery eye which may become infected from time to time. By 9 months the obstruction has spontaneously cleared in the vast majority. Gently massaging the corner of the eye against the side of the nose, pressing on the tear duct, may speed up the process. When a yellow discharge develops antibiotic drops or ointment should be given. Very rarely it may be necessary to prise open the tube under a general anaesthetic, but this is probably not necessary before 18 months.

Sticky eyes

About 1 in 10 newborn babies has sticky eyes in the first days of life. The reason for this is not entirely clear but appears to be due to irritation caused by blood, amniotic fluid and antiseptics entering the eye as the head passes through the birth canal. Because there are no

tears to wash away these irritants they cause inflammation of the surface (conjunctiva) of the eye. In most children all that is required is
for the eyes to be flushed with sterile saline drops 3–4 times per day.
When there is a yellow or green discharge which persists swabs are
taken and antibiotic drops or ointment are prescribed. The bacteria
causing sticky eyes come from the mother, attendants and the environment. Two infections which come exclusively from the mother
are gonococcus (gonorrhoea) and chlamydia; both require special
swabs and treatment. When there is no response to the usual eye antibiotics (chloramphenicol or neomycin) these infections are usually
considered. In Britain, gonococcal infections are rare; in the USA,
although they are also uncommon, preventive treatment of the eye is
still widely administered immediately after birth. Chlamydia infections are common in both countries and many hospitals are now
checking all sticky eyes for chlamydia. Both infections require systemic treatment as well as eye treatment, in the case of chlamydia it is
to prevent pneumonia developing subsequently (p. 210). The parents
of children with these infections also require treatment.

Conjunctivitis (red eye)

It is common for children to develop red sticky eyes which discharge
and with lids which are stuck together on awakening in the morning.
Conjunctivitis, inflammation of the outer layer of the eye is usually
caused by bacteria or a virus. If the eye does not appear to be clearing
after a day or two antibiotics (drops or ointment) are usually prescribed.

Styes

Styes are common in children and are sometimes recurrent. A stye
looks like a small boil on the eyelid and is caused by an infection of
the root of an eyelash and its oil producing (sebaceous) gland. It is
tender and unsightly but causes no harm. Styes, like boils, will
eventually get better without any treatment. The process can, however, be speeded up by applying warmth. The best way of doing this
is to wrap some lint or cotton wool around a wooden spoon. The lint
is dipped in hot water and then applied to the stye until it feels cold.
This should be repeated at half-hourly intervals for a few hours.

Make sure the water is not too hot. Children with styes should not share face cloths.

ALLERGIC RHINITIS/CONJUNCTIVITIS

Allergic rhinitis (inflammation of the nose) and conjunctivitis (inflammation of the eye) affect as many as 1 in 10 children at some time. Many of these children will have asthma or eczema as well and frequently another member of the family will have had one of these 'allergic' illnesses. The lining of the nose (mucosa) and the eye (conjunctiva) are similar to the lining of the lung. It thus follows that the same things that irritate the lung to cause asthma can also irritate the nose and eye. Other than allergic substances, common irritants of the nose and eye are cold air, tobacco smoke, perfume and newspaper ink. When nose and/or eye symptoms are present all year round the constant 'cold' is referred to as perennial rhinitis/conjunctivitis. When symptoms are only seasonal the condition is called hay fever. The allergic substances causing perennial symptoms are similar to those causing perennial asthma, the house dust mite being the most common. Hay fever is caused by pollen and occasionally by moulds. Many children with multiple allergies and perennial symptoms are worse in the pollen season and may also be said to suffer from hay fever. Interestingly, perennial symptoms may be obvious within a few months of birth while the hay fever pattern does not become obvious until the child is of school age. The number of children presenting with hay fever for the first time increases during the teens to reach a peak at about 21, the symptoms tending to disappear in middle age. Perennial symptoms like asthma tend to improve in the late teens.

What are the main symptoms?
The main symptoms are runny nose, blocked nose, sneezing and itching of the nose and throat. The ears may also itch and many children have a 'popping' sensation. Mouth breathing and snoring are common. Speech may have a 'nasal' quality. Nose itching may cause rubbing and twitching which may become a habit and continue even when the nose is all right. Many children look pale and develop a bluish swelling of the lower eyelids, 'allergic shiners'. Smell sensation is affected and, in consequence, some may lose their appetite.

When symptoms are severe children may feel depressed or isolated because of incessant taunts of 'use your handkerchief' or 'blow your nose'. Common associated complications of allergic rhinitis are:

1. frequent nosebleeds
2. sinusitis causing headaches
3. deafness due to 'glue ears'.

Common allergic eye symptoms are redness, watering and itching. There may also be a 'gritty' feeling. When the eyes are rubbed, swelling of the eyelids sometimes develops. Although eye and nose symptoms frequently co-exist, most children seem to be troubled more by one than the other.

When is the hay fever season?

While grass pollen allergy occurs classically in June and July, children may be allergic to tree pollen which occurs in April and May, or flower pollen which is prevalent in August. Those who have hay fever in September are almost certainly allergic to moulds.

How is allergic rhinitis/conjunctivitis diagnosed?

The diagnosis is made by the history and examination of the nose or eyes. A history of asthma or eczema in the patient or his relatives will support the diagnosis. If there is any doubt a smear of the nasal discharge is taken and sent to the laboratory where it is stained and examined under the microscope. Provided the discharge is not infected an abundance of cells known as eosinophils confirms the diagnosis of allergic rhinitis. As in asthma allergy tests may be done but I have not found them helpful. Neither do they help with the diagnosis nor do they affect the way the condition is managed.

How is it treated?

Allergy avoidance measures – these are listed in more detail on page 201. Although worth trying, the benefit, if any, is likely to be minimal.

Desensitisation – only worth trying when there is allergy to a single allergen, for example, grass pollen. A course of injections is generally given yearly for 3 years in the period preceding the pollen season. This treatment is inconvenient, expensive and not without risk. It would be fair to say that most paediatricians regard the small improvement in symptoms that may accrue not to be justified by these drawbacks.

Drug treatment – in many children a definite diagnosis and subsequent explanation of the condition will be sufficient and no drug treatment will be needed. A doctor is only able to advise and the decision about the need for drug treatment depends on the parents and child.

Drugs for the nose

This group of drugs is the treatment of choice. They are extremely effective, without side-effects and can be given twice daily.

STEROID SPRAYS

Approved Name	Trade Name
beclamethasone dipropionate	Beconase (aerosol or liquid)
budesonide	Rhinocort (aerosol)
flunisolide	Syntaris (liquid)

Sodium cromoglycate (Rynacrom or Lomusol): although very effective for asthma it does not appear to be equally effective in the treatment of allergic rhinitis. It has the disadvantage of requiring four doses per day to be fully effective.

Drugs for the eye

Sodium cromoglycate (Opticrom): this is the treatment of choice for allergic conjunctivitis. Available as drops or ointment. It is very effective and has no side-effects.

Steroid eye drops or ointment: these bring about a dramatic improvement but, because of side-effects, should *never* be used for more than a few days unless under the direct supervision of an eye specialist.

Drugs for both nose and eyes

Antihistamines: these may be very helpful and are taken by mouth. They have the advantage of being effective for both nose and eye symptoms. In the past their use was limited because they produced drowsiness which caused learning problems and often interfered with summer exams. There are now new antihistamines which have the advantage of causing much less drowsiness. These drugs can be used by themselves or in combination with other treatments. The main

effect of antihistamines is on sneezing, a runny nose and conjunctivitis; they have little effect on a blocked nose. If, in addition to the
above symptoms, a blocked nose is a prominent symptom then it may
be helpful to combine antihistamine treatment with a steroid spray.
Two of the new antihistamines are listed below.

Approved Name	*Trade Name*
astemizole	Hismanal
terfenadine	Triludin

Astemizole is taken once daily and terfenadine twice daily. Because
terfenadine acts rapidly it is the drug of choice for intermittent treatment when symptoms are severe.

Steroids (tablets or injections): because of their side-effects these
drugs are seldom used. When hay fever is very severe, however, and
does not respond to the measures outlined above then a short course
of oral steroids or a long-acting steroid injection (methylprednisol-
one) can be very beneficial. This form of treatment is particularly
useful for teenagers taking their exams during the hay fever season.

Chapter 12

Skin Problems

ECZEMA (ATOPIC DERMATITIS)

Childhood eczema is one of the atopic diseases, others being asthma and hay fever. The word atopic means 'strange' and all affected children have in common an allergy to a wide variety of substances, the commonest being house dust, house dust mite, pollen and feathers. Eczema is indeed strange for, unlike asthma or hay fever, which are caused by allergy, the cause of eczema is unknown. Both environmental and genetic factors play a part. As yet it is not known precisely which environmental factors are responsible. It is, however, known that eczema is much more common when one or both parents were similarly affected.

As many as 5% of children may be affected and about half will develop hay fever and/or asthma as well. The rash presents in the first year in most children and virtually never starts after age 5. Although it can begin anywhere it classically starts on the face between 3 and 6 months. Within a few months it may extend to the front of the elbows, back of the knees and areas of friction such as the neck, ankles and wrists (Fig. 12/1). Occasionally there is a 'reverse pattern', the back of the elbows and the front of the knees being involved. Children have a dry skin and from time to time inflamed, moist patches develop. These are intensely itchy and chronic scratching produces thickening of the skin. When the scratched areas become repeatedly infected, enlarged glands may develop and these are easily felt in the armpits and groin. Scalp involvement produces profuse dry scales. Why the rash migrates from the face to the body and hands is a mystery; this is however the usual pattern. Another strange feature of eczema is its tendency to fluctuate widely in severity, often for no apparent reason. Eczema, like other atopic diseases, improves with

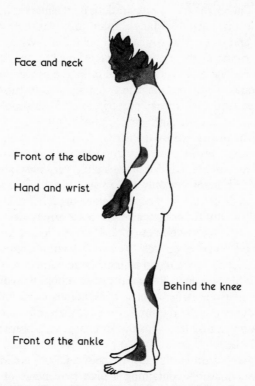

Face and neck

Front of the elbow

Hand and wrist

Behind the knee

Front of the ankle

Fig. 12/1 The most common pattern in childhood eczema

age. More than half outgrow it by age 10 and it is rarely seen after 20. The vast majority of children will become well-adapted adults.

The principles of management are as follows:

1. Keep the skin well hydrated. Oil should be added to the bath and at least one bath per day should be taken. The bath water temperature should be comfortable but not too hot. Oil clings to the bath surface after the water has been drained and the bath may become very slippery and dangerous. Always warn other members of the family about this, particularly the elderly. Soap has a drying action and should be avoided, the cleansing action of bath oil being just as good. I normally recommend using a bath oil, emulsifying ointment or Unguentum Merck ambiphilic cream as a soap although 'superfatted' soap such as Oilatum soap and most baby soaps are also suitable. The skin should be regularly

oiled. There are various preparations on the market which can be
used for this purpose. Many contain additives such as urea, gly-
cerine and lactic acid which help the outer layer of skin retain
water. Some of these additives occasionally cause 'stinging' of
the skin. The main action of the oil is the prevention of water
evaporation from the skin. Many parents find it embarrassing to
ask frequently for repeat prescriptions. This problem can be
avoided by issuing large prescriptions, for example, bath oil
should be prescribed by the litre.

2. Prevent itching. This is a very important part of the treatment. A
persistent intense itch can make a child very miserable. Prevention of itch helps not only the eczema but also has a profound
psychological benefit. The medicines used for itch prevention
are called antihistamines and all cause drowsiness as a side-
effect. New antihistamines (p. 234) which do not cause drowsiness have no effect on itch. To avoid daytime drowsiness many
paediatricians recommend a single large night-time dose. If the
child is 'dopey' on wakening the dose should be reduced or the
medicine given earlier. For antihistamines to be fully effective
adult doses may be required. Because their effect may wear off
with use you may find your doctor changes the preparation from
time to time.

3. Wear the correct clothing. Pure cotton fabrics are ideal but expensive; mixtures containing a high percentage of cotton are
cheaper and also acceptable. Both wool and nylon garments
should not be in direct contact with the skin. Wool fibre irritates
the skin and pure nylon causes perspiration, both making the
itch worse. Cotton bedding may also be helpful and both clothing and bedding should be thoroughly rinsed after washing.
When eczema is severe use a 'pure' soap powder (Lux flakes)
rather than powders containing 'enzymes', bleaches and fabric
softeners. Children with foot eczema should wear loose-fitting
leather shoes which allow the foot to 'breathe'. Plimsoles (trainers, sneakers) should be avoided.

4. Treat inflamed skin with hydrocortisone. It is seldom necessary
to use anything stronger than 1% which, unlike stronger
steroids, can be used on the face with safety. Moist areas are best
treated with a cream or ointment. Cream, which contains less
water and is less oily than ointment, is preferred by many children and their parents. On the other hand ointment, being greas-

ier, does work better and needs less frequent application because it is not easily removed. Ointment is also less likely to become contaminated by bacteria and has a longer shelf life. When scooping ointment or cream out of a container, always wash your hands thoroughly first or use a clean spatula (stick) on each occasion; this reduces the chance of contamination. Hydrocortisone need not be used on the scalp. This is best treated 2–3 times a week by rubbing in well 2% salicylic acid in emulsifying ointment at bedtime and shampooing with a tar shampoo in the morning. Dry scales of skin are removed and scalp appearance will be dramatically improved. Those children who find tar shampoo irritating should use a non-tar shampoo such as Cetavlon PC. An even more effective scalp preparation, but very messy is Ung. Cocois Co. It is a mixture of salicylic acid, tar and coconut oil and is used in the same way as salicylic acid in emulsifying ointment. The coconut oil melts, thereby helping to spread the tar and salicylic acid.

5. Treat dry, thickened (lichenified) skin with tar. Tar is a very effective treatment for dry, thickened or scaly skin and is widely used both for eczema and psoriasis. The effect on the skin can be quite dramatic, but in a few children it can cause quite severe irritation. It is best to avoid applying it to raw areas. Tar may be applied in combination with hydrocortisone (Tarcorten) or separately as a paste or a tar impregnated bandage. I have found tar-impregnated bandages extremely useful, particularly on the limbs. Not only do they provide effective treatment but they also prevent the child from scratching. The bandages are usually applied at night and are covered with 'Coban', a self-gripping elasticated bandage which allows air in but prevents the tar from seeping out. 'Coban' is very expensive and a crepe bandage would suffice. A calamine-impregnated bandage is sometimes used for wet inflamed eczema; children find it very soothing.

Children with eczema usually have both sides of the body affected to the same extent. It is often beneficial, when evaluating a new skin treatment, for only one side of the body to be treated initially. This will enable you to compare the two sides and observe the effect of treatment.

6. Control skin infections. The bacteria most commonly infecting eczema are known as streptococcus and staphylococcus. An antibiotic which is effective against both bacteria may be required

from time to time. Erythromycin and Augmentin (amoxycillin with clavulanate) are two commonly used antibiotics. The child's nails should be kept short and clean. It may be necessary to have the child sleep with mittens so that the skin is not scratched.

Certain viral infections produce a very severe illness in children with eczema. One such virus is herpes, the cause of 'cold sores' (p. 70). Children with bad eczema should avoid contact with anyone with cold sores. Although seldom required now, smallpox vaccination should never be given. Eczema is not a contra-indication to any other vaccination.

7. Avoid excessive heat. Heat aggravates the itching and makes the child very uncomfortable. Simple advice is as follows: avoid too many jerseys; if the blankets are kicked off during the night leave them off; do not leave the central heating on all night; do not sleep with the child in your bed; energetic games immediately before bed should be avoided.

8. Keep exposed parts of the body covered in cold winter winds. Compared with warm air cold air is dry (has a low humidity). The effect of the cold dry air blowing on the exposed skin is to remove further water from the already dry skin making the eczema worse.

9. Avoid stress. It should be emphasised that eczema is not primarily a psychological illness, but anxiety makes itching worse. Children with eczema should be treated no differently from other children. Unfortunately there is widespread ignorance of this condition and these children are often singled out and treated differently. Parents are advised to have a discussion with the teacher about the child and his eczema. In this discussion it is important to emphasise that eczema is not infectious. Persistent teasing and bullying by schoolchildren should be dealt with. Indeed, it is part of the education of all children to learn compassion for those with physical disabilities.

10. Apply oil to skin before and after swimming. Swimming is a normal recreational activity of all children and should not be discouraged. Both pool and sea water may be harmful but on occasion sea water may even be beneficial. To prevent the harmful effect all the skin should be thoroughly coated with emulsifying ointment or some other oily preparation before entering the water. If you wish to use emulsifying ointment ask your doctor to prescribe it by the kilogram. Many swimming pools have chlo-

rinated water in the showers and a shower at the pool should be followed by an oil bath at home.

11. Join the Eczema Society (p. 352). This society sends out information about eczema and parents often obtain useful 'tips' about its management which may not have been given by the paediatrician or dermatologist (skin specialist). The Society publishes a quarterly magazine called *Exchange* which contains interesting and useful information about eczema.

As mentioned previously, children with eczema are usually allergic to a variety of substances. The number of these substances is too numerous to make allergy tests worth while and they are seldom performed. It can sometimes take days for eczema to become worse after exposure to an allergen, making it very difficult to identify the cause accurately and, indeed, know what to avoid. Avoidance measures are generally unhelpful unless a specific factor can be shown on *repeated* occasions to cause worsening of the eczema. For example, if eczema becomes worse on each occasion a cat is stroked then it would seem wise to avoid cats. In general I do not recommend getting rid of family pets where children have eczema or asthma.

A few children benefit from special diets. Many dietary substances may make eczema worse; the most common are eggs, milk, colouring agents and preservatives. A diet avoiding these foods should be undertaken only in close co-operation with a paediatrician and dietitian. The diet is complicated and unpleasant and there is no guarantee of success. It is only worth trying in the most severe forms of eczema; in less severe forms parents and children will often complain that the taste and inconvenience are worse than the eczema itself. Avoidance of single foods such as milk or eggs may be more convenient but not as effective.

Does breast feeding protect against eczema?

At the present time this issue is unresolved for there is no firm proof for or against breast feeding.

What is the risk of the next child having eczema?

The risk is about 1 in 4. Where 2 children in the family have eczema the risk for the next child is about 1 in 2. It should, however, be borne in mind that the severity need not necessarily be the same; a child with severe eczema may have a brother or sister with very mild eczema.

In conclusion, all cases of eczema, however severe, can be improved. At present we do not fully understand the cause and there is no cure. Effective management is time consuming and often frustrating but unfortunately there are no short cuts. The knowledge that things can only get better should allay despair and provide some incentive to bring the child through this difficult period emotionally unscathed.

SCABIES

Scabies is caused by a mite (insect) called *Sarcoptes scabei*. It has a rounded body, four sets of legs and is about 0.4mm long. The male is about half the size of the female. Males and females mate on the surface of the skin, then the pregnant female spends the rest of her life constructing a winding burrow in the surface layer of the skin (Fig. 12/2). Saliva from the mite partially digests and softens the skin making it easier to eat and tunnel through.

The male lives only a day or two. The female lives about 30 days, eventually dying at the end of the burrow. At times she may live as long as 2 months, when her burrow may be as long as 3cm. During this time she lays 2–3 eggs a day. These soon hatch to form larvae, which develop into adults and make their way to the skin surface at the same time. The whole cycle then starts again. Fortunately, less than 10% of eggs actually give rise to adults; the number of adult female mites per child is about 11 or 12.

Scabies can affect all ages, but is more common in adults. It characteristically affects certain parts of the body: the sides of fingers and webs between fingers, wrists, elbows, armpits, female breasts, and the areas around the umbilicus, penis and lower buttocks. The rash is

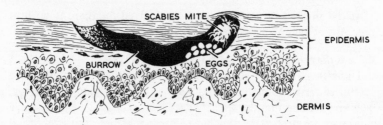

Fig. 12/2 Scabies, showing the mite and eggs in a burrow

very itchy, particularly at night, and consists of red bumps and lumps (papules and nodules) a few millimetres in diameter. In young children the disease is often missed because the mites can involve unusual sites such as the scalp, face, neck, palms and soles. These children may also have a fine blister (vesicular) rash. The intense itch causes the child to scratch so that burrows are only occasionally seen. Instead, sore, weepy (eczematous) areas are formed, sometimes leading to the mistaken diagnosis of eczema. These areas soon become crusted over and may get infected.

The itch in scabies is thought to be caused by an allergic reaction to the saliva of the mite; the child first develops the rash and becomes itchy about 4 weeks after infestation. In a few children there may be an 'allergic rash' (urticaria) which may cause confusion and delay the diagnosis of scabies. After a child has been treated for scabies his allergy persists so that reinfestation at a later date causes an immediate allergic reaction. Within a few hours the child becomes very itchy and the mites are destroyed, by scratching or the allergic reaction in the skin. It is therefore not possible to get scabies twice.

Scabies is caused by prolonged skin contact which frequently occurs when young children lie in bed with their infested parents. It may be spread when children hold hands during games. The female mite has spines on her back which she uses to bore directly upwards through the skin as she transfers to the skin of the new host. The process obviously takes time, hence the need for prolonged contact. Scabies never leaves the skin except to transfer to another human host. Contrary to public belief clothing and bedding do not transmit scabies and do not require any special treatment. Mites found on these items are either dead or dying and incapable of spreading to a new host. Within 24 hours of completion of treatment it is no longer possible for scabies to be transmitted from one person to another.

The diagnosis is usually made by finding an intensely itchy rash in sites typical of scabies, particularly when a close contact has a similar rash. The diagnosis can be supported by taking a skin scraping of a non-scratched bump or burrow and examining it under the microscope. The presence of the mite, its eggs or faeces will confirm the diagnosis.

When the child is treated, all close personal contacts are treated at the same time so that spread can be prevented. Because the rash and itch take a month to develop, close family members who have no rash should also be treated. There are three insecticides commonly used to treat scabies. The most widely used in Britain is benzyl benzoate, and gamma benzene hexachloride in the USA. Neither is used on the face; young children with facial scabies are usually treated with crotamiton (ointment or lotion) which is less irritating. When using benzyl benzoate it is desirable but not essential to take a warm bath before applying the lotion. This facilitates skin penetration of the insecticide. It is best for young children not to have a bath before applying gamma benzene hexachloride. This preparation is normally rapidly absorbed into the bloodstream and there has been concern about the safety of large amounts in the blood.

Benzyl benzoate (25%) is safe and effective but unpleasant to use. The liquid is thick and sticky with a characteristic odour and may be irritating to the inflamed skin. A half-strength application should be used for children (quarter-strength for infants). A suitable regimen is as follows:

1. After a warm bath the child should be dried.
2. The entire body below the neck should be completely covered and allowed to dry.
3. A second application is given after 24 hours. The child should *not* bath before this application but should wait a further 24 hours before bathing. A 4–5cm paintbrush is often used for painting on the liquid in older children and adults.

Gamma benzene hexachloride (1%) lotion is found to be more acceptable than benzyl benzoate by most older children and adults. It has a pleasant odour and requires only one application. It is applied to the whole body below the neck and washed off after six hours. There is, however, a question mark over the safety of this preparation in children, particularly infants. Most recent evidence suggests that it is safe with the following provisos:

1. Excessive amounts should not be used.
2. It should be washed off at the recommended time.
3. Care should be taken to make sure the skin is not licked or sucked.

Crotamiton (10%) is applied to the face when there is a facial rash. Like benzyl benzoate a second application is given after 24 hours. Care must be taken to avoid the eyes. Crotamiton does not appear to be as effective as the two preparations already mentioned. Unlike the other treatments it is very effective in relieving the itch.

It is most important to realise that itching can persist for 2–4 weeks after treatment and often becomes worse immediately afterwards. Persistent itching does *not* require further applications of insecticide. Local application of crotamiton on the itchy areas may provide some relief, or the itching may be helped by taking antihistamines by mouth. When the scabies rash is raw and inflamed (eczematous) it is sometimes treated with hydrocortisone ointment. This is very helpful but the hydrocortisone should only be used *after* the insecticide part of the treatment is complete. An infected rash is usually treated with antibiotics by mouth.

Can a child get scabies from a dog?

Yes, this can occur when a child has prolonged contact with the infested animal, usually a puppy. It is an uncommon problem but when it does occur both the child and the animal need treatment with insecticide.

THE HEAD LOUSE (PEDICULOSIS CAPITIS)

The incidence of head louse appears to be increasing and in Britain the number of children affected each year is about half a million. The peak age incidence is between 4–6. Each year in September thousands of children at school medical examinations are found to have lice. Unfortunately the way the 'discovery' is handled often leaves a lot to be desired, causing shame or distress among families and over-reaction and panic in the schools. As the news spreads like wildfire through the community, countless numbers of parents turn to the family doctor for advice. It is to be hoped that the information provided here will dispel some of the common myths about lice and aid in its eradication.

A louse is an insect which is a grey-tan colour and little larger than a pinhead, the length being 2–3mm (Fig. 12/3a). The lice make their home in the warm semi-dark areas of the scalp and the average number per child is between 12 and 25. They derive their nourishment (blood) by biting the scalp. A child with just 12 lice will suffer more than 50 bites each day.

The lifespan of a louse is about 40 days during which females lay about 5 eggs daily, each firmly glued to the base of a hair. The eggs actually touch or are close to the scalp, the warmth of which is required for hatching. The eggs take about a week to hatch leaving an empty eggshell (called a nit) still attached to the hair (Fig. 12/3b). As

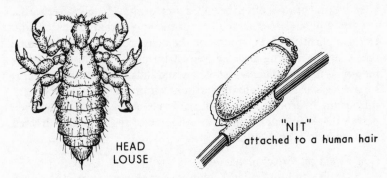

Fig. 12/3 (a) Head louse; (b) 'Nit' attached to a hair

the hair grows the nit moves away from the scalp. Hair grows about 1cm a month, and it is therefore easy to estimate the age of infestation by measuring the distance between the scalp and the most distant nit. The average British school child has had the infestation for 4 months. The number of lice is kept down by combing or scratching; such actions injure the louse, preventing its laying eggs.

Contrary to public belief, having lice is not a 'dirty' disease. It is common in *all* social classes and is in no way connected with the frequency with which the child baths or washes his hair. Long hair does not make louse infestation more likely, on the contrary, lice seem to prefer short hair. Interestingly, infestation seems to be slightly more common in girls than boys.

What are the clinical effects of lice?

The first few thousand louse bites cause no reaction, leave no mark and pass unnoticed. Eventually the louse saliva (spit) causes an allergic reaction and the head becomes very itchy. Infestation with many lice for a long time may make the child feel unwell and, rarely, an allergic rash develops on the body. The intense itch causes the child to scratch and the scalp skin may become severely irritated and infected. Oozing septic sores and scabs on the back of the scalp and behind the ears together with enlarged glands at the back of the neck are sometimes seen.

How are lice diagnosed?

It is often very difficult to see lice. When the hair is parted the light causes them to move very quickly and they are soon hidden from view. The diagnosis is usually based on finding nits in the hair. Nits are shiny grey oval-shaped specks which unlike dandruff are firmly attached to the hair and will not fall off. Examination with a magnifying glass is also helpful. Dandruff is an irregular shape and encircles the hair while nits are round and attached to the side of the hair.

What is the treatment?

In Britain there are two commonly used insecticides, malathion and carbaryl, both highly effective in killing both the louse and the eggs. These agents are available in 2 forms, lotions and shampoos. Unlike shampoos lotions require only a single application and are to be preferred. With the exception of Derbac, all lotions contain alcohol. Not only are the alcohol containing preparations more irritating to the skin, but they are also inflammable so that the hair should always be allowed to dry naturally. Hair dryers or any form of heating should be avoided. The following regimen is the one I recommend:

1. Apply lotion (malathion or carbaryl) to roots of hair and scalp at night. Rub gently into the scalp making sure that all hair on the scalp, around the ears and back of neck, is covered. Try to avoid getting the lotion in the eyes.
2. Leave to dry naturally and wash in ordinary shampoo the next morning.

All the lice and eggs are killed within 2 hours of exposure, but it is desirable that the lotions be left on for 8–12 hours. This will allow the insecticide to bond to the hair. Alcohol containing solutions bond particularly well and malathion does this better than carbaryl. Bonding of the insecticide to the hair prevents reinfection of a treated head because any louse reinvading that head will rub off insecticide on to its body; the insecticide may not kill the louse but will impair its reproductive ability.

In the USA, malathion has recently been withdrawn from the market. Two commonly-used preparations are gamma benzene hexachloride (Lindane; Kwell) and 1% permethrin which is marketed under the name of 'Nix'.

Since the nit is an empty eggshell, it cannot cause re-infestation and need not be removed. Removal is difficult and uncomfortable and is only desirable if an improvement in the cosmetic appearance is sought. Nits are best removed when the hair is wet. Applying a 1:1 vinegar:water rinse prior to removal helps. A fine steel comb with teeth close enough together to allow the eggs to be caught is necessary. Plastic combs are unsuitable. After combing the comb can be cleaned with soap and water.

Scalp infections are treated with antibiotics either applied to the scalp or taken by mouth.

How can the spread of lice be prevented?

For obvious reasons all members of a family should be treated at the same time. Lice are normally spread by direct head-to-head contact as they can neither jump nor fly. Contrary to public belief lice cannot be spread by brushes, combs, hats, scarfs, bedding or chairs. A louse is happiest on the head and does its best to stay there. Only those which are injured and therefore unable to reproduce are dislodged from the head and found on these objects.

MISCELLANEOUS SKIN, MOUTH AND TONGUE DISORDERS

Harmless spots

MILIA

These are tiny yellow or white spots on the cheek, nose, chin or forehead of newborn babies. They are very common and usually go after 3 weeks, but may last as long as 4 months.

MILIARIA (SWEAT RASH)

These are spots or small blisters which occur on the sides of the neck, upper chest, in the groins or armpits of infants. A sweat rash is caused by overheating. The treatment is to make sure the child does not get too hot. Sweat rashes sometimes get infected and require antibiotic treatment.

ERYTHEMA TOXICUM (URTICARIA NEONATORUM)

This is usually seen soon after birth. White spots surrounded by a red area come and go during the first 10 days. They may be confused with septic spots, but they can be easily differentiated by examining the contents of the spot under a microscope. These spots have a characteristic cell called an eosinophil. The cause of erythema toxicum is not known; it is seldom seen in premature infants.

Harmless marks

SALMON PATCHES

These are present at birth in well over a quarter of infants. They are pink marks over the eyelids, forehead and base of nose and nape of neck (stork mark). Except for the stork mark, which often persists but will probably be covered by hair, other marks disappear by the first birthday.

STRAWBERRY MARK (CAPILLARY HAEMANGIOMA)

This is particularly common in premature infants. It is usually not present at birth but starts as a red spot which rapidly enlarges in the first months to look like a strawberry: the speed with which it enlarges sometimes causes parents alarm. After the first 18 months there is no increase in size. At about 2½ it gradually fades from the centre so that by school age almost all will have disappeared.

Nappy (diaper) rash

Most infants have nappy rash to some extent. There are 3 types.

1. IRRITANT DERMATITIS

Prolonged irritation of the skin by a moist nappy which contains urine and stools is the cause. The rash is usually limited to the margins of the nappy with sparing of the flexures (creases). Sometimes areas of broken skin, which look like burns, are seen. Irritant nappy rash is commonly infected with thrush (a fungus). The skin can be protected by applying zinc and castor oil or petroleum jelly to the nappy area each time the child is changed. Where possible the bottom should be kept exposed but if nappies are worn they should be changed frequently and plastic pants avoided. Cotton nappies should be thoroughly rinsed. If there is no response to this regimen an antifungal cream should also be prescribed.

2. THRUSH

This fungal infection causes a dark red rash which is often slightly scaly. Unlike irritant dermatitis it usually involves the flexures (creases), there are often patches (satellite lesions) extending beyond the main area of the rash. Thrush is treated with nystatin or an imidazole antifungal cream; the cream should continue to be applied for a few days after the rash has subsided. Many children will also have thrush in the mouth for which treatment may be required.

3. INFANTILE SEBORRHOEIC DERMATITIS
(also called napkin psoriasis)

The cause of this rash is not known; about 20% later develop eczema. The rash, which is usually red and scaly, starts in the first weeks of life but can occur later in infancy. The napkin area or the scalp (cradle cap) are the first areas involved, the rash then spreads to the face, neck, top of chest, armpits and rest of trunk. The child is generally healthy and not in any discomfort. The rash responds dramatically to daily oil baths and regular applications of a cream containing a very mild steroid and antifungal agent.

Miscellaneous conditions

CHILBLAINS (PERNIOSIS)

They are caused by exposure to cold and occur mainly on the fingers, toes, nose, ears, and occasionally on the legs in girls with short dresses and no tights. The chilblain is a blue or red patch, which may have areas of broken skin. Toes and fingers may be swollen and itchy, occasionally painful. Cold, swollen hands are common in infants. Treatment is to avoid exposure to cold, after which the chilblains go in 1–2 weeks.

THE SACROCOCCYGEAL (PILONIDAL) DIMPLE

It is quite common to find a skin dimple in the midline at the lower end of the spine over the sacrum. The dimple sometimes opens into a blind tract (sinus). This abnormality is permanent and of no significance. In adults, however, infections do occasionally occur in the tract, antibiotics and surgical treatment may be required.

Allergic and infective rashes

It is thought that these rashes are caused by an allergy or an infection. The allergy is usually caused by a food or drug rather than something the child has inhaled.

THE HENOCH SCHÖNLEIN SYNDROME
(also called anaphylactoid or allergic purpura)

It commonly affects children between 2–10. The cause is not known but is thought to be due to allergies to foods, drugs and infections. In the vast majority it is not possible to establish the cause. The main features of Henoch Schonlein syndrome are a rash, joint pain, abdominal pain, and blood in the urine (haematuria). The rash, which is characteristic, is always present, other features need not be present.

The rash is found on the back of the limbs, particularly the ankles and buttocks. Small red areas of skin haemorrhage (purpura) join together to give larger areas of haemorrhage and bruising. Bleeding under the skin of the eyelids and scrotum may occur. The rash has a tendency to occur over areas of pressure such as underneath the elastic at the top of the socks. It may come and go over a period of many months. Some children, particularly the young ones, develop swelling of the face, hands and feet.

Joint involvement may be pain only (arthralgia) or painful swelling (arthritis) (p. 257). Ankle and knee swelling is most common. Abdominal pain may be accompanied by diarrhoea and vomiting. Occasionally blood is seen in the stool or vomit.

A small quantity of blood in the urine is common, but in only a third is it obvious (macroscopic). Blood may appear in the urine several months after the rash. Generally, symptoms do not occur in any order, usually they occur within a week of each other and sometimes recur over a period of several weeks. There is no treatment. A few children with blood in the urine do require follow-up to make sure the blood clears and that there is no lasting kidney disease.

ERYTHEMA MULTIFORME

It is a 'target-like' rash which mainly occurs on the hands, feet, back, elbows and knees and may be itchy. A red ring surrounds a purple centre, which at times forms a small blister. When the rash fades the purple centre often persists for a few days giving the impression of bruising. The child may have a temperature and be off colour. Arthralgia (p. 258) and swelling of the feet are common. No treatment is required other than calamine lotion, which is applied to the skin if the itch is severe.

A more extensive form of the illness is known as Stevens–Johnson syndrome. Children with this syndrome have mouth, eye and genital involvement and may be very ill. They are admitted to hospital where they are treated with antibiotics and steroids.

HIVES (URTICARIA)

Rubbing against nettles produces hives, hence the descriptive term 'nettle rash'. It is a common problem affecting about 1 in 10 children at some time. It is more frequently seen in girls and is particularly common in children with allergies. The rash appears as raised, well-demarcated red or pink areas. These areas which may be itchy join up with one another and are known as wheals. Although allergy or infection are thought to be the most likely cause, the real cause cannot usually be found. Other causes of urticaria are emotion, exercise, heat or cold. In some children the condition persists for months or years, when it is called 'chronic'. It may sometimes be associated with swelling of the eyes, lips, tongue and throat. The vast majority of children do not have any problems, but very rarely when there is throat swelling the airway may be blocked, requiring urgent attention. Any child with lip or face swelling who is having breathing difficulty should immediately be taken to an accident and emergency department where adrenaline (epinephrine) steroids and antihistamines will be given.

There is no treatment for urticaria other than antihistamines or calamine lotion applied to the skin to relieve itching. Allergy tests for chronic urticaria are not helpful. A short trial of a diet which excludes aspirin, preservatives and colouring agents is worth trying but is seldom of much use.

Viral skin problems

MOLLUSCUM CONTAGIOSUM

These are pearly 'pimples' which are common in infants and young children, particularly those with eczema. The 'pimples' which have a central depression may occur singly or in groups anywhere on the body. They are most common on the face, buttocks and trunk. No treatment is required, almost all go within a year.

WARTS

These are acquired by direct contact or by contact with something contaminated with the virus. They are usually seen in children over

4, can occur anywhere but are most common on the fingers (common warts) or soles. Those on the soles are flat and are called plantar warts or verrucae. Plantar warts are usually painful while other warts are not painful unless infected. Virtually all warts go within 3 years, some disappearing in months rather than years. It is best not to treat warts unless they are causing pain or embarrassment.

Below are outlined two schemes, one for treating the common wart and the other for plantar warts.

Common wart

1. Rub the surface of the wart with an emery board or pumice stone until the wart becomes flat.
2. Apply a drop of Salactol (USA Duofilm) – salicylic acid and lactic acid in collodion – to the centre of the wart and allow to dry.
3. Repeat nightly until the wart has disappeared. Treatment may need to be continued for a few months.

Plantar wart

1. After soaking in the bath, pare away as much of the overlying skin as possible. Use a pumice stone or emery board.
2. Apply a piece of 40% salicylic acid plaster to the area over the wart and hold in place with a wide adhesive bandage. It is *very* important to make sure that the salicylic acid plaster is only in contact with the wart and not normal skin.
3. Leave the plaster on for 2–3 days during which time the foot should be kept dry.
4. Repeat the procedure until the wart has disappeared completely, which usually occurs after a few weeks.

In the interests of public health children should not use public swimming pools until plantar warts are treated. Those children who have warts which do not respond to the regimens detailed above should be referred to a dermatologist (skin specialist).

Skin conditions of the foot

The following conditions all cause itching and are helped by avoiding trainers (sneakers), wearing cotton socks and leather shoes and thoroughly drying the feet and toes after bathing.

1. *Juvenile plantar dermatosis* is a recently described condition. Chil-

dren are usually between 5 and 13. The forefoot has a red, glazed, slightly scaly appearance and may be intensely itchy. The cause of the condition is thought to be synthetic materials in the manufacture of shoes or socks. Many of these children have a history of allergy. Treatment consists of paying particular attention to footwear: cotton socks and leather shoes should be worn. A steroid or tar preparation applied to the sole may help.

2. *Tinea pedis (athlete's foot)* is a fungal infection which is uncommon before puberty. It is best treated with an imidazole antifungal agent.

3. *Foot eczema* occurs at any age; usually eczema is present elsewhere (p. 236).

Conditions of the mouth and tongue

ORAL THRUSH

This is very common in newborn babies and is caused by a fungus called *Candida albicans*. White elevated patches which resemble curdled milk appear on the tongue, lips, inside the cheeks and in the throat. Unlike curdled milk it cannot easily be scraped away; such attempts may cause bleeding. Thrush is usually of no significance, but when it is extensive it may make the mouth sore causing difficulty with feeding. It is treated with nystatin or an imidazole antifungal agent. Treatment is given after feeds. Contrary to the belief of many parents, the presence of thrush does not suggest poor hygiene. Many infants with thrush in the mouth also have a thrush napkin rash. Thrush develops more commonly in infants given antibiotics.

HALITOSIS (BAD BREATH)

This problem often causes parents and children concern but is not easily remedied. It is frequently difficult to determine the cause of halitosis. Foods which cause smelly breath are easily recognised and can be avoided. Halitosis can be caused by dental caries and disease of the gums, nose, throat, sinuses or lungs. When no cause is obvious the best remedy is to use sweet-smelling mouth washes.

WHITE TONGUE

A furred white tongue is seen in some young infants and is of no significance. Unlike thrush, the tongue is uniformly involved; there are also no white patches elsewhere in the mouth.

BLACK TONGUE

Some children develop a black/brown patch on the tongue. This is of no significance and is likely to persist for a number of years.

GEOGRAPHIC TONGUE

Smooth, flat, grey patches move across the tongue and join up giving a maplike appearance, hence the name geographic tongue. The patches may come and go over many months or years. Occasionally children experience discomfort and a bland diet or steroids applied to the tongue may help. The cause is not known.

TONGUE TIE (ANKYLOGLOSSIA)

Many parents wrongly attribute feeding problems or slow speech to tongue-tie, which is the inability to protrude the tongue or lick the upper lip. It is rarely, if ever, necessary for an operation to be performed, and never before the first birthday.

DENTAL HYGIENE

Parents are advised to start brushing a child's teeth towards the end of the first year when a reasonable number of teeth have erupted. Teeth should be brushed twice daily after the morning and evening meals. Fluoride toothpaste should be used, the amount on the brush no larger than a pea. Other dental advice and dosage recommendation for oral fluoride are shown on page 186. Before starting fluoride check the fluoride content of the water in your area. This information should be available from your paediatrician or dentist. The first visit to a dentist should be made when the child is 2½–3. Regular 4–6 monthly check-ups should be arranged throughout early childhood.

Chapter Thirteen

Bone and Joint Problems

GROWING PAINS

'Growing pains' is the name used for recurrent limb pains. It is the commonest cause of limb pain in childhood, affecting about 5 in every 100 children in the UK. It is slightly more common in girls and occurs between 6 and 13. Although called 'growing pains' the cause is unknown and has nothing to do with growth. The reason for this misnomer is unclear and illogical because most children experience a growth spurt (period of rapid growth) after age 13.

Two-thirds of children have pains in the legs only while in the remaining one-third pain may be in the arms, trunk and legs, either at the same or different times. It is most unusual for growing pain to be only in the arms. The pain is not in the joints; it is typically found in the calves, thighs and behind the knees and is always bilateral (both sides). It may be made worse by excessive exercise during the day. Some children may have headaches and abdominal pain at the same or at different times. The pain, which is usually described as a 'deep ache' or 'heavy', comes on during the day or evening and in 25% occurs only at night. Pain at night is almost always only in the legs and may be severe enough to waken the child from sleep. Typically, severe pain during the night will have gone completely by morning; occasional children complain of heaviness in the limbs the next day. I have seen children with night pain so severe that they have been unable to walk, yet by morning they are perfectly well.

Children with growing pains are healthy, and examination of the child, both during and after the painful episode, does not reveal any abnormality. The diagnosis is made by the history and no blood tests are required. Growing pains cause much parental anxiety; many find it hard to accept that there is no rational explanation for the severe discomfort. Parents are usually told that there is nothing seriously wrong and that the child will eventually grow out of it, although it may persist intermittently for a few years. It is a common source of friction between parents and doctor. Distressed parents often feel frustrated by the unsympathetic doctor who repeatedly examines the child and, on finding no abnormality, does no more than call it 'psychological'. In some children and their families there are emotional problems, but the majority of children I see with growing pains are well adjusted and from happy families. Interestingly, other members of the family often have 'rheumatic' complaints. A number of parents also suffered from bellyaches, headaches or limb pains as children.

In my experience analgesics (painkillers) do not appear to have any effect in treating growing pains. During the day most children are kept occupied and learn to tolerate the pain. At night the pain is eased by rubbing and will pass off after a short while when the child falls asleep. Hot water bottles (covered) placed over the painful areas also give effective pain relief.

ARTHRITIS

Arthritis means joint inflammation, arthralgia is the term used for joints which are painful but do not appear to be inflamed. Arthritis can be divided into acute and chronic: acute has a sudden onset and rapid recovery while persistent arthritis is called chronic.

Acute arthritis

In general, this can be divided into conditions affecting single joints or many joints.

SINGLE JOINTS

The most common cause of single joint inflammation is a bacterial infection of the joint, this being called septic arthritis and sometimes septic osteomyelitis when the bone around the joint is also infected. Children with this condition have a painful swollen joint, a high fever and are generally unwell. They require intravenous antibiotics for at least 1–2 weeks. If the child does not show much improvement in the first day or two pus may need to be removed from the joint or bone by insertion of a drain (fine rubber tubing) under general anaesthetic. Intensive antibiotic treatment and drainage of pus is usually followed by complete recovery.

MANY JOINTS

The cause of arthritis in many joints is usually a virus or an allergy. There are several viral infections, including rubella, mumps, chicken-pox and glandular fever which may be associated with arthritis. This form of arthritis is usually mild and gets better without treatment within a few weeks, sometimes being followed by arthralgia for a few weeks. Occasionally aspirin, which provides pain relief and reduces inflammation, may be helpful if the joint pain is severe. Viral arthritis, especially when it follows a sore throat, may mimic rheumatic fever. This may cause concern to parents, particularly grandparents who may still have memories of rheumatic fever. In industrialised countries like Britain there is now no cause for concern; I have yet to see a case of rheumatic fever in Britain.

Allergy, the other cause of arthritis affecting many joints, is associated with characteristic skin rashes, the skin conditions being known as anaphylactoid (Henoch Schönlein) purpura (p. 250) and erythema multiforme (p. 251). The arthritis in anaphylactoid purpura involves mainly the knees and ankles and symptoms seldom persist for more than a few days, but may recur. The arthritis in erythema multiforme is mild, arthralgia probably being more common.

What is an 'irritable hip'?

This is also called observation hip or transient synovitis of the hip. It is the commonest cause of hip pain in children under 10, being particularly common in those under 6. Boys are more affected than girls. The onset is usually sudden, but may come on slowly; the child will complain of pain in the hip (sometimes knee as well). He may walk with a limp or pain may be so severe that he is unable to bear weight. He is generally well, although there may be a slight fever. The cause is unknown; it is thought that the joint lining (synovium) may be transiently inflamed following an injury or viral infection. Hip x-rays are usually normal. A second episode sometimes occurs in the other hip. There is no treatment: the joint usually recovers after a few days' rest. Perthes disease, a serious hip disease of unknown cause in which the head of the femur fragments, may start as an irritable hip. To exclude Perthes disease an x-ray of the hip should always be done at the time of diagnosis of irritable hip and again 3 months later.

Chronic arthritis

How common is it?
It affects about 1 in 1000 children.

What is the cause?
There is no known cause. There is no clear evidence of inherited factors in most children with chronic arthritis.

Is it the same condition as adult rheumatoid arthritis?
About 90% of children with chronic arthritis have a totally different disease. The few children with the adult form of the disease have 'juvenile rheumatoid arthritis'. It usually affects girls and seldom before age 11. Joints of the hands are mainly affected and serious damage may arise if the condition is not recognised and properly treated.

How is 'juvenile rheumatoid arthritis' recognised?
This is the only form of arthritis in children in which a blood factor called rheumatoid factor (RF) is found.

What is the main type of chronic arthritis?
Of the 90% who are RF negative the vast majority (about three-quarters) have 'juvenile chronic arthritis' (Fig. 13/1).

What is juvenile chronic arthritis?
It is defined as an arthritis of more than 3-months' duration before the 16th birthday where no cause has been found. Depending on which joints are involved and whether other signs or symptoms exist it can be subdivided into 3 categories; pauci-articular (60%), polyarticular (20%) and systemic (20%).

What is pauci-articular arthritis?
Pauci means few. It is the name given when only a few (4 or less) joints are swollen; a single swollen joint is called monarticular arthritis. It affects mainly young girls and older boys.

The form that affects girls occurs under 5. The joints most commonly involved are ankles, knees and occasionally hips. There is little disturbance of general health. A third develop inflammatory eye disease (chronic uveitis), which is particularly common in those with a blood factor known as antinuclear factor (ANF).

The pauci-articular arthritis in boys usually occurs after 9. Knees are most commonly affected followed by hips and ankles. They, too,

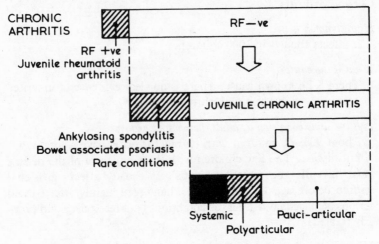

Fig. 13/1 Types of chronic arthritis and their distribution

are well but occasionally develop an eye complaint (acute iritis). Unlike the eye problem in the young child this is usually obvious as a painful red eye: the need for a close watch of the eyes is therefore unnecessary.

What is polyarticular arthritis?

It is an arthritis involving more than four joints which affects mainly girls at any age. They usually have symmetrical (both sides) involvement of the hands and fingers but any joint can be involved including the jaw (temporomandibular) and neck joints (cervical spine). Other than pain there may be little effect on general health. Knee pain and swelling is common, stiffening in a mechanically bad position (contracture formation) will occur unless care is taken to prevent this.

What is systemic onset arthritis?

This form of arthritis is also known as Still's disease. It is the name given to the arthritis in which the child has a persistent fever, is ill, and has many features other than pain in the joints. It affects boys and girls equally and usually occurs between 1 and 5. It starts with a fever, which tends to be very high at night and falling by midday, like an infection, but it may persist for days or weeks. A rash which is

most apparent at the height of the fever and fades when the temperature falls is one of the most distinctive features. Red blotches which
may be itchy come and go. Glands in the neck, under the arms and in
the groins commonly enlarge. Abdominal organs (liver and spleen)
may enlarge. Occasionally there may be inflammation of the lining of
the heart (pericarditis) and less often the lungs (pleurisy). At first
there may be no pain in joints, a mild arthralgia, or one or two painful
swollen joints; occasionally many joints are affected right from the
start. When the temperature is high the child will be listless and
unwell, not wanting to take notice of anything. He may brighten up
by midday as the temperature falls, only to become unwell again in
the evening as the temperature rises. If the systemic illness continues
for many weeks or months the child will lose weight, become pale and
anaemic and progressively weaker.

How is juvenile chronic arthritis diagnosed?

It is diagnosed on clinical grounds. The characteristic fever pattern
and the rash which comes and goes are particularly helpful pointers to
the systemic onset type. Routine blood tests usually include antinuclear factor (ANF) or RF. These do not diagnose the condition but
are of use in categorising the type.

What of the future?

It is not possible to predict accurately the outlook for an individual
child. It can be said, however, that the outlook is very good: as many
as three-quarters will eventually grow out of the disease. Of those that
do not grow out of it, a few will have joints going out of shape and not
working properly. Even for them, better management improves the
outlook.

What are the principles of management?

Because there is no cure, management is really a 'holding operation' to achieve the best functional and cosmetic affect until such
time as the child grows out of it. Joint function and appearance can be
maintained by provision of medication to prevent pain and suppress
joint inflammation and by regular physiotherapy.

How can parents help?

Parents can help by playing an active role at home in all aspects.
The outlook depends to some extent on the ability and co-operation
of parents who may need considerable support themselves during the
often protracted course of the illness. Adaptations to the home may

be required but only for those few children who are very severely affected. Financial assistance for these adaptations can usually be obtained from the local authority social services. The organisation responsible for the provision of 'aids for daily living' varies from area to area but may be the province of the physiotherapist, occupational therapist or social worker.

What does physiotherapy involve?

The physical management of a child is just as important as any medication and possibly more important. Physiotherapy involves keeping the joints moving so that they do not stiffen up and become permanently fixed in an abnormal position which is both unsightly and mechanically unsound. The physiotherapist will ensure that the joints are exercised each day and that during rest they are immobilised in a straight position. Exercise is an important part of the management and should become part of the child's normal activities. Non-weight-bearing exercises such as swimming and cycling are particularly useful and should be encouraged. The physiotherapist may supervise swimming in a warm water pool (hydrotherapy). It allows muscles to relax and permits movement of joints with minimal discomfort. Arthritis is almost always worse in the morning: a hot bath as soon as the child wakes provides relief and is a good time to put his joints through their movements. At home, hot water bottles applied to painful joints before physiotherapy may also help. Make sure that they are not too hot! During the active phase of the disease contact sports such as rugby, football and hockey are best avoided as trauma can cause sudden 'flare-ups'.

Rest in bed is rarely necessary and should be reserved only for those children who are very ill with systemic disease. Bed posture during sleep is very important: the physiotherapist will provide advice about this. Pillows should *never* be placed under the knees even if the child complains of pain, as this encourages a bent knee deformity. The physiotherapist may provide 'rest splints', which when worn during rest prevent or correct bent joint deformities (contractures) by keeping the legs straight. Most modern splints are made of a plastic-like material which is moulded to fit the individual child. Very occasionally 'working splints' are required for wear during the day to provide support for weak joints. Should there be serious involvement of the hips or knees the child should be encouraged to stretch them out by lying on his front (prone) for an hour or two each day. Most children are quite happy to lie on the floor watching television.

What is the medical treatment?

The medical treatment aims at providing pain relief and reducing inflammation to prevent muscle spasm around the joint. Some children, particularly young girls with single joint involvement, may require no treatment. The drugs usually used are known as non-steroidal anti-inflammatory drugs (NSAIDS). These include aspirin, naproxen, indomethacin, ibuprofen, diclofenac and tolmetin sodium. It is important to spread doses so as to provide full relief around the clock: your paediatrician will give you precise advice. These drugs are given by mouth, but suppositories which act slowly are often used last thing at night to alleviate early morning stiffness.

For those children whose arthritis does not improve after several months or years on NSAIDS, or who are developing joint damage, shown on *x*-ray, special anti-rheumatic disease modifying drugs with a prolonged effect are used. Anti-rheumatic drugs include gold, penicillamine and chloroquine. These drugs may have serious side-effects and their use is best supervised by a paediatrician with a special interest in arthritis.

Corticosteroid drugs such as prednisolone are occasionally used. The only indication for their use is when systemic illness is severe.

Will he go to a normal school?

Most children are able to live at home and attend a normal school, their treatment being supervised on an outpatient basis. Only a few children are educated at schools for the physically handicapped, where both their physical and educational needs can best be met by expert facilities on the premises and specially trained teachers.

How often should the eyes be checked?

Chronic uveitis occurs in about 10%. Unfortunately, unlike acute iritis the child will be completely unaware of the problem in its early stages when it is curable. It can, however be recognised in the early stage by examination by an ophthalmologist (eye specialist) using a special instrument called a slit lamp. Because delay in treatment may lead to serious eye damage or blindness, all children with pauci-articular arthritis and antinuclear antiobodies (ANA) should have slit lamp examination every 3–4 months. All other types should be checked at least yearly. It is important to remember that the eye checks should continue for many years even if the arthritis has settled.

What about surgery?

This is sometimes necessary to repair damaged joints and to conserve joint function.

What are the other types of chronic arthritis?

These comprise about a quarter of all RF negative arthritis (Fig. 13/1). They can be divided into 4 categories; juvenile ankylosing spondylitis, bowel associated arthritis, psoriasis and rare conditions.

Ankylosing spondylitis: there is a considerable overlap with boys in the pauci-articular group, hips, knees and ankles being most commonly affected. There is also a strong family history and most carry the genetic factor HLAB27; the latter may also be carried by normal family members. A quarter develop acute iritis. The first x-ray changes of ankylosing spondylitis occur in the bottom part of the spine where it joins the hip girdle (sacro iliac joints); eventually the process extends upwards causing stiffening of the spine. The outlook for children is better than for those who develop it in later life.

Bowel associated arthritis: an arthritis may develop in bowel conditions such as ulcerative colitis, Crohn's disease and dysentery.

Psoriasis: it is a scaly skin disease which often runs in families and can occur with arthritis. The psoriasis first becomes apparent at about 9 or 10 and in some children the arthritis may precede the skin signs.

Rare conditions: arthritis may occur in a disease known as systemic lupus erythematosis (SLE), in sickle cell anaemia – a disease mainly of Afro–Caribbean people – and in Mediterranean fever, a disease which affects people living in countries around the Mediterranean.

When your Child has Arthritis, by Barbara Ansell, is a helpful book and is available from the Arthritis and Rheumatism Council (p. 351).

THE UNSTABLE/DISLOCATED HIP

The hip joint is a ball and socket joint. The top of the thigh bone (femur) is called the head; it is rounded like a ball and fits snugly within a socket which is part of the pelvis. The outstretched leg is able to rotate by movement of the ball in the socket. In the newborn, when the hips are examined, they are called unstable when gentle pressure on the thigh bone is able to move the head out of the socket. When the head lies outside the socket, even though it can be temporarily placed in the socket, it is called dislocated.

Very occasionally the socket is underdeveloped, enabling the head to slip out, but the vast majority of unstable and dislocated hips are normally formed. The main cause for the extra moblity of the head appears to be laxity of the ligaments which normally hold the head firmly in the socket.

How common is it?

The incidence is generally found to be between 0.75–1.5/1000 births.

What causes it?

We do not know for certain but there are probably several causes. It runs in families, affects girls more than boys and over a third have been in the breech position in late pregnancy. Either or both hips may be dislocated but in about half it is the left. The association with breech positions and girls has led to speculation that there may be a mechanical cause, or alternatively, an excess of female hormones may cause ligament laxity.

Are dislocated hips sore?

There is no pain at all; she will be totally unaware that her hips are dislocated.

How are dislocated hips diagnosed?

You will probably have seen the doctor examining your child. The thighs are gripped firmly and by movement and pressure an attempt is made to manipulate the head in and out of the socket. In the newborn, x-rays are not very helpful, the diagnosis being based almost entirely on clinical examination.

Why do we need to know the hips are dislocated?

For every 6 children, 5 will correct themselves spontaneously. If not treated, those that do not correct will eventually become permanently damaged, causing leg shortening, limping and severe pain in the hip joint. To prevent this serious situation from developing screening newborns has become routine since the middle 1960s. If detected early and treated properly virtually all dislocated hips can be put right. Although it was originally hoped that all dislocated hips would be detected and treated this has not been the case; the reason for failure of detection is not clear.

Because it is not possible to know which hip will resolve spontaneously, it has become necessary to treat all dislocated/unstable hips. The only side-effect of treatment is damage to the femoral head which it must be emphasised is very rare.

What is the treatment?

The treatment is splintage. The purpose of the splint is to keep the legs wide apart so that they cannot be brought together, ensuring that the head of the femur is firmly positioned in the socket. The hips remain splinted until they are stable. The length of time depends to a certain extent on whether the hips were unstable or dislocated, and may be as little as 6 weeks or as long as 9 months (average 6 months).

There are many splints used to treat this condition, the type depending on the preference of the orthopaedic surgeon (doctor who specialises in treating bone and joint diseases).

There is no urgency about fitting splints; they are usually fitted within a week or two of birth. Depending on the custom of the orthopaedic surgeon some infants may be admitted for a short stay on a children's orthopaedic ward.

What about follow-up?

This varies widely with the surgeon and the type of splint.

What about double or triple nappies?

This is a most unreliable form of treatment, one I would never recommend. If the hips are truly unstable or dislocated then *proper* splintage is required.

What about baby slings and baby walkers?

A baby sling to carry the child does no harm but choose one that keeps the legs wide apart. It is best to avoid baby walkers as they put an unnecessary strain on the hip, which is only just recovering.

What is the treatment for a dislocated hip which is not detected at birth?

It depends on the age of the child. Over 8 treatment is generally not recommended as hip damage has already occurred. Over 6 months the child will require hospital admission during which traction will be given. The joint ligaments will be stretched by attaching a pulley and weights to the leg. After this procedure, known as traction, the head of the femur will be manipulated into the socket under general anaesthesia and immobilised by splinting. Where this is not possible then surgery will be undertaken. Interestingly, the number of children having surgery nowadays is no different from the number before screening was introduced.

CLUB FOOT (TALIPES)

This is a common abnormality affecting about 1 in 1000 births. It can affect one or both feet. The feet are twisted inwards so that if the child were able to stand he would not stand on the sole but on the side of the foot. The calf muscle and foot are usually smaller than normal. It is twice as common in boys and there is a strong familial tendency.

What is the treatment?

Treatment should start as soon as possible after birth and no later than 3 days. The foot will be splinted by an orthopaedic surgeon or physiotherapist; it will be gently moulded towards the desired position with adhesive strapping and felt pads to protect the skin at pressure points. The child will be reviewed weekly, on each occasion the straps will be adjusted as the foot is moulded a little further. At about 6–8 weeks progress will be reviewed and an x-ray taken. In about half, the treatment will not have worked, in which case surgery is required. Whether or not surgery is required, splintage will continue at least until the child starts walking. The splints will be gradually adjusted at fortnightly and then monthly intervals until they are removed.

What about follow-up?

Most children with club feet continue to be observed throughout childhood by an orthopaedic surgeon. Despite early and careful treatment some feet revert to their former position necessitating splintage for many years. Further operations may also be necessary.

What are the chances of the next child having club feet?

Genetic advice depends on the sex of the child with club feet, whether the parents are normal, and their race. The incidence varies between races, it is particularly high in Polynesians (about 7/1000) and low in Chinese (about 0.4/1000). In whites, if the parents are normal and the child with a club foot is a boy, the risk is 2% for the next child; 5% if the child with a club foot is a girl. If both a parent and a child (either sex) have club feet the risk rises to 25%.

What is postural club foot?

It is quite frequent for normal feet to resemble club feet in the newborn. The distorted appearance arises from pressure on the feet as they are positioned in the womb. Postural club feet can easily be distinguished from true club feet by the fact that they can be manipulated easily into the correct position. No treatment is required, the feet will appear normal within a few weeks of birth.

IN-TOEING (PIGEON TOES)

There are 3 causes of in-toeing:

1. femoral anteversion
2. outward curved tibia
3. 'comma shaped' foot.

1. Femoral anteversion – the most common cause. The head of the femur is attached to the shaft by a segment of bone called the neck. Femoral anteversion means that the neck is angled forward so that when the leg is straight ahead (extended) outward rotation of the foot is limited and inward rotation increased. The normal range of movement compared with that of an anteverted femur is shown in Figure 13/2.

These children are most comfortable with their feet pointing inwards; standing, the legs appear bowed and the knee caps (patellae) point inwards. When they run their heels throw out to the sides in a characteristic and clumsy looking manner. Some sit with the inside (medial part) of the thighs touching the chair and their feet splayed out at the side, the so-called 'television position'. About 80% improve by the age of 8 and no treatment is required. Surgery after that age is uncommon and is reserved for only the most severe form. A mild degree of in-toeing is cosmetically acceptable and does not warrant surgery.

2. Outward curved tibia – the tibia is the main bone below the knee. In infancy the tibia is normally bowed, but in this form of in-toeing it is both bowed and twisted so that the foot is turned inwards (Fig. 13/3). One or both legs may be affected, left leg involvement being more

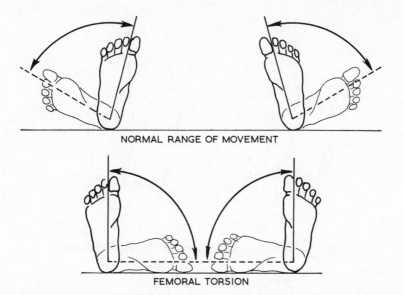

NORMAL RANGE OF MOVEMENT

FEMORAL TORSION

Fig. 13/2 Range of rotational leg movement from the hip with the leg extended: *above*: normal range; *below*: femoral anteversion

common. Parents are concerned about the fact that the legs do not point in the same direction; some actually worry about the normal leg turning outwards. Bow legs can also be caused by rickets and a rare bone condition called Blount's disease in which the bowing occurs at an acute angle in the upper part of the femur. There is no treatment for outward curved tibia; almost all have normal shaped legs and gait by 4.

3. 'Comma shaped' foot (metatarsus varus) (Fig. 13/5). This usually affects both feet, the foot curves inwards from heel to toes in the shape of a comma. The abnormal shape can look very alarming; anxious parents often feel that something should be done, and sooner rather than later. There is no treatment: in 90% the feet will have straightened by 4. It is not possible to predict accurately which ones will not straighten, but there is absolutely no harm in waiting until the child is 4, when abnormal feet will be corrected by moulding in plasters and only occasionally will surgery be required.

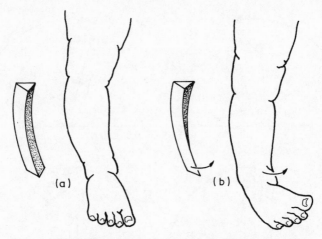

Fig. 13/3 (a) Normal bowed tibia. (b) Outward curved tibia

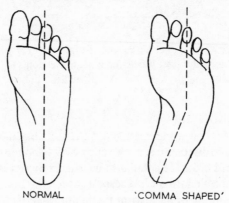

NORMAL   'COMMA SHAPED'

Fig. 13/4 Normal and 'comma shaped' feet

OUT-TOEING

The opposite of in-toeing is out-toeing or 'Charlie Chaplin'-like gait. In this case the neck of the femur is angled backwards. It is common in the first two years and is most frequently found in infants who lie on their front (prone). Because of extreme out-toeing these children often appear to have flat feet. The feet begin to look normal as the legs move into the correct position within a year of established walking. No treatment is needed.

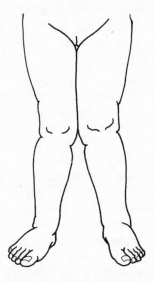

Fig. 13/5 A typical example of knock knee which corrects spontaneously

KNOCK KNEE (GENU VALGUM) (Fig. 13/5)

Three-quarters of children between 2 and 4½ have some degree of knock knee, often associated with loose joints. With the child lying with the legs together, a distance between the inner ankle bones (malleoli) of 9cm is quite normal. There is no treatment. Well over 90% correct themselves, the rare few that do not may require surgery in their teens. Shoe wedges serve only to protect the footwear, but do not improve the appearance.

FLAT FEET

All infants and toddlers start life with flat feet, this being more apparent than real. The arch is well-formed but is obscured by a pad of fat on the inside edge (medial side). Parental concern arises when they notice that on standing the child's inside arch touches the ground, or when walking with wet feet no arch is apparent in the footprint. As soon as the child can stand on tiptoe or raise his big toe an arch will be apparent. An arch will be apparent in normal stance by the 3rd birthday; it may take a little longer in children who walk very late. The shape of the foot in older children and adults is largely determined by genetic factors, some families having flat feet and others high arches.

When is flat foot a problem?

Almost all the children I see do not have a problem, the arch being apparent by 3 without any treatment. In the older child a flat foot which otherwise looks normal, with the child standing, requires no treatment. The only time treatment may be required is when the foot becomes pronated (heel and sole turn outwards). An imaginary line should normally run from the centre of the knee through the heel (Achilles) tendon to the centre of the heel. By standing behind the child you will be able to see if the foot is pronated, in which case the line will not run to the centre of the heel but to the inside (medial edge). When there is a marked degree of pronation the foot bones may grow abnormally and produce pain in adulthood. The aim of treatment is to maintain normal bone growth; the flat foot appearance which is caused by weak muscles and joint supports (ligaments) is not likely to be altered. There are various treatments, the most common being arch pads and heel wedges or special insoles.

TOE WALKING

There are three causes of toe walking, the most common being a habit. This will eventually correct itself, but encouraging the child to walk heel/toe or playing games walking on heels may be helpful. The other causes of toe walking are cerebral palsy (see p. 297) and tightening of the heel tendon.

CURLY TOES

This is a common problem: usually the fifth toe overlaps the fourth or lies beneath it. Occasionally the third toe lies below the edge of the second. Curly toes do not require any treatment. Strapping is useless. Surgery is only required when there is difficulty with shoe fitting or shoe irritation causes pain.

Choosing children's shoes

Shoes serve two purposes, first to keep the foot warm and second to protect the foot against sharp objects. There is no ideal age at which shoes should first be worn. While there is little need for shoes until the child walks, giving the child shoes earlier does no harm. Parents sometimes ask which is the best shoe for a child learning to walk. A soft shoe without a heel is most appropriate; it will enable the child to feel the contours of the ground without the risk of the heel's catching on objects. Contrary to the belief of many parents, a cheap pair of plimsoles (sneakers) are as good as anything. For the older child leather shoes which mould to the foot and allow the foot to 'breathe' are best.

It is most important that the shoes fit properly. An experienced shoe fitter can be very helpful. A simple rule is to make sure that when the child stands the distance between the big toe and the end of the shoe is about equal to the breadth of the child's thumb. The shoe should also be wide enough so that a pinch of leather can be squeezed between the fingers at the broadest part.

There are two common postural abnormalities seen in children.

CONGENITAL TORTICOLLIS (WRY NECK)

It is caused by shortening of the main neck muscle (sternocleido-mastoid) which is attached to the side of the head and the chest. In this condition the head does not face straight ahead but is lopsided, being inclined to the side with the shortened muscle. It is usually first apparent about 2–3 weeks after birth. Most have head tilting to the right and about a third have a palpable lump (like a small olive) in the middle of the shortened muscle. The lump, which is harmless, can usually not be felt before the first week and may be palpable for as long as 6 months. The cause of wry neck is unknown; it can occur after any delivery, but is more commonly associated with difficult forceps or breech delivery. In time, flattening of the face on the side of the shortened muscle may occur, probably due to pressure on the face as it is pressed against the mattress during sleep. About a fifth have dislocated hips; the reason for the association is not clear.

Without treatment, well over two-thirds recover spontaneously,.

but many orthopaedic surgeons do recommend neck 'stretch' exercises which are usually supervised by a physiotherapist. Surgery on the muscle to correct the deformity is sometimes necessary but seldom before 2 or 3.

Other causes of torticollis in children are tonsillitis: the inflamed neck gland causes the neck muscle to go into spasm (spastic torticollis) and vertical squint (p. 228). Spastic torticollis corrects itself with recovery from the throat infection, and squint correction results in normal head alignment.

SCOLIOSIS

It is a descriptive term signifying lateral (sideways) curvature of the spine and is the most common spinal abnormality seen in children. It is quite common for parents to consult a paediatrician about their teenager's posture. Most of these children slouch because they are at an awkward age, moreover they know it irritates their parents. Postural curving of the spine may occur quite naturally just before puberty and disappear with growth, no treatment being required. All children with spinal curvature should be made to bend forward – a postural curve will straighten whereas a structural abnormality of the spine will produce a rib hump, mostly on the right. The cause of the structural abnormality is unknown, it is called 'idiopathic'. It runs in families and affects girls more than boys, usually starting at the onset of puberty (adolescent idiopathic scoliosis). It probably affects about 2/1000 schoolchildren. The importance of detecting this condition is that it nearly always gets worse without treatment. Children should be referred as soon as possible to an orthopaedic surgeon with an interest in spinal disease. He will keep the child under close observation; a spinal support (brace) or surgery may eventually be required.

A similar condition rarely occurs in the first 3 years of life, being most common in the 1st year (infantile idiopathic scoliosis). Unlike the adolescent form boys are more affected than girls and about 80% resolve spontaneously.

Other causes of scoliosis are congenital (birth) defects of the spine, nerve and muscle diseases and a tilted pelvis due to shortening of a leg.

USEFUL BOOKLETS

Your Baby's Hips. A Parents' Guide to Congenital Instability or Dislocation of the Hip, by D. Stratton. Available from Cow and Gate Limited, Trowbridge, Wiltshire, UK.

Your Child's Feet. Available from the Health Education Council, London.

Chapter 14

Neurological Problems

EPILEPSY

The word epilepsy is a Greek word meaning 'to seize upon' or 'take hold of'. In the past, because of ignorance and social prejudice, there has been a reluctance to use the word epilepsy. Children with epilepsy have been said to be suffering from convulsions, seizures, fits or 'turns'.

What is epilepsy?

This is best explained by comparing the brain with a computer. The brain has various parts which perform specific functions and information to and from these specialised areas is transmitted by electrical circuits in the brain cells (neurones). Occasionally there is a 'short circuit' in the neurones and messages become distorted. The resulting physical aberration depends on the site of the electrical disturbance and varies considerably from a mild abnormality of sensation to bizarre behaviour. There may be slight twitching or violent jerking of the limbs. Loss of consciousness may vary from seconds to hours. Most 'short circuits' repeatedly occur in the same area producing sudden symptoms, which are usually a repetition of those which occurred on previous occasions.

Is a fit or seizure the same thing as a convulsion?

No, they are not always the same. The term convulsion is reserved only for those seizures in which jerking, shaking or twitching occurs. All convulsions are seizures but not all seizures are convulsions.

How common is epilepsy?

Epilepsy can occur at any age and about 90% of epileptics first develop symptoms during childhood and the teens. During this time about 2 in every 100 children will develop an epileptic fit and the number with recurring fits (epilepsy) is about 7 in ever 1000.

What is the cause of epilepsy?

The vast majority of epileptic fits have no known cause. When the cause is known it is usually brain injury or some factor affecting brain function. Common causes of brain injury are birth difficulties and head trauma. The brain may also be injured by infections, the commonest being meningitis. Very rarely deposits or growths form in the brain damaging the surrounding tissue. Brain function is affected by changes in blood chemistry. For example, a common cause of fits in the newborn is a low blood sugar. The reason why neurones 'short circuit' suddenly and unexpectedly from time to time remains a mystery. The tendency to 'short circuit' (to fit) is increased by fever, fatigue (lack of sleep), excitement or severe emotional stress. In some children 'short circuits' may be induced by flickering lights, certain noises or strong smells. Fits are more common during menstruation in teenage girls.

What are the common types of epilepsy?

The most common types in their order of frequency are grand mal, temporal lobe, benign epilepsy and petit mal. More than half are grand mal and petit mal accounts for less than 5%. A few children have more than one type. A brief description of each type is as follows:

Grand mal – also called tonic-clonic seizures. Although present in young children it is more common after age 5. After loss of consciousness there are usually jerking movements of limbs and eye rolling. Breathing may be noisy and irregular, sometimes causing a blue–grey appearance. The child may pass urine, but only rarely does soiling occur. After the fit he slowly regains consciousness and is typically confused and sleepy. When fully awake he may complain of headache and is unable to remember what happened. Some children develop a 'strange feeling' (aura) immediately before the fit and it is common for parents to notice a change in mood or behaviour hours or even days before a fit.

Temporal lobe – also called psychomotor or complex partial seizures. Usually develops in late childhood and adolescence. In addition to controlling smell, speech, hearing and memory, the temporal lobe receives messages about sensations from various parts of the body.

During a fit these sensations are altered and the variety of strange sensations may lead to quite bizarre behaviour. Because the level of consciousness is altered, it is usually not possible to get through to the child who is behaving quite inappropriately. The child may hear or see frightening things and may be terrified by these strange sensations. Speech disturbances sometimes occur. What the child with a temporal lobe attack feels is unnatural and beyond normal experience and, in consequence, is often impossible to describe to the family or doctor.

A classic example is the child who gets a feeling of discomfort in the abdomen, suddenly loses consciousness and stops talking. He may fidget and move objects without any sense of purpose. His behaviour may be regarded as quite inappropriate and there may be smacking of the lips. The episode may last a couple of minutes and, on recovery, the child may have to be gently restrained because of confusion. Temporal lobe epilepsy is sometimes confused with a condition of pre-school children known as *benign paroxysmal vertigo*. In this condition the child suddenly becomes unsteady on the feet, frightened and may clutch at a parent. Preservation of normal alertness during the attack is the most important way of distinguishing it from epilepsy. Benign paroxysmal vertigo is a self-limiting condition, children grow out of it within 2–3 years.

Benign epilepsy – usually affects children between 4 and 13. It occurs in both sexes with boys predominating. The typical story is that parents hear a noise at night and find the child awake but making gurgling noises, salivating and twitching down one side of the face or body and unable to speak. After a few minutes the fit ends, and if asked the child will be able to remember what happened and often describes a prickly feeling in the mouth and a feeling that the tongue was too large. He may describe a variety of weird sensations involving the tongue, mouth or throat. Occasionally after these fits there is a transient weakness of one side of the body. Benign epilepsy can occur during the day but occurs mainly during sleep, particularly in the first two hours after going to sleep or shortly before wakening.

Petit mal – also called absence seizures. Most commonly affects girls between 5 and 12. During a petit mal fit the child goes 'blank' for a few seconds during which the face may be pale or flushed with flickering of the eyelids. The child is unable to remember what happened. These fits may be brought on by overbreathing.

There are two very rare types of fit which occur in the child under 6. These are called infantile spasms (West's syndrome) and myo-clonic epilepsy. Both are associated with a high incidence of mental retardation.

What is the difference between a fit and a faint?

Most children with faints feel lightheaded and can feel the faint coming on. Faints, which commonly occur in teenage girls usually occur while standing in a warm atmosphere such as school assembly or in church. They can also be brought on by emotional causes such as the sight of blood, needles, injections, etc. In fits there is often no warning and they just occur without any obvious cause. After a faint, recovery is rapid without confusion, sleep, headache or vomiting, whereas all these are common after a grand mal seizure. Jerking and passing urine can occur with both fits and faints. The EEG does not help in distinguishing a fit from a faint; the only way this can be done is to get a clear and concise story.

Does epilepsy run in families?

Yes, this is particularly evident in families with benign epilepsy and petit mal. Although epilepsy may be influenced by genetic fac-tors, the risk is small and should *not* be taken seriously when planning further family.

How is epilepsy diagnosed?

Epilepsy is diagnosed by the history. Unless the paediatrician is given precise details it is extremely difficult to make an accurate diag-nosis. Information should be obtained from friends or a school teacher or anyone who may have seen what happened.

What investigations are required?

In an otherwise healthy child when the diagnosis is obvious no tests are necessary. The electro-encephalograph (EEG) is a brain wave trace which records electrical activity of the brain. The test causes no discomfort and is even suitable for very young children. It may be requested when there is uncertainty about the diagnosis or when some guidance about the choice of treatment is required. It is *not* a diagnostic test for epilepsy. There are many epileptics with a normal EEG pattern as well as many 'normal' people with epileptic EEG pat-terns. Seizure patterns are more easily detected while the child is asleep; occasionally an EEG during sleep is arranged. x-ray studies of the skull or brain are sometimes requested by paediatricians. Information derived from these studies is of most help in a child who, besides suffering from fits, also has another abnormality of the nervous system.

Will epileptic drugs affect the EEG pattern?

Epileptic drugs do not affect the EEG pattern and should not be stopped before the test, except drugs known as benzodiazepines: diazepam, clobazam, clonazepam and nitrazepam. They will make an abnormal pattern look normal and should be discontinued about 2 weeks before the EEG. If your child is on one of these drugs *never* stop the treatment without first discussing it with your doctor.

Do children grow out of epilepsy?

This obviously depends to a major extent on the cause. In general all children grow out of benign epilepsy and three-quarters grow out of grand and petit mal. About a third grow out of temporal lobe epilepsy but the outlook is very much worse in children suffering from infantile spasms and myoclonic epilepsy. It is fair to say that the outlook for epileptic children is best when they are both mentally and physically normal and there is a short history of fits which are well controlled by drugs.

Is it necessary to treat a child after a single convulsion?

The answer is usually no because many children would be treated unnecessarily. Only about a third have a recurrent convulsion and this usually occurs within the first 3 years.

Are fits harmful?

Short fits, no matter how frequent, do *not* cause brain damage. Indeed, it is only when they last many hours or even days that there is any possibility of brain damage.

Why do we treat epilepsy?

As mentioned earlier many children eventually grow out of their epilepsy.

Drug treatment should not be seen as a 'cure' but rather a way of preventing convulsions. Besides the social advantage of not having fits, the main aim of prevention is the freedom from danger while going about normal activities.

What about drugs for epilepsy?

The drugs which prevent fits are called anticonvulsants. The choice of a particular drug is based on the type of fit; the dose is calculated according to the child's weight. Each drug does have side-effects, but these are uncommon. Children do *not* become addicted to anticonvulsants. A small dose is chosen initially and then gradually increased until such time as the fits are controlled or side-effects arise. If there is failure of control or side-effects the level of the drug in the blood maybe checked before trying another drug. Drug changes and dosage modifications are usually based on information given by the parent or child. Details about fits or side-effects should be carefully recorded on a diary card and brought to the clinic at each visit. Table 14/1 shows anticonvulsants commonly used and the fits for which they are used.

Table 14/1 Drugs commonly used to treat epilepsy

Type of epilepsy	Drug
Grand mal	carbamazepine sodium valproate phenobarbitone phenytoin primidone
Petit mal	sodium valproate ethosuximide
Temporal lobe	carbamazepine phenytoin sodium valproate
Infantile spasms	ACTH prednisolone benzodiazepines
Myoclonic	sodium valproate benzodiazepines

What are the most common side-effects of drugs?

About 3% who take carbamazepine develop a rash, which soon goes when the drug is discontinued. Sodium valproate may cause excessive weight gain and patchy hair loss. A number of children on phenobarbitone become hyperactive, they have abnormal behaviour, insomnia, mood changes and sometimes aggression. The most common side-effects of phenytoin are cosmetic; it causes gum enlargement, acne, abnormal and excessive hair growth (hirsutism) and sometimes coarsening of the features. The main side-effect of benzodiazepines is sedation; this improves with time. Ethosuximide may cause loss of appetite, nausea, vomiting and headaches but is generally very well tolerated.

How long should drug treatment continue?
There is no satisfactory answer to this question, suffice to say that most paediatricians would withdraw treatment after a fit free period of 1½–4 years. Never suddenly stop epileptic drugs without reducing the dose over a few days as the sudden stoppage may cause withdrawl fits.

Will he come to harm if he forgets to take his tablets?
Forgetting the odd tablet here or there probably causes no harm, but regular lapses of memory will certainly put him at great risk of having fits.

How many children respond to anticonvulsants?
About 60–70% have no further fits, 15–20% have a considerable reduction in fits and fit frequency is unaltered in the remainder. Rarely, in severe epileptics who have not responded to drugs a special diet (ketogenic diet – a complicated diet consisting predominantly of fat) or brain surgery may be tried.

After drugs have been withdrawn how long need parents wait before they can be certain that the child has grown out of epilepsy?
Two-thirds of children who have further fits do so within 2 years and 85% within 5 years.

How should a convulsion be managed?
The child should be placed on the side in a safe place. Nothing should be placed in the mouth. Most children do *not* bite the tongue or cheeks during a fit, but if this does happen regularly then a *soft object* such as a piece of leather should be placed between the teeth. After the fit the child should be placed in a comfortable position and allowed to sleep. It is now possible to stop fits immediately while at home with an anticonvulsant given in the rectum from a convenient dispenser. Stesolid (rectal diazepam) should be used strictly under medical supervision and can be obtained from a paediatrician or

family doctor. The usual dose is 5mg for those under 3, and 10mg over 3.

Can children with 'flickering light' induced fits watch television?

Yes, but the room should be well lit and the distance between the child and the television not less than 3 metres. When approaching the set the child should look away or close one eye. A remote control is ideal in that it obviates the need to approach the set to change channels. This type of fit is also called 'photosensitive epilepsy'. It affects about 1 in 4000 children. Flashing lights in discotheques, especially white light, may cause a problem for teenagers. If treatment is required sodium valproate is the drug of choice. Children with this type of fit can quite safely work with a computer visual display unit. However, when watching a computer programme on a domestic television set there is a risk of a fit. The risk is greater than normal because of the closer proximity to the set. It is best to use a small set both for watching television and for computer games.

What about immunisations?

A child who has a history of fits should not be given whooping cough vaccination but should have all the others. A *family* history of fits is *not* a contra-indication to whooping cough or any other vaccination. The answer to this question is controversial. See page 77.

What other problems may children have?

Some children with fits have behaviour and learning difficulties. These children are often hyperactive or clumsy and have poor concentration. If educational problems arise remedial education may be required. About 100 000 children in England and Wales have some form of epilepsy, the vast majority attend normal schools. There are, however, a disproportionate number of epileptics in schools for the mentally handicapped. This is not surprising as epilepsy is found in many abnormal brain conditions. In Britain there are 5 special schools for children with epilepsy. Details about these schools can be obtained from The Epilepsy Association (p. 352).

How much independence should epileptic children be given?

It needs emphasising that the majority of children with epilepsy are normal and must be taught to regard themselves as normal. The child can take part in all recreational activities, although swimming should be supervised. The child should not feel restricted or overprotected, although a certain amount of common sense should prevail. It is best to take each activity in turn and ask the fundamental question, could it be harmful if a fit occurs? If the answer is yes then the activity should be modified to render it safe. For example, a child may have a fit in a bath but bathing would be relatively safe if the bathroom door were not locked.

It is always a good idea for older children with epilepsy to carry some form of identification which states that they are epileptic and gives the name of their family doctor or hospital they attend. The SOS Talisman (bracelet or pendant) or Medic-Alert identification (bracelet or necklet) are ideal (see pp. 350–1 for the addresses).

Should the school be informed?

For reasons of safety it is essential that the school be informed and know how to deal with a fit should it occur at school. The school should be told that it is not necessary for a child to be sent home each time a fit occurs. Punishment, both physical and other, does not bring on fits and epileptic children can be punished. The school also has an important educational role in fostering healthy attitudes towards epileptics.

Are there any jobs which exclude epileptics?

Certain jobs by the nature of their danger are unsuitable for epileptics. At the present time epileptics are prevented from making a career in the police and armed services; in the UK, although there is no official bar to an epileptic person's training as a nurse, there is likely to be difficulty in being accepted for training. Similarly, it may not be possible to train for certain specialist areas of teaching such as physical education. Further information should be sought from the relevant professional organisations.

Is it possible for an epileptic to obtain a driving licence?

A driving licence for a public service vehicle or heavy goods vehicle is *not* given to anyone who has had a fit after age 5. The regulations concerning private vehicles were revised in 1982. These allow a patient with a history of epilepsy to drive if he has been free of attacks for 2 or more years, or in the case of attacks occurring in sleep if such attacks have been confined to sleep over the previous 3 or more years. There are many problems with the interpretation of these regulations and any difficulties that may arise should be referred to the Medical Adviser, Driving and Vehicle Licencing Centre, Swansea. All motor insurance companies load their insurance premiums for epileptics owing to the greater risk. Epileptics would be well advised to shop around for the best deal.

Does the teenage girl with epilepsy have an increased chance of producing an abnormal baby?

Yes, there does seem to be an increased risk; it is not known why but does not seem to be related to any particular drug. The risk is 2–3 times greater than normal. For every 1000 babies born 20 are abnormal; this figure rises to 40–60 if the mother is epileptic. Put another way, the risk is indeed very small, at the very least 940 of 1000 babies would be normal.

Further information about epilepsy can be obtained from The British Epilepsy Association (p. 352).

FEBRILE CONVULSIONS

Parents experiencing a febrile convulsion in their child for the first time find it very distressing. Their feelings are perfectly natural as many parents say that during the fit they thought their child was dying and minutes seemed like hours. This section has been written to give them some information about febrile convulsions and, hopefully, relieve some of their anxiety.

Febrile fits occur when a young child gets a fever. Although epileptic fits can be brought on by fever, febrile convulsions are *not* epilepsy. About 3 in 100 children between 6 months and 5 years have febrile fits, hence it is one of the commonest causes of admission of children to hospital in the UK. Most convulsions occur at about 18 months and although slightly more common in boys (ratio 1.5:1), girls both develop and grow out of them at a younger age. Fits usually last less than 15 minutes and generally involve the whole body. When breathing is affected the child may develop a blue-grey colour.

The cause is not clear, it is not the height of a temperature but probably the sudden change of temperature or the rate of rise which induce fitting. Although many children have viral infections causing the temperature, the virus is not thought to be responsible for the fit. In addition to temperature there is a strong genetic factor. About 1 in 10 children have parents or a sibling who experienced febrile convulsions. Convulsions are not caused by children becoming hot due to the weather, getting excited or running around.

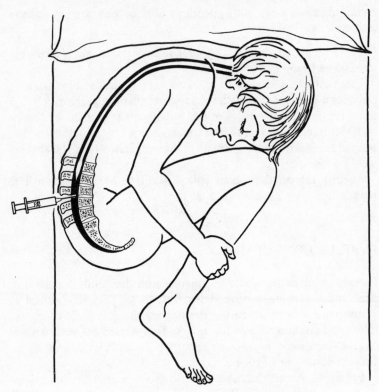

Fig. 14/1 Positioning for a lumbar puncture

Hospital admission is usually not more than 48 hours and may not be necessary for second and subsequent convulsions. If the child is still fitting on arrival at the hospital an anticonvulsant injection (drug which stops fits) is given into a vein. After taking the history the admitting doctor will usually have made the diagnosis, the examination being mainly to find the cause of the fever. When the cause is not obvious a lumbar puncture (Fig. 14/1) blood or urine culture (test for growing bacteria) may be required. Despite no evidence of its value in preventing convulsions, most paediatricians do prescribe paracetamol to bring down the temperature. Some treatment may also be prescribed for the cause of the temperature.

The overall risk of further convulsions is about 30–40% and depends on age. About half the children under 18 months and a third of those over 18 months have a further convulsion. Three-quarters of second convulsions occur within a year and about 10% have more than two convulsions. An EEG (brain wave trace) is of no value in predicting the risk of further convulsions or epilepsy. The outlook for children with febrile convulsions is excellent. The subsequent risk of epilepsy (non-febrile fits) is about 2–3%, which is slightly higher than the risk (0.5%) in children who have never had febrile fits. The risk is not influenced by the number of fits. When there is a family history of epilepsy, developmental delay or abnormality of the nervous system the outlook is not as good. Other poor risk factors are very long convulsions (hours) and focal fits (when only one side or part of the body is affected). Even when more than one of these poor risk factors are present only about 10% develop epilepsy.

There is no proof that prevention of febrile fits will reduce the very small risk of subsequent epilepsy and, with rare exceptions, there seems no justification for daily drug treatment to prevent convulsions. Two drugs, phenobarbitone and sodium valproate, are effective in preventing fits, however neither is free from side-effects. In as many as a quarter of children phenobarbitone causes hyperactivity, behaviour and sleep problems. Although sodium valproate is widely used and is generally regarded as safe, rare serious side-effects have been reported.

After the first convulsion, management of further fevers and fits usually concerns parents and advice from the paediatrician should be obtained before discharge from the hospital. Below age 5, in an unwell child with fever, a drug which brings down temperature – paracetamol (acetaminophen (USA)) – should be given as soon as possible. There is *no* need to remove clothing, tepid sponge or fan the child. In a well hydrated child fever is not harmful. Furthermore, these measures which are of unproven value make the child uncomfortable. Placing the child in bed with the parents, as often happens, is a controversial issue. It may cause the child's temperature to rise but does relieve parental anxiety in that it facilitates better observation.

During the fit the child should lie on the right side and *no* attempt should be made to place anything in the mouth. I have yet to see a child with a bitten tongue following a febrile convulsion, however, I have seen children with teeth knocked out by hard objects forced into the mouth. A fit lasting a few minutes requires no further action other than a visit from your family doctor to see if the cause of the fever requires treatment. A fit lasting longer can be stopped by taking your child to a hospital accident and emergency department. If you do not have transport phone for an ambulance (999) and be sure to mention that your child is fitting. Many parents find it reassuring to have in the home a drug which they can use to stop the fit. If you feel it could be of help discuss this with your paediatrician or family doctor; the drug 'Stesolid', diazepam, is marketed in a small, toothpaste-like plastic tube with a long nozzle which is inserted in the child's bottom. The tube is squeezed and then removed and the fit stops within minutes. It is very effective and your doctor will give you advice about dosage. When preventive treatment is deemed necessary Stesolid is very effective in preventing convulsions in those at high risk. Many parents find this method of prevention far more acceptable than having children on regular anticonvulsants for sometimes as long as a few years. Preventive treatment is usually recommended as soon as the temperature rises above 38.5°C; doses (maximum 4) are repeated 12-hourly while the temperature remains high.

Finally, children with febrile fits are at an age when they would normally be supervised. There is, therefore, no need to stop visits to swimming pools or any other normal childhood activities.

What about aspirin?

In June 1986 the Department of Health in Britain withdrew the licence for the use of aspirin or aspirin-containing medicines in children under 12, unless specifically indicated as, for example, in children with arthritis. The reason for the withdrawal was the link between aspirin use and Reye's syndrome, a very rare but serious illness. In Britain, Reye's syndrome occurs in 3–7 of every million children under 16; it affects mainly the brain and liver, more than half die or end up brain damaged. Studies in the USA in the early 1980s first reported an association between aspirin use and Reye's syndrome. These studies generated much controversy, nevertheless the USA Food and Drug Administration and the manufacturers of aspirin-containing medicines warned parents against giving aspirin to children and teenagers with influenza or chicken-pox, the viral illnesses most commonly linked with Reye's syndrome. As a result of this warning fewer children received aspirin for these conditions producing a significant decline in the incidence of Reye's syndrome.

The evidence to date does not prove beyond doubt that aspirin causes Reye's syndrome, although it does suggest that it may have a part to play in this tragic illness. Paracetamol, which is just as effective for temperature control as aspirin and is free from side-effects at normal doses, must be the drug of choice for treating febrile convulsions.

MIGRAINE

Contrary to popular belief, migraine is a common cause of headaches in children. Although present in the pre-school child, the incidence is unknown in view of difficulty of diagnosis. At 7 about 3% have migraine and there is a slight increase throughout childhood so that by adulthood about 10% of the population are affected. In young children sex incidence is similar but in older children and adults more females are affected. Migraine is genetically determined, the vast majority of children have a parent or sibling who suffer from 'headaches'.

What is migraine and how is it diagnosed?
The diagnosis of migraine is based entirely on the history. Headaches occur at periodic intervals (a few days to months) and generally last 2–8 hours but never more than 2–3 days. During the headache there is a lack of appetite, a feeling of nausea and sometimes vomiting. A minority will have visual disturbances immediately before the onset of the headache. These are commonly blurred vision, tunnel vision, 'blind spots', transient blindness, flashing lights or coloured lines. A few may have 'pins and needles' and a numb feeling in the limbs or around the mouth. During the attack the child looks tired and pale and may have dark rings around the eyes. Irritability and a dislike of light and noise are common. Many prefer to lie in a darkened bedroom and eventually fall asleep. Characteristically, on waking from a long sleep the headache is gone. In the adult the headache is on one side but in children is more often on both sides, usually involving the front of the head or temple. Although the pain is throbbing, most children describe it as an 'aching pain'.

The above description of migraine is both common and typical, but the signs and symptoms and severity can vary considerably from the occasional mild discomfort to the frequent debilitating ache. There are also very rare forms of migraine which can be quite alarming. In addition to the usual symptoms there may be unsteadiness of the feet, double vision, slurred speech together with loss of consciousness (basilar migraine). There may be temporary paralysis of one side of the body (hemiplegic migraine) or a dilated pupil with drooping of the eyelid and squint (ophthalmoplegic migraine). There is always complete recovery from these rare forms within a day or two.

Are there any warning signs of a migraine attack before it develops?

Most just occur without any warning, however, many parents are able to predict the signs of an impending attack hours before. The most helpful sign is a change in mood; some children become excitable and others depressed, anxious, irritable, withdrawn and generally low. There may be inappropriate tiredness and yawning. Appetite, particularly a desire for sweet food is sometimes increased.

What causes migraine?

The cause is not known. We do know what can bring on an attack. These so-called 'trigger factors' are an important part of the management of migraine. The commonest of these is irregular or missed meals. Others are alteration of sleep pattern, interrupted sleep, too little or too much sleep, vigorous exercise – especially competitive sports; environmental factors such as bright light, noise or strong smells. In teenage girls hormone changes can trigger a migraine. It is quite common for migraine to develop just before menstruation. Stress can bring on migraine but, interestingly, the pain only starts after the stress when the child is relaxing. The 'post-exam' or 'after-school' headache is common among teenagers.

The relationship of allergy to migraine has long been controversial and at present this relationship remains unresolved. Almost every food has been incriminated as causing headache and much attention has been given to this by the media. When evaluated scientifically it is evident that food related attacks are very rare indeed. The foods most commonly implicated are as follows: chocolate, cheese, citrus fruit, tea and coffee, pork and seafood. Certain individuals are very sensitive to a food preservative, monosodium glutamate, which is used in abundance in Chinese cooking. This headache, as well as other symptoms, has led to the well-known 'Chinese Restaurant Syndrome'. As well as type of food and additives the temperature of food may also produce a headache. Drinking or eating very cold foods may cause the so-called 'ice cream headache'.

What are the other causes of headaches in children?

When a child is unwell with a feverish illness a headache is common and will usually subside within a few days. Persistent or intermittent headaches are usually 'emotional'. In my experience sinus or eye problems are very seldom the cause of headaches in children. Very rarely a high blood pressure or brain tumour can cause persistent headaches. A paediatrician can quickly exclude these conditions by a thorough physical examination.

Why does the head ache?

Blood vessels (arteries) taking blood from the heart to the brain have a muscular coat which enables them to change diameter. The walls of these vessels also contain pain sensors which respond to stretch. Normally the migraine starts by the vessels narrowing and causing a reduced blood flow to the brain which in turn produces the visual symptoms. The narrowing phase is followed by a widening phase during which the vessel wall is stretched causing pain. There are many chemical changes in the blood during a migraine attack; the precise causes of changes in vessel diameter are not known.

Is there a particular personality associated with migraine?

The answer is no. Children with migraine do, however, frequently suffer from motion sickness. Sleep walking is also more common in children with migraine.

How should migraine be managed?

A most important way of preventing migraine is by avoiding 'trigger factors'. This can best be done by keeping a diary and recording the time and frequency of attacks together with relevant information in the period immediately preceding the attack. Recorded information should include times of meals, type and amount of food eaten; sleep pattern, exercise and stress. Environmental factors such as excessive heat or noise, bright or flashing lights and strong smells should be noted. Having pinpointed a 'trigger factor' then every effort should be made to take appropriate action where possible. For example, if you find that migraine always develops on the morning after a late night movie, particularly when breakfast has been omitted, then migraine can be avoided by having more sleep and a wholesome breakfast. Keeping a diary is very helpful to the paediatrician who will be able to advise you accordingly and so bring about much improvement. The fear and anxiety caused by migraine is a cause of stress for many children and their parents and can easily be relieved by explanation and reassurance.

Drug treatment is usually given for an attack or on a continuous basis. Every effort must be made to give treatment *early* in the attack. If parents suspect that the child is going to have an attack because he is tired, pale, quieter or more irritable, then at the first sign of the headache a painkiller, paracetamol (acetominophen (USA)), should be given and repeated as necessary. For mild, infrequent attacks no other treatment is required. In more severe attacks these painkillers should be combined with metoclopramide (by mouth or injection). This drug is unique in that, in addition to preventing nausea and vomiting, it renders the painkiller more effective. Severe headaches *with preceding visual disturbances* can be treated very effectively by a drug called ergotamine. To be fully effective the drug must be given at the onset of the visual disturbance and is best given by suppository in a young child or inhalation in an older child. If your child is given an inhaler ask your doctor to check that he is using it properly. Tablets are available but are less effective. Excess ergotamine itself may cause headache and vomiting and should only be taken under strict medical supervision. Always check the dose and frequency with your doctor. These should not be exceeded.

Parents of school age children should inform the teacher that the child suffers from migraine and every effort should be made to avoid the child being sent home. Older children can carry their drugs and take them as necessary but the young child will need to ask for drugs which should be kept at school. Most schools are very willing to co-operate.

Continuous drug treatment to prevent attacks is seldom required in children. Most respond to 'trigger factor' avoidance and the drugs previously mentioned. However, when attack frequency is sufficiently distressing to interfere with ordinary life or education then continuous drug treatment should be tried for a few months. There are various drugs for continuous use, each having a different action. Those most commonly used are pizotifen, propranolol, clonidine and methysergide.

Do children grow out of migraine?

By the onset of puberty about half the children with migraine will have less attacks or no attacks. It is difficult to predict the outlook in an individual child but, in general, children with very frequent severe attacks are less likely to grow out of migraine.

In this section I have provided a short résumé of migraine and its management in childhood. Should you require further information this can be obtained from The British Migraine Association (p. 352).

MENINGITIS

Meningitis is an uncommon illness of childhood, but a potentially serious one. It is caused both by bacteria and viruses. Based on hospital laboratory reports, on average about 750 children under 15 develop bacterial meningitis each year in England and Wales. The number of reports of viral meningitis is similar. It is, however, generally estimated that 80% of cases of meningitis are viral; the low number of reports suggest that most viral meningitis is mild and does not warrant hospital admission, alternatively, viral meningitis may be under-reported. The only time bacterial is more common than viral meningitis is in the first month of life, when the incidence is about 1 in 2500 births.

What is meningitis?

The brain and spinal cord are surrounded by a clear fluid, cerebrospinal fluid (CSF). The fluid is encased by a thin membrane known as the meninges. When the membrane becomes infected and inflamed the illness is called meningitis.

How do the meninges become infected?

The most common source of infection is the blood. The meninges contain numerous fine blood vessels. Infected blood passing through these vessels causes inflammation by spreading out bacteria and virsuses on to the meninges.

Direct exposure of the membrane to infection can also cause meningitis. This may happen with spina bifida, skull fractures, and rarely with ear or sinus infections.

Which bacteria and viruses cause meningitis?

In the newborn the two most common bacteria are *E. coli* and *Group B streptococcus*, the latter recently becoming the more common. Haemophilus is the most common in the pre-school child. Most infections in the school age child are caused by meningococcus followed by pneumococcus. Viruses most commonly causing meningitis are echovirus, coxsackie and mumps.

What are the signs and symptoms?

These depend on the age of the child. In the newborn they are often non-specific requiring a high degree of clinical skill and suspicion to make the diagnosis. Poor feeding, vomiting, lethargy, irritability, convulsions, bulging fontanelle (dimple on front of skull) are some of the most common signs and symptoms. Temperature may be normal, raised or depressed.

Older children may have fever, headache, vomiting, dislike of light (photophobia), irritability and convulsions. Neck stiffness which is frequent in older children is often absent in the first 1–2 years.

The symptoms of viral meningitis are usually milder and of slower onset, however, clinically it may be extremely difficult to distinguish viral from bacterial meningitis. Of the types of bacterial meningitis haemophilus has a slow onset. A typical story is that of a child who a few days after a respiratory or ear infection has a rise in temperature, becomes irritable and drowsy. Pneumococcus and meningococcus have a rapid onset, the latter sometimes associated with shock. As many as half the children with meningococcal meningitis have a rash which is usually first apparent on the back and buttocks before spreading to the rest of the body.

How is meningitis diagnosed?

It may be suspected by the history and examination but it can only be diagnosed with any degree of certainty by lumbar puncture. There are several other medical conditions which produce *meningismus*, the name given to signs and symptoms which mimic meningitis. A lumbar puncture involves passing a thin needle between the lumbar vertebrae in the back (see Fig. 14/1); the membrane around the spinal cord is punctured and a few drops of fluid (CSF) are removed. The procedure is uncomfortable but necessary. By examining the fluid in the laboratory it is possible to confirm whether meningitis is present and the type. In the case of bacterial meningitis the antibiotics likely to be effective can also be established.

Blood samples are usually taken to see if bacteria can be cultured (grown). Meningitis frequently causes biochemical abnormalities in the blood; samples may be sent for chemical tests (electrolytes).

What is the treatment?

Treatment may be given for symptoms such as headache, vomiting and convulsions. If the child is unable to feed or retain feeds a 'drip' (intravenous fluid) is used and any biochemical abnormalities are corrected at the same time.

There is no specific treatment for viral meningitis. Bacterial meningitis is treated with antibiotics which are given as soon as the lumbar puncture has been done, particularly if the CSF is cloudy, which is highly suggestive of meningitis. On occasions when there is no doubt about the diagnosis antibiotics may be given before the lumbar puncture if the child is very ill. There are many antibiotics currently being used. In the early stage (first 24–48 hours) of treatment it is sometimes not possible to determine which bacteria are involved and which antibiotics will be effective against them. The initial choice of antibiotic or combination of antibiotics is therefore based on those which are most likely to be effective against all the common bacteria causing meningitis. This treatment may be amended accordingly when the bacteria and their antibiotic sensitivity are known.

The choice of antibiotic also depends on those most likely to reach a high concentration in the fluid around the brain. Most antibiotics are at their highest concentration when the meninges are inflamed. In the early stages of meningitis antibiotics are always given intravenously to maintain a high concentration in the blood and in turn the CSF. When the child is getting better it may be difficult to maintain a drip in a restless child. At this stage parents may request that the antibiotics be given by mouth. This is most unwise as it is very important that high antibiotic levels in the blood should be maintained at a time when meningeal inflammation is receding and in consequence less antibiotic is able to enter the CSF. The length of time the child requires antibiotics varies but is mostly between 10–14 days, after which the child should be ready for discharge.

It is customary in many paediatric hospitals to repeat the lumbar puncture during or at the end of treatment to gauge the response in the CSF. This is probably not necessary provided the temperature has settled and the child is generally well.

What is the outlook?

Meningitis, particularly bacterial, can be a very serious illness. Anxious parents expect answers to their questions about the short- and long-term outlook. Unfortunately at times it is extremely difficult for a paediatrician to give a definite answer with any accuracy. If you find your doctor will not commit himself do not fear the worst; the reason is probably that he does not know.

The outlook depends on the age of the child, the type of meningitis and the speed with which treatment is given. Meningitis is a paediatric emergency; best results are obtained when it is diagnosed and treated early. The age at which meningitis is most serious is in the first month, particularly when *E. coli* bacteria are the cause.

Of all meningitis, viral meningitis has the best outcome. While the outcome of bacterial meningitis is not quite as good, most children make a complete recovery, the results being best for haemophilus and meningococcal infection. Impairment of hearing seems to be the most common complication of meningitis. It is prudent for children to have hearing tests a few months after they have recovered from meningitis.

Can meningitis be prevented?

Vaccines against haemophilus (USA only) and pneumococcus are available and effective in children over 2. The small number of children affected by pneumococcus has not led to its routine use for the prevention of meningitis. In parts of Africa where meningococcal disease is very common vaccines are currently widely used. The meningococcal vaccine is not completely effective below age 4; most children require more than one vaccination to be fully protected.

Is meningitis contagious?

Yes, both meningococcal and haemophilus are contagious, but it must be emphasised that the bacteria can only be acquired by *very close* contact. It is quite safe for these children to be nursed in open paediatric wards. Special precautions are not necessary for doctors and nurses working closely with the child.

Most paediatricians are agreed on the need for treatment of close contacts (brothers, sisters and parents) of children with meningococcal meningitis. The antibiotic of choice is rifampicin in a dose of 10mg/kg/twice daily (maximum 600mg per dose) for 2 days. It can be taken as capsules or syrup and may cause an orange-red colour in the urine. Despite the fact that the child with meningitis has recovered he may continue to harbour the bacteria and should also be treated with rifampicin at the same time as other family members.

The treatment with rifampicin of all household contacts where one member of the household is under 4 is controversial in haemophilus meningitis. The American Academy of Paediatrics has recommended such treatment, but a lack of proof of benefit has led most British paediatricians not to subscribe to this view.

CEREBRAL PALSY (CP)

What is cerebral palsy?

The brain has a movement and a thinking part. CP is the name used to describe an abnormality of movement following damage to the movement part of the developing brain. The damage is permanent and, although there is no further damage to cause deterioration, the extent may only become apparent with time as the child develops and the abnormal movement becomes more obvious. The severity of CP shows a wide variation, some children may be so mildly affected that no special treatment is required. A number of children also have damage to the thinking part of the brain. Many parents may find that after the diagnosis is made their paediatrician will provide noncommittal answers to their questions about the likely severity of the handicap. There is a good reason for this; in the early stages it is often very difficult to be certain and he would rather give no answer than the wrong one.

What does spastic mean?

In most children with CP the muscles of the affected limbs have an increased tone so that the arm or leg will feel stiff. This increased tension or stiffness is called spasticity.

How common is CP?

Between 1 and 3 children in every 1000 births will develop CP. In the USA there are about 300 000 children with it. Boys are affected as often as girls.

What is the cause of CP?

There are many causes of CP, all have in common their ability to cause brain damage, which may occur before, during or subsequent to birth. In half damage has occurred before birth and about a third are connected with events surrounding birth, most infants in the latter group weighing less than 2.5kg. The cause may not always be obvious: this point is important to bear in mind, as parents not unnaturally feeling guilty blame themselves and imagine all sorts of causes, which are usually totally unconnected.

Are there different types of CP?

Yes, the type depends on the cause and the part of the brain most damaged. There are four types – spastic, athetoid, ataxic and mixed. The spastic type is most common, accounting for about 70%; the spasticity can involve 1 or all 4 limbs. The medical terms used to signify which limbs are involved are as follows:

Hemiplegia	disability of one side of the body. This is the most common form of spasticity, which affects about two-thirds.
Quadriplegia	disability of all 4 limbs.
Monoplegia	disability of 1 limb.
Triplegia	disability of 3 limbs.
Diplegia	disability of the upper and lower limbs of both sides, usually meaning that the legs are more severely involved. Most children with diplegia were premature births.
Double hemiplegia	disability of the upper and lower limbs of both sides, usually meaning that the arms are more severely involved.

Unlike the spastic type, children with other types of CP may have a reduced muscle tone and appear quite floppy. Some of these children make purposeless jerking movement (athetoid type) while others (ataxic type) are unsteady on their feet and may have a tremor (fine rhythmic movements of the hands). Children with features of more than one type are said to have a mixed type.

How is cerebral palsy detected?

Most children with CP are diagnosed because of a delay in their development, the movement aspect in particular. Others are detected when parents note that all limbs do not move to the same extent. Occasionally children are admitted to hospital for other causes such as fits and are noted to have CP.

How is it diagnosed?

There is no special test to diagnose CP. The diagnosis is made by a thorough medical examination. During this examination the doctor will check for spasticity and any abnormality of posture which has resulted. Limb movement and reflexes may also be tested. Children with spastic legs often have a crossed over appearance (scissoring), while spastic arms are associated with a clenched thumb (fisting). The latter is however quite normal in the first 3 months of life.

What about a CT scan?

A computerised tomographic (CT) scan is a very specialised *x*-ray of the head which is able to show the brain in 3 dimensions. A scan is occasionally performed but does not make the diagnosis of cerebral palsy. The main reason why the paediatrician will do a scan is to find out, if possible, what the cause for the cerebral palsy might be. Areas of underdeveloped brain (atrophy) where damage has occurred are the most common scan finding. In my experience when brain changes are apparent it is rarely possible to know the precise cause for these changes, and when the cause is known little can be done. I therefore do not see much point in doing a CT scan as a routine procedure.

Do children with CP have any other problems?

Yes, the most common problems are:

1. Fits – occur in about 25%.
2. Eye problems – occur in about 50%, squint being the most common.
3. Hearing impairment – not as common as eye problems but should always be excluded.
4. Orthopaedic abnormalities – these arise as a result of stiff muscles. Limited joint movement (contractures) and shortening of tendons occur, especially the Achilles tendon at the back of the ankle joint. Limb shortening, dislocation of the hips and altered spinal curvature (scoliosis) may develop.
5. Feeding, drooling and speech problems. Feeding difficulty in early life and drooling are common. Speech problems occur in 50%. These are caused by weak inco-ordinate movement of the tongue, lips and muscles at the back of the throat (pharynx). Expert help of a speech therapist is very useful when faced with these problems.
6. Gastro-oesophageal reflux (p. 136) is common in those with a severe handicap, the vomiting of 'coffee grounds' (altered blood) usually indicates that reflux is occurring.
7. Behaviour problems. These are more common than one would expect and are found in both those with normal intellect and those retarded. The reason for this is not clear, but does not appear to be

related to the severity of the handicap or how the parents handle the children.

Will he walk?

This is usually one of the first questions I am asked. It needs emphasising once again that every child is different. Suffice to say that most children with cerebral palsy do walk, albeit later than usual.

Will a baby walker help?

There is no evidence that a baby walker is beneficial, indeed there is some suggestion that it may actually impede progress. The lack of proof of the benefit and probable harm in addition to the fact that baby walker accidents do occur would lead me to recommend strongly against their use.

Will he be mentally retarded?

About 20% have an IQ (intelligence quotient) of average or above and some are well above, but 50% are educationally subnormal. These have particular difficulty with visual perception. This means that although their eyes may see normally the brain interprets what they see in an abnormal way. This leads to poor concentration and difficulty with reading and mathematics in particular.

Will he go to a normal school?

This obviously depends on the extent of his physical or mental handicap. Some children with CP do go to normal schools and make good progress. On the other hand schools for the handicapped are there specifically to meet the needs of the child who requires extra help. These schools are now equipped with advanced technological aids which can facilitate communication and bring out the best in the child. They have staff who have specialised in teaching handicapped children and physiotherapists are based on the premises. In Britain free transport is provided to and from these schools.

How is CP treated?

As mentioned earlier brain damage is permanent and there can therefore be no cure. We can, however, minimise the handicap by concentrating on all aspects of development so that ability is exploited to its maximum potential. The aims of treatment can be summarised as follows:

1. To develop independent daily living activities such as feeding, dressing, washing and toileting.

2. To develop some form of communication whether it be speech, gesture, symbols, writing, sign language or typing.
3. To develop some form of mobility.

Most children with CP are treated by a team of experts, the paediatrician acting as a co-ordinator and treating fits if they occur. Other members of the team may be a physiotherapist, speech therapist, occupational therapist, psychologist, teacher, social worker, orthoptist (squint specialist), ophthalmologist (eye specialist), audiologist (hearing specialist), otolaryngologist (ear, nose and throat surgeon) and orthopaedic surgeon.

While the paediatrician may be the co-ordinator the physiotherapist is, in my view, the leader. She is the member of the team who will work most closely with the child and his parents. She will get to know them well and will often become a friend and confidante of the family. While there is little objective evidence of the benefit of physiotherapy or occupational therapy in CP almost all paediatricians feel that they do help particularly when started early. There are various physiotherapy techniques for the treatment of CP, each has its enthusiasts but there is no reason to believe that one is better than another. Two popular methods in Europe at the present time are those of Bobath and Peto.

There is much overlap between the work of the physiotherapist and the occupational therapist. In many centres their combined duties are undertaken by a single therapist. The occupational therapist will help with many of the activities of normal life, which parents of non-handicapped children take for granted, since their child will learn from imitation. These activities include feeding, dressing, writing and control of fine movements to reduce clumsiness. The occupational therapist will also provide help and advice about those domestic aids which are available to make life safe and comfortable for both parents and child. She will provide advice about the most suitable clothing and shoes so that the child can dress unaided. The social worker will be able to supply you with information about the benefits to which you are entitled as a parent of a handicapped child. She will be someone you can turn to at times of crisis and she will help you plan for your child's future.

Are there any drugs which reduce spasticity?
Two drugs, baclofen and diazepam, are occasionally used to reduce spasticity on a short-term basis. Both drugs need to be intro-

duced very slowly to minimise side-effects which may be quite distressing.

What about his teeth?

Dental work is often more difficult in handicapped children and in order to minimise the amount of dental work you should take extra care with his teeth and give him fluoride drops or tablets in areas where the water is not fluoridised. See dose on pages 186–7.

What are the chances of the next child having CP?

If your child has spastic quadriplegia and there does not appear to be any obvious cause then the reason may be genetic, in which case there would be an overall risk in the next pregnancy of 1 in 8. If your child has asymmetric involvement, for example hemiplegia, then the risk is indeed low, probably less than 1 in 200.

What about the future?

The outlook for the future and the chance of employment depend on the degree of handicap. Studies have shown that about 25% of children with CP will eventually hold normal jobs in the community. The needs of the adult with cerebral palsy have in the past been poorly met, but the situation now appears to be improving.

What is the Spastics Society?

The Spastics Society is the leading organisation in the world for the care, treatment, education and training of children and adults who suffer from cerebral palsy. It was founded in January 1952 by a group of parents who were concerned about the neglected needs of their disabled children. Since its inception the Spastics Society has established 60 national schools and centres of various kinds to cater for the wide variety of needs among spastic children and adults. The Society also offers advisory and supportive services to anyone with cerebral palsy who approaches them. They provide an excellent series of pamphlets for parents. (See page 351 for address.)

DUCHENNE MUSCULAR DYSTROPHY (DMD)

What is a muscular dystrophy?

It is an inherited disease of unknown cause in which muscle fibres gradually die over several years being replaced by scar tissue and fat.

The more the muscle fibres are replaced, the weaker the muscles become. Some muscles are selectively involved before others, the type of muscular dystrophy being determined by which muscles are first involved.

What is the Duchenne type?

This is the most frequent and severe, affecting about 1 in 3000 male births. About 100 new cases are diagnosed in Britain each year. Females who carry the disease are normal. Muscle weakness starts in the thighs and next involves the shoulders.

What are the clinical features?

Affected boys are usually normal for the first 2 years, the only abnormality may be a delay in walking. Between 2–5 the child may appear to walk clumsily and be unable to run properly. He may be noted to fall frequently. Later there is increasing difficulty in running, climbing stairs and standing up after a fall. Medical advice will then be obtained, when it will be noticed that the child has excessively large calf muscles (pseudohypertrophy). The child usually walks on his toes, feet widely apart and spine curved producing a hollowed area in the lower back. The characteristic walk is known as a 'waddling gait'. Another typical sign (Gower's sign) is that of the child pressing on his thighs as he attempts to lever himself upwards from the floor after a fall.

What is the outlook?

The muscle weakness slowly progresses so that between 8–11 he becomes unable to walk, requiring a wheelchair. For a time after this little change may be noticed but the arms slowly become weaker and such actions as wheeling the chair, brushing the teeth and hair and eventually drinking and eating become successively more difficult then impossible. At the same time joints such as the ankles, knees and hips become stiffened and deformed, stiffening in the sitting position so that lying in bed becomes awkward and uncomfortable, often requiring frequent turning. Weakness of the spinal muscles causes the spine to become distorted and deformed (kyphoscoliosis) severely limiting movement of the chest. Eventually muscles of the face, hands and respiration become involved. The heart muscle which is also affected becomes progressively weaker. Chest infections become more frequent and more difficult to treat so that most children eventually die of a chest infection between 16–25.

How is the diagnosis made?

The diagnosis is usually obvious from the history and typical appearance, but can be confirmed by measuring in the blood creatine phosphokinase (CPK), a muscle enzyme normally released from dying or damaged muscle fibres. Children with DMD have very high levels.

What is the management?

As there is no cure the aim is to make life as happy and as comfortable as possible. His potential should be exploited to the full. He should not be overprotected but instead a sense of independence should be actively encouraged while he is mobile. There are different aspects to the management; these will be dealt with under separate headings.

Physical aspects   The child should be encouraged to get as much exercise as he is comfortably able. This will ensure that those muscles which are working normally are maintained in good working order. Muscle weakening causes joint stiffening and deformities known as contractures. These can be slowed down by regular stretching exercises supervised by a physiotherapist. However, contractures become inevitable after the child is confined to a wheelchair. Walking may be prolonged for a year or two by the use of long leg calipers. This often has a beneficial effect on the child's morale. When the spine starts to bend a lightweight spinal brace is usually used to support the spine.

Aids and other equipment   Ordinary and electric wheelchairs, home aids and home alterations can usually be arranged through the hospital occupational therapy department or through the Social Services Department. In Britain a charitable trust, The Rowntree Trust, based in York, will usually provide financial help to families with a handicapped child. They frequently provide money for washing machines, driving lessons for a parent and help towards a holiday.

Emotional aspects   There may be a natural reluctance of the family to have a social worker involved in their affairs. While this is understandable any such feelings should be shelved in the interest of the child and the emotional well-being of the family as a whole. The role of the social worker is to counsel, support, and to provide information about benefits to which the family may be entitled.

The three times of major crisis when a social worker may be very helpful are:

1. When the diagnosis is made. At this time the child is usually only mildly affected, causing disbelief and difficulty in coming to terms with the diagnosis. The realisation that the condition may have been transmitted causes feelings of guilt and recrimination.
2. When the child stops walking. This provides firm evidence of a deterioration and a realisation of what is likely to happen.
3. When death is approaching, the death itself, and the subsequent months.

Parents are greatly helped by getting to know other parents who are going through, or have recently been through a similar experience. Should parents desire, the social worker will usually make these arrangements. She will also attend to the emotional needs of the siblings, who should not be forgotten.

The diagnosis with all its implications will gradually need to be explained to the child. He will eventually need to be told that death will be neither painful nor uncomfortable and will most likely occur during a chest infection. These and very many other issues will need to be discussed and brought out into the open. Although the prospect of what is likely to happen may cause the child much anger and frustration he seldom becomes depressed. Parents not unnaturally do sometimes become very depressed and require help.

Education   Only about half the children with DMD have an IQ (intelligence quotient) in the normal range. The choice of school will depend on the child's intellect, his physical disability and the school facilities in his area. Many children start their schooling at a normal school before transferring to one which specifically caters for physically handicapped children.

General measures

1. Avoid unnecessary bed rest. For example, if the child has a temperature and a sore throat, do not keep him in bed.
2. Establish a sensible diet and eating habits from a young age and watch his weight. Children with DMD have a tendency to put on weight through lack of exercise when they become confined to a wheelchair. Chest infections are more difficult to overcome when children are obese.
3. Treat chest infections early with antibiotics and physiotherapy.
4. Have him immunised. All routine immunisations should be

given. The teenage child should also have influenza immunisation each year (p. 82).

How is DMD inherited?

Although this is an inherited disease in a third there is no family history. When the condition arises without a family history it is said to be a 'fresh mutation'. When it is inherited it is always inherited through the female, who is known as a carrier. It is now possible to identify about 80% of carriers by two blood tests (DNA probe test and CPK). All parents of a child with DMD should have genetic counselling. Blood will be taken from the mother and if she is a carrier blood will also need to be taken from her daughters and sisters to determine their carrier status.

What about the next child?

Women who are carriers have a 50% chance of having a boy with DMD or a girl who is a carrier. It is rarely possible to diagnose DMD by DNA probe test or a chorion biopsy (p. 335). If the fetus is affected the pregnancy can then be terminated at an early stage, if the parents wish.

In most pregnancies the sex of the fetus is determined by chorion biopsy or amniocentesis (p. 335) and a male fetus can be aborted. It has the disadvantage of a 50% chance of aborting a normal fetus. This predicament has led to the use of fetoscopy (p. 314) in some centres; blood is removed from the male fetal umbilical cord for testing and only an affected fetus is aborted. Explicit details of the various techniques and their risk can be obtained from the genetic counsellor in each centre.

What is Becker Muscular Dystrophy?

This is a rare form of muscular dystrophy which has the same pattern of inheritance and clinical features as DMD. The only difference is that it has a later onset (late teens) and a longer life expectancy.

Useful booklets

Help Starts Here – for Parents of a Handicapped Child. This is obtainable from the National Children's Bureau (address on p. 353).

Children with Neuromuscular Disease: A Layman's Guide to Neuromuscular Diseases and their Management, by D. Gardner-Medwin.

Everybody's Different, Nobody's Perfect, by I. M. Siegel.

The above two titles are obtainable from the Muscular Dystrophy Association (address on p. 352).

The Toy Libraries Association, Seabrook House, Wyllyots Manor, Darkes Lane, Potters Bar EN6 2HL can also supply helpful literature.

Chapter Fifteen

Jaundice and Other Blood Disorders

JAUNDICE

What is jaundice?

It is a term used to describe a yellow colour of the skin and the white of the eyes. Another cause of a yellow skin in infants is benign carotenaemia, which is caused by eating a diet high in carotene such as carrots. Unlike jaundice the white of the eyes is not discoloured.

What causes jaundice?

Red cells, the oxygen carrying cells of the blood, normally have a lifespan of about 120 days. When the cells break up they form a yellow-green pigment called bilirubin which, in excess, causes yellowing of the skin and eyes. The bilirubin in the blood binds to a protein, albumen, and is transported to the liver and other parts of the body. In the liver the bilirubin is removed and enzymes alter it to a form known as conjugated bilirubin which is excreted into the bowel. The main reasons why an excess of bilirubin accumulates in the blood are:

1. The liver enzymes are not sufficiently developed to cope fully with the conversion of bilirubin to the conjugated form.
2. Any increase in red cell destruction causes excess bilirubin which overwhelms the capacity of the liver to excrete it.
3. Bilirubin may be removed by the liver and converted to the conjugated form, but is prevented from being discharged into the bowel by an obstruction. The conjugated bilirubin which is trapped in the liver then returns to the blood.

What is physiological jaundice?

The liver of almost all newborn infants is not working at full capacity at birth so that large numbers of newborn infants have a yellow tinge which is apparent at 3–4 days and may persist as long as 10 days. The term used for this 'normal' jaundice is physiological. The liver of premature infants is less developed so that jaundice becomes apparent a day or two later than in the term baby and is more intense and may persist as long as a fortnight. Physiological jaundice is harmless; no treatment is usually required, but some babies are given light treatment (phototherapy).

When is jaundice not physiological?

Jaundice, which becomes apparent within the first day of birth, is very intense, or which persists longer than normal, is not physiological.

What are the causes of non-physiological jaundice?

These can be categorised as causes of a raised unconjugated bilirubin, and causes of a raised conjugated bilirubin.

Causes of a raised unconjugated bilirubin

1. Increased red cell destruction – the most common cause is a blood group incompatibility in which the mother's blood group is different from her newborn baby. The mother produces antibodies (protein substances) which attach themselves to the red cells of the fetus causing their destruction before and immediately after birth. Blood group incompatibility arises when the mother is Rhesus negative and the infant Rhesus positive, or when the mother's group is O and the infant A or B. Unlike the latter, jaundice from Rhesus incompatibility usually does not affect firstborn infants.

A reduced lifespan of red cells also occurs when there is an inherited defect in the red cell wall rendering the cell more fragile. Most of these defective cells which are of abnormal shape can easily be detected by examining the blood under a microscope.

2. Breast milk jaundice – about 1 in 100 breast fed infants develop jaundice, the cause is not known. It usually starts a few days after birth and may persist for a month or two. If breast feeding is discontinued it may take as long as 5 days for the jaundice to disappear. Interestingly, when breast feeding is restarted the jaundice does not return. It must, however, be emphasised that breast milk jaundice is harmless, there is no need whatsoever to discontinue breast feeding.

In areas where thyroid screening tests are not routinely done on new-born infants, a blood test to exclude thyroid deficiency (cretinism) should be arranged. Thyroid deficiency, which occurs once in 4000 births, requires urgent treatment to avoid the risk of brain damage. It may mimic breast milk jaundice in that the only early sign may be persistent unexplained jaundice.

Causes of raised conjugated bilirubin

There are two uncommon causes of a raised conjugated bilirubin in the first months of life. They are hepatitis (inflammation of the liver) and biliary atresia. The cause of hepatitis is usually an infection or an inherited abnormality of liver function. Biliary atresia is a condition of unknown cause in which the tubes (ducts) both inside and outside the liver may be obstructed, impeding the normal excretion of conjugated bilirubin. Unlike breast milk jaundice the persistent jaundice of hepatitis and biliary atresia is associated with pale stools and dark urine. Clinically it is not possible to distinguish biliary atresia from hepatitis. Hepatitis usually improves within a few months and does not require treatment. On the other hand the outlook for biliary atresia is very poor unless an operation is performed within 60 days of birth. For this reason all children with persistent jaundice, which is not breast milk jaundice, require urgent referral to a paediatrician.

Is jaundice harmful?

Jaundice is seldom harmful, but there is little doubt that very high levels of unconjugated bilirubin can cause brain damage, a condition known as kernicterus. Another complication is high tone deafness. Children with severe jaundice need their hearing kept under close observation. The precise bilirubin level at which these very rare complications are likely to occur is unknown.

What is the treatment?

For the vast majority 2–3 days of treatment under lights is all that is required. Because we do not know at what level bilirubin is harmful the decision to use lights is made rather empirically and will probably vary from one doctor to another. Light exerts its effect on bilirubin in the skin which is altered to a form readily excreted by the liver. Both white and the slightly more effective blue lights are widely used on post-natal wards; admission to a special care unit is seldom necessary. The child can be fed and cared for in the usual way while under the lights. He should, however, not be clothed or covered up. In some hospitals exposure to light is continuous, in others the lights are switched on and off at intermittent intervals.

Is light treatment safe?

It is completely safe. Occasional infants develop loose stools or may have a 'flea bite' rash. Light treatment causes increased fluid loss from the skin, so it has become customary in many hospitals for extra fluid to be given during treatment.

Why are the eyes covered during light treatment?

The effect of prolonged light exposure on the eye of a newborn is not known, but it would be very surprising if there was any harm. A study in the human in which the eyes have deliberately been exposed to prolonged light and the consequence evaluated has never been done. Because of the uncertainty, the light manufacturers and paediatricians recommend that the eyes be covered. This is usually achieved by means of a disposable eye mask or by placing the infant's head under a smoke coloured Perspex screen. The screen has the advantage of reducing eye infections and facilitating visual stimulation.

Is there any other treatment?

Occasional infants with severe jaundice require more than just phototherapy and are given an exchange transfusion. This too is generally regarded as a safe procedure in a child who is otherwise healthy. Over a period of 2–3 hours small volumes of the infant's jaundiced blood are removed and replaced with donor blood. Sometimes two or more exchange transfusions are required.

Are there any drugs which a jaundiced infant should not have?

Most drugs can be given to jaundiced infants, however some should be avoided, the most notable being sulphonamides. By binding with albumen these drugs facilitate the movement of bilirubin into the tissues increasing the risk of brain damage.

IDIOPATHIC THROMBOCYTOPAENIA

Platelets are blood cells which are essential for normal clotting. When there is a deficiency of platelets the condition is known as thrombocytopaenia. Idiopathic means of unknown cause, but in most cases the cause is a viral infection such as German measles or measles in the previous month. It usually affects children between 2–7. For some unknown reason the child suddenly starts to bruise easily. Nose-bleeding may also occur. A blood test will usually show a platelet count of less than 10 000/mm^3 (normal – more than 150 000/mm^3). The body produces antibodies (protein substances) which cause platelet destruction. These antibodies are platelet specific, the number of red and white cells is normal. The only test needed is a blood test to confirm that platelets are reduced and that red and white cells are normal.

No treatment is needed, bruising stops as platelet levels return to normal within 3 months in most children. If the child is bleeding heavily or if platelet numbers do not correct spontaneously, steroids or intravenous gamma globulin may be given to cause a rapid rise in platelets: both block the action of the antibodies. Some paediatricians treat all children with steroids in the 1st month.

While the platelet count is depressed the child may return to the school or nursery, but it is *very* important that he does not rough-house in the playground or at home. Contact sports must be avoided. If the child has a bleed he should be taken to the nearest accident and emergency department. In a very few children the platelet count does not rise despite the measures outlined previously, in which case the spleen, an abdominal organ, may need to be removed.

HAEMOPHILIA

Haemophilia is an inherited bleeding disease. For clotting to occur both platelets and blood clotting factors need to be present in sufficient number. There are three types of haemophilia: (1) Haemophilia A – this is caused by a deficiency of factor 8 and accounts for about 80%; (2) Haemophilia B or Christmas disease is caused by a deficiency of factor 9 and accounts for about 15%; (3) Von Willebrand's disease which is usually much milder and improves with age. It affects males and females, a parent is frequently similarly affected.

There is a wide variation in the severity of haemophilia, the severity being related to the degree of clotting factor deficiency. Only severe haemophiliacs (less than 5% of normal factor) have the typical signs and symptoms of the disease. Severe haemophilia affects about 1 in 10 000 boys; there are about 25 000 in the USA. The first signs are that the child bruises very easily when he walks or crawls. Prolonged bleeding after a minor injury or circumcision may occur, sometimes lasting several days. These are followed at 3–4 years by bleeds into muscles and large joints such as the ankles, knees or elbows. In von Willebrand's disease bleeding into joints is uncommon but nosebleeds are very common. All children with bleeding diseases have difficulty with dental extractions which, if necessary, should be performed in hospital.

The treatment of haemophilia has improved dramatically over the last 15 years and is continuing to improve. The treatment given will vary from one child to the next. All children should be referred to a haemophilia centre, where the child and his family will have sophisticated tests performed and will be given genetic and other advice about haemophilia by experts.

The mainstay of treatment is prompt replacement of the missing factor at the first sign of a bleed. The factor is given at the centre, but where possible parents are taught to inject the child so that the factor can be stored in the fridge at home and used as necessary. This saves much time and inconvenience. Von Willebrand's disease is usually treated with a form of factor 8 known as cryoprecipitate. Unlike other factors it must be stored in a freezer. All factors are extracted from blood. At present some children with mild haemophilia and von Willebrand's disease are treated with a non-blood product DDAVP (desmopressin) which works by causing a rise in factor 8. This drug is, however, not sufficiently effective for the treatment of severe haemophilia and it is anticipated that it will not be long before non-blood factors will be commercially available. It must however be emphasised that the risk of AIDS (acquired immune deficiency syndrome) is now rare since all blood is screened for the AIDS virus. The risk of hepatitis has also diminished since the development of an effective vaccine against hepatitis B.

Joint haemorrhages may be painful and pain relief can be obtained from paracetamol (acetominophen (USA)). Aspirin should *never* be used. Needless to say, haemophiliacs should not have intramuscular injections. Repeated joint swelling and pain cause muscle weakness, joint stiffness and eventual deformities. These can be prevented by prompt factor administration and close supervision by a physiotherapist and orthopaedic surgeon. Short episodes of joint immobilisation may be required from time to time.

The vast majority of haemophiliac children live at home and attend normal schools, but for obvious reasons do not partake in contact sports. Very few need to attend residential schools for haemophiliacs. There are two such schools in Britain.

What about the next child?

Any mother who has a child with haemophilia can be tested to confirm that she is a carrier. If a carrier, there is a 50% risk of a male child having haemophilia. Should this be desired, blood can be taken at 18–20 weeks from the fetal umbilical cord to determine whether the fetus is affected. The procedure, which is known as fetoscopy, does not cause any discomfort and is similar to amniocentesis (p. 335), except that the fetus is visualised directly through a fine fibre optic light in the womb rather than on a screen.

THALASSAEMIA

This is a severe form of anaemia which becomes evident in the first months of life. If not treated these children suffer ill-health, poor growth and frequently die. Although uncommon in Britain (less than 500 children), it is a common problem in certain Mediterranean, Asian and Far Eastern countries. It is inherited in an autosomal recessive pattern like cystic fibrosis (p. 126). The anaemia is caused by an inability to make red cells; those that are made are abnormal, reducing their lifespan. Thalassaemics also have a tendency to absorb excessive iron from the diet. Because the bone marrow is overactive some bones eventually assume an abnormal shape giving the face a characteristic appearance. Many have a slate grey appearance from a combination of anaemia and mild jaundice. The outlook has improved dramatically in recent years so that thalassaemics should now not only look normal, but should have a considerably improved life expectancy.

The treatment consists of regular 2–4-weekly blood transfusions for life. By maintaining the haemoglobin, the oxygen carrying part of the red cell, in the normal range bone deformities will be avoided and normal growth will ensue. The haemoglobin should *not* be allowed to fall below 12g/dl. In the recent past children who were maintained on regular blood transfusions eventually died from the accumulation of excessive iron in the heart muscle and other body tissues. Excessive iron accumulation can now be avoided by giving an iron excreting drug, desferrioxamine (Desferal) as soon as the blood transfusions start. Vitamin C also assists iron excretion. The important point about desferrioxamine is that for it to be fully effective it needs to be given by a slow injection under the skin over a number of hours. Most children now sleep with a small portable syringe injector attached to them at night. If started at an early age they soon get used to it. Bone marrow transplantation for thalassaemia is currently being evaluated.

Carriers of thalassaemia usually have a mild anaemia but are otherwise well. Carrier status can be determined by a blood test (electrophoresis). An antenatal test (chorion biopsy (p. 335)) is now available.

SICKLE CELL ANAEMIA

It is an inherited condition that affects red blood cells. These are normally round, doughnut shaped, very pliable and capable of squeezing through the smallest blood vessels. Children who have sickle cell anaemia have some red cells which form a 'sickle' or half moon shape when they release their oxygen in the body tissues. These abnormal cells which are very rigid are unable to pass through small blood vessels. By clumping together they block the flow of blood causing pain and other complications.

The inheritance pattern is similar to cystic fibrosis (autosomal recessive, p. 126). Those people who carry the gene (carriers) are said to have sickle cell trait and are perfectly healthy. About 1 in 10 people of Afro-Caribbean origin have the trait which interestingly seems to offer some protection against malaria. About 1 in 300 babies of Afro-Caribbean origin are born with sickle cell anaemia. Although primarily an Afro-Caribbean condition it does occur in Asian, Mediterranean and Arab countries.

Episodes during which large numbers of cells suddenly become sickled are called 'crises'. These can be brought on by infection, chills, strenuous exercise, anaesthetics; often for no apparent reason. Symptoms rarely start before 6 months, and may include swelling of the hands and feet in young children. There may also be frequent episodes of joint pain, abdominal pain or pain anywhere in the body. Clumping of red cells in the lungs may produce a condition indistinguishable from pneumonia. Other problems which may arise are mild jaundice, a big spleen (an abdominal organ), strokes, leg ulcers, blood in the urine, eye problems, and delayed growth. Children who are very anaemic become tired and breathless on exertion. Sickle cell anaemia causes a lowered resistance to certain infections causing pneumonia, meningitis and osteitis (bone infection). Between 'crises' most children appear well and are able to lead a normal life.

There is no cure. During crises it is often necessary for children to be admitted to hospital. Treatment consists of giving drugs for pain relief and extra fluids, which are given by mouth or an intravenous infusion (a drip). Infection is treated with antibiotics. It is usually only necessary to give a blood transfusion if symptoms are severe, anaemia is worsening or in preparation for a general anaesthetic.

Carrier status can be determined by a blood test (electrophoresis). An antenatal test (chorion biopsy, p. 335) is available. In some parts of the world babies are screened at birth for sickle cell anaemia. Those found to have the condition should have daily penicillin throughout childhood and longer.

Chapter 16

Some Birth Abnormalities

SPINA BIFIDA AND HYDROCEPHALUS

What is spina bifida?

The spine is composed of a number of small bones one on top of the other, called vertebrae. The back part of each vertebra has a cavity through which passes the spinal cord surrounded by fluid and enclosed in membranes. Spina bifida occurs at the end of the fourth week of pregnancy when a gap in the formation of the vertebrae occurs. In its most mild form (occulta) it may not be apparent, in the most severe form (myelomeningocele) there is a large midline swelling of the back which is covered by membranes, not skin. Spina bifida is one of the most common handicapping conditions of childhood. The incidence in Britain is about 1 in 2000, but appears to be falling.

What are the types of spina bifida?

There are two types:

1. *Spina bifida occulta* – these children have vertebral defects usually involving the lower back. There may be no noticeable abnormality or a slight swelling, a tuft of hair or a vascular or pigmented mark over the affected vertebrae. In most children spina bifida occulta calls for no further action, but occasionally a small cosmetic operation to the back is required. Very rarely there is an abnormality of the spinal cord (diastematomyelia) in which there may be difficulty with bladder control and leg movement.

2. *Spina bifida cystica* – when only the membranes and fluid protrude through the gap in the vertebrae and the lump in the back is covered by skin it is called a menigocele. When in addition to fluid and membranes, the cord also protrudes through the defect and the

lump is covered by a combination of skin and membrane it is called a myelomeningocele.

What is hydrocephalus?

Hydrocephalus literally means water in the head. The cavities (ventricles) of the brain normally contain fluid which is produced and removed in the brain, continually flowing from point of production to point of removal. When an obstruction occurs fluid continues to be produced but cannot be removed, causing enlargement of the brain and head, the condition being known as hydrocephalus. Hydrocephalus can occur without spina bifida, but is frequently encountered in this condition. About 1 in 10 children with a meningocele develop hydrocephalus and 9 in 10 with a myelomeningocele.

What is the cause?

We do not know, but there are probably many causes. It seems in part to be influenced by genetic and environmental factors, there is a tendency for it to run in families and it occurs with greater frequency in certain geographical areas.

What are the implications of the diagnosis?

These *may* include the following:

1. Paralysis and absent sensation of the lower limbs.
2. The immobility of the legs is often associated with orthopaedic abnormalities such as dislocated hips, club feet, or fractures.
3. Damage to the nerves of the bladder may mean that the child is unable to pass urine normally; when it becomes full urine will overflow causing dribbling. The stagnant urine in the bladder causes frequent urine infections and back pressure on the kidneys may ultimately cause kidney damage.
4. Damage to the nerves of the bowel may cause abnormal bowel function so that these children may have chronic constipation and uncontrolled defaecation.
5. Most school age children have IQ (intelligence quotient) within the normal range, the level generally being higher in those without hydrocephalus.

What is the management?

The initial decision on how to manage a child with severe spina bifida is never easy for either doctor or parents. It is influenced by emotions, attitudes, personalities and ethics. The important point for parents to realise is that whatever course of action is eventually taken there is never a need for an urgent decision; any decision should be taken in the cool light of day.

In the case of a meningocele an operation soon after birth to repair the back and avoid rupture of the fluid-filled sac is usually all that is required, the outlook generally being good. In the case of a myelo-meningocele, where the outlook is very different, a decision to operate is not so straightforward.

The decision to operate is usually taken after careful consideration of the individual child. Ultimately the parents have the final say, but their decision is usually helped by frank and detailed discussion with a paediatrician or surgeon. Although this is probably the most heart-searching decision parents will ever need to make it should be pointed out that a decision not to operate can subsequently be revoked with little harm to the child.

What is the operation?

Immediately after birth the swelling on the back is kept moist and protected by covering it with sterile saline dressings. This is routinely done for all children. Those children who are selected for surgery usually have the back closed within 1 or 2 days so as to avoid the risk of infection. After the operation the child is carefully observed for signs of meningitis and if the wound is infected antibiotics may be prescribed. When he is well enough he will be discharged and further follow-up will be undertaken in the outpatient department, where he will be reviewed by a team of experts well acquainted with the many problems likely to be encountered.

Who are in the team?

Children with severe spina bifida require lifelong follow-up. Visits to the various specialists will be very frequent initially but will eventually be no more than 2 or 3 times a year. The team is usually made up of a paediatrician, surgeon, orthopaedic surgeon, physio-therapist, social worker and occupational therapist. The paedia-trician is usually the team co-ordinator whose function is to liaise with other specialists. The team as a whole will deal with all the many problems likely to be encountered and will at the same time provide comfort and support for the child and his family. They will also arrange for the various aids such as calipers, wheelchairs, etc., to be provided. There are a number of approaches to the management of various aspects of spina bifida, each approach being individually tailored to the child and his family.

What is the management of the child who has no surgery?

This child, too, will be reviewed from time to time by a paediatrician and a social worker. At these visits the paediatrician will be able to assess whether the child is comfortable and will give the parents an opportunity to discuss aspects of the management. Should the help of another team member be required the paediatrician will arrange this.

How is hydrocephalus treated?

When hydrocephalus seems to be progressing or there is leakage of fluid from the wound a small operation is performed. A shunt, a plastic tube with a one-way valve, is inserted in the neck so that fluid can drain from the brain to the heart or to the abdomen, where it is absorbed. Sometimes medication is given as a temporary measure to reduce the fluid until such time as the shunt is inserted.

What problems may occur with a shunt?

The two main problems are:

1. A blocked valve – this may cause headache, vomiting, drowsiness and sometimes a fit.
2. Infection – this may cause fever, vomiting, irritability, poor appetite and sometimes neck stiffness. If problems with the shunt are suspected urgent medical advice should be sought.

What about school?

If possible it is hoped that children will be able to attend a normal school. Where the child attends will obviously depend on the severity of the handicap and the facilities of the school. Most children attend schools for the physically handicapped.

What happens after school?

This is very difficult to predict. If the child has been able to manage in an ordinary school there is a good possibility of his holding down a job in the open market. Females are able to conceive and have children, males are not able to father children.

Will it happen again?

The chance of a recurrence is about 1 in 20, after 2 affected children it rises to 1 in 10.

Can it be diagnosed antenatally?

Yes, about 85% including all the severe forms can be diagnosed by amniocentesis (p. 335) at 16–18 weeks by measuring the alphafeto-protein (AFP) and/or acetylcholinesterase. Because it is neither practical nor desirable to perform an amniocentesis on all pregnant women a screening test measuring alphafetoprotein in the blood has been developed and is now widely used throughout the world. After high blood levels have been obtained an amniocentesis is done to confirm the diagnosis. It may be possible to avoid the risk of amniocentesis by first doing an ultrasound test, which may be able to detect the defect in the fetal back.

Can spina bifida be prevented?

There is some evidence to suggest that folic acid given early in pregnancy may prevent some. As spina bifida occurs within the first 6 weeks of pregnancy folic acid needs to be given from the time the pregnancy is planned and *not* after it is diagnosed.

Useful booklet

Your Child with Spina Bifida, by J. Lorber. This is available from the Association of Spina Bifida and Hydrocephalus (address on p. 353).

CLEFT LIP AND PALATE

The birth of a child with cleft (split) lip or palate causes parents considerable distress. They should find some comfort in the knowledge that the appearance, which many find grotesque, will eventually be no different or very similar to other children and adults. This dramatic change will come about by surgery and close supervision by a team of experts.

How common is it?

One in 700 newborn babies has a cleft of the lip, with or without a cleft of the palate. One in 2000 has a cleft of the palate only. About 1500 children are born with cleft lip and palate each year in Britain. Half have a cleft of the lip and palate, the other half have a cleft of only the palate or only the lip. The cleft may be unilateral (one side) or bilateral (both sides). Cleft lip is more common in girls; cleft palate more common in boys.

What causes it?

Early in pregnancy parts of the body are formed in segments which eventually join up. Where perfectly formed parts fail to unite a cleft arises. The reason for the failure of fusion is not known; there is no way the abnormality could have been prevented.

What is the treatment?

The major part of treatment is surgery. It is difficult to detail the treatment because the extent of the cleft varies considerably. The information about treatment will be generalised and does not apply to every child. The treatment is always individualised, various procedures are undertaken according to the preference of the team and needs of the child and his family.

Which specialists are in the team?

All children with these abnormalities are seen at some time by most, if not all members of the team. The team consists of a paediatrician, a plastic surgeon, an orthodontist, an oral (mouth) surgeon, an ear, nose and throat surgeon (otolaryngologist) and a speech therapist. An orthodontist is a dentist who has specialised in the growth and development of the face, jaws and teeth.

What are the aims of treatment?

The aims are threefold:

1. To achieve the best cosmetic result.
2. To have perfect speech.
3. To have normally situated, healthy teeth.

What happens after the birth?

The first specialist to examine the child and meet the parents is usually the paediatrician. To provide comfort and reassurance he will probably show them other children's photographs taken before and after surgery so that parents quickly realise the dramatic effect of treatment. One major anxiety at this time is whether the baby will be able to feed. The paediatrician will endeavour to keep mother and baby together and with the help of the nursing staff will give advice on feeding. I would not wish to pretend that feeding is always easy; it may be very difficult and extremely frustrating. With persistence and willingness to be flexible by trying different feeding methods to find the most suitable, these difficulties can eventually be overcome. The palate, which has a hard (bony) and a soft (muscular) part forms the roof of the mouth. It is quite common during feeding for milk to pass through the cleft into the nose. Sucking is often not possible or difficult because the sucking muscles of the soft palate do not function properly.

How should the child be fed?

It is always best to try conventional methods first. Breast feeding may be possible, but if not the milk may be expressed and given by another method. There are a variety of special teats (nipples) available for feeding children with a cleft palate; these may not be necessary, a large hole in an ordinary teat or a soft teat used for feeding premature babies may suffice. Cleft palate teats are usually wide or flanged so that the hole in the roof of the mouth is 'plugged' as the child sucks. A lamb's teat which is long and soft seems to work very well and is widely used, particularly in the USA. When the child is not able to suck a teat he will be fed with a cup and small spoon or alternatively from a feeding bottle with a spoon attachment (Fig. 16/1). This makes feeding easier; the milk flows on to the spoon as the child feeds. Details about special teats and a spoon attachment together with a list of manufacturers can be obtained from the Cleft Lip and Palate Association (CLAPA) (p. 351). Some children are fitted with a dental plate, particularly when the cleft is bilateral. An impression of the palate will first be made before the plate is fitted on the roof of the mouth. A dental plate is made of plastic and is held in place by fixing it to the skin on the outside of the mouth with elastoplast. It is specially designed so that in addition to helping with feeding it brings the separate segments of the lip and palate closer together, making future surgery easier.

When is surgery performed?

The cleft lip is usually repaired at about 3 months. In some hospitals the lip is repaired within 48 hours of birth. This is of great psychological benefit to parents, but does have the disadvantage of requiring further lip surgery more often than the operation at 3 months. Some surgeons also close the soft palate at the initial operation.

The next operation to close the palate is now usually done between 6 months and a year when speech is starting to develop. The length of time in hospital on each occasion is usually between 1–2 weeks. After the lip repair the child may be nursed on his side to protect the oper-

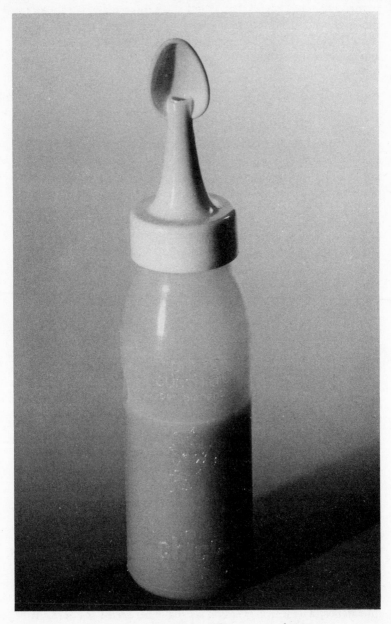

Fig. 16/1 Feeding bottle with spoon attachment

ation site. He may not like this if he is used to sleeping on his front. It would be best to get him used to sleeping on his side soon after birth. Almost all hospitals undertaking cleft palate surgery have facilities for mothers to room in.

How is he fed after the lip operation?

When you see your surgeon, ask him how he prefers the baby to be fed following the lip operation. Your hospital may have its own procedures to follow. As a general rule, if a baby is breast feeding, it is possible to continue breast feeding soon after the lip operation. With some operations this is not possible so a feeding bottle with spoon attachment should be tried. If your child is feeding from a bottle, it may be necessary to spoon feed immediately after the lip operation so that the lip is not put under too much pressure by sucking from a teat. In which case it is a good idea to let him get used to spoon feeding just before the operation, so he is not too upset by the change. After a few weeks you can go back to bottle feeding if you wish.

How is he fed after the palate operation?

It is sometimes advisable to get the baby off bottle feeding before the palate repair. This is because the bottle can't be used immediately after the operation and the baby will miss the bottle. The same applies to a dummy (pacifier).

It is usual to give a diet of liquids or 'soupy' foods for the first 10 days, e.g. fresh orange juice, milk, yoghurt, thin cooked cereals and strained soups. The ward staff will advise you on feeding when your baby is allowed to go home.

What are the common problems associated with a cleft lip and palate?

The two main problems are connected with hearing and speech.

Hearing problems – children with a cleft palate have a very high incidence of glue ear (p. 215). The tendency to glue ear is not affected by palatal closure. The effect of hearing impairment may cause worsening of a co-existent speech impediment. Children with cleft palates require prompt diagnosis and treatment of ear infections. A large number will eventually require grommet insertion. Some otolaryngologists insert grommets routinely.

Speech problems – normally when we speak air moves up from the lungs into the back of the throat (pharynx). The muscles of the soft palate pull the palate upwards so that the back of the nasal part of the throat (nasopharynx) is 'sealed'; air unable to enter the nose is forced through the mouth. Cleft palate repair does not always produce a perfect seal so that some air escapes into the nose. Speech therapy, encouragement and stimulation may be required so that the child learns to talk normally. Tonsillectomy or adenoidectomy may cause a severe and permanent deterioration in speech and the advice of the child's speech therapist and otolaryngologist should always first be obtained.

What other procedures may be necessary?

It is important to realise that not all children need further procedures after lip and palate closure in infancy. Some procedures that may be needed are listed below. At about four years a pre-school 'touch up' operation may be required for the lip. Despite intensive speech therapy some children continue to experience difficulty with speech because of air that escapes into the nose. A 're-seal' operation called a pharyngoplasty may be necessary between 6–9. Between 9–11 orthodontic procedures and some dental extractions may be needed so that teeth are brought into perfect alignment. In the late teens when the face is fully grown final operations may be done on the nose and facial bones to achieve the best cosmetic result.

What is the risk of the next child's having a cleft lip and palate?

The risk depends on whether the parents are normal and the abnormality the child has. With normal parents and a child with cleft lip, with or without cleft palate, the risk is about 4%, with cleft palate only it is 3%. With one parent affected and a child with cleft lip, with or without cleft palate, the risk rises to about 17%, with cleft palate only it is about 15%.

What is the risk that an adult who had a cleft lip and palate will produce a child with a similar abnormality?

Where the adult had a cleft lip with or without a cleft palate the risk is about 3%, an adult with cleft palate only has a greater risk, about 7%.

What is the Pierre Robin syndrome?

This is the name given to a child with a cleft palate and breathing difficulty. In addition to the cleft palate there is a small jaw and the tongue attachment to the jaw is situated further back than usual. The tongue, which is too large for the space provided, acts as a ballcock falling back and blocking the airway during inspiration. This causes severe breathing and feeding difficulty which is apparent soon after birth, particularly when the child lies on his back (supine). These children are nursed and fed on the front (prone) to prevent the tongue from falling back. Tube (gavage) feeding is often required. After the first 6–12 months as the jaw enlarges and the size of the mouth and throat increase the risk of obstruction from the tongue recedes. The cleft palate is repaired at the usual time. By the 1st birthday almost all are perfectly healthy and look normal.

DOWN'S SYNDROME

Most parents of a child with Down's syndrome find out shortly after the birth of the baby. Many have never heard the term before. Much of the information given in the first interview will not be remembered, but the manner in which the information is presented will be remembered for ever. At this interview there are only two points which I emphasise in the hope that they are grasped and retained. These are: first, that the child is going to be intellectually impaired and second that the cause is an 'accident of nature' for which neither parent is to blame.

The way parents react to this information varies. Most are immediately shocked and baffled as to why it should happen to them. There may even be disbelief as to the correctness of the diagnosis. Feelings may then range from over protection to rejection, some parents experiencing both. They not only grieve the loss of the normal child they had wanted but also start forming an attachment to the new baby. 'Postnatal blues' (depression) are common; many mothers develop a low self-esteem and question their ability to cope. Family support may not be forthcoming as some parents are reluctant to tell their relatives. Coming to terms with what has happened takes time. While parents are adjusting to the new situation feelings of denial, anger, guilt and sadness may be experienced. Not only are these feelings common, but they are quite normal.

What is Down's syndrome?

It could best be described as a combination of characteristic physical features associated with intellectual impairment. It is named after J. Langdon Down who first wrote about it in 1866. He wrote that the facial appearance resembled mongols (inhabitants of central Asia), hence the term 'mongolism' sometimes used. It was in 1959 that J. Lejeune and co-workers first reported that Down's syndrome was always associated with a genetic abnormality.

How common is Down's syndrome?

The incidence is about 1 in 700. About 1000 children with Down's syndrome are born in the UK each year.

What are the characteristic features of Down's syndrome?

There are well over 100 physical features that may be associated with Down's syndrome. It is important to realise that not all are present in every child; some occur in normal children. As in the rest of us features change as the child ages, but not to the extent that the condition will no longer be obvious. It is usually quite easy to distinguish an adult with Down's syndrome. Most children are undergrown at birth (average birth-weight = 2.9kg) and continue to grow slowly throughout childhood. The adult is usually a lot smaller than the normal adult. At birth all Down's infants are floppy (hypotonic). Muscle tone improves with ageing. The skin which may be moist at birth eventually becomes dry. The common features are:

1. Upward slanting eye slits (palpebral fissures)
2. On the inner (medial) aspect of the eye slits there are prominent folds (epicanthic folds).
3. The coloured part of the eye (iris) may be speckled with yellow-white spots (Brushfield spots).
4. They have a flat nasal (nose) bridge.
5. The shape of the back of the head is flat (brachycephalic).
6. The neck appears short and excessive folds on the nape are often seen.
7. The ears are small and may appear underdeveloped.
8. The mouth is small giving the false impression of a large tongue which protrudes and often has a grooved (fissured) appearance.
9. The hands are short and broad (spadelike) and the little finger curves inwards (clinodactyly). The palms may show a single palmar crease (simian crease).
10. The feet show a wide gap (sandal gap) between the first and second toes. There may also be a large plantar crease between these toes.

Although these features may be obvious to the 'trained eye', it may be some weeks before parents become convinced that the child looks abnormal. At the first interview, when I have told mothers that the new baby looks abnormal, the response has sometimes been 'but he looks just like his father'.

What causes Down's syndrome?

We do know what Down's syndrome is and how it happens, but we do not know the cause.

The reason why we are all different is because every cell in our body contains unique information about us. This information is stored in an envelope (nucleus) and is coded on chainlike structures called chromosomes. Each chain can be broken into small segments called genes. Man has 46 chromosomes, in Figure 16/2 the chains have been separated and arranged in order, the picture being called a karyotype. When we reproduce we pass half our genetic code to our offspring, 23 chromosomes going in the sperm and 23 in the egg. When the sperm and egg meet (fertilise) they join together to form the first cell of the new person. This cell then divides into millions and millions of identical cells as the developing fetus grows into a fully grown baby with 46 chromosomes.

In Down's syndrome a chromosome abnormality occurs around the time of conception when cells have started to divide, the net result being an extra chromosome or bit of chromosome in each cell. There are 3 types:

1. Trisomy 21 (also called non-disjunction type). About 95% are of this type. They have an extra chromosome 21, the total number of chromosomes being 47 (Fig. 16/3).
2. Translocations. About 4% are this type. These have 46 chromosomes but have an extra bit deposited (translocated) on either chromosomes 14, 21 or 22.
3. Mosaics. About 1% are this type. Some cells are normal (46 chromosomes) and others have 47 chromosomes.

It needs to be emphasised that in all types the extra chromosome material can come from the mother or father.

How is Down's syndrome diagnosed?

Almost all are diagnosed at birth by a careful physical examination. The lines on the skin of the palm have an abnormal pattern (dermatoglyphic pattern) and the pelvis is an abnormal shape. In the past palm patterns and pelvic x-rays were used to help make the diagnosis, but nowadays the diagnosis is confirmed by chromosome analysis.

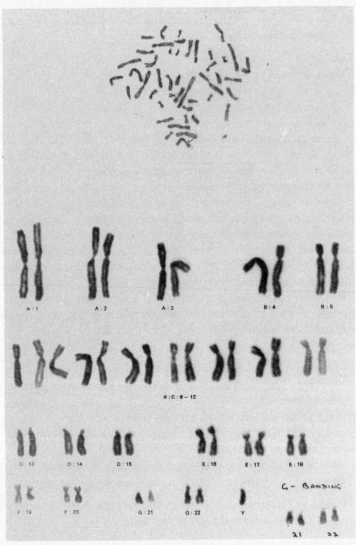

Fig. 16/2 Chromosomes of a normal male: *above*: all the chromosomes in a single cell; *below*: a karyotype showing how these chromosomes are arranged

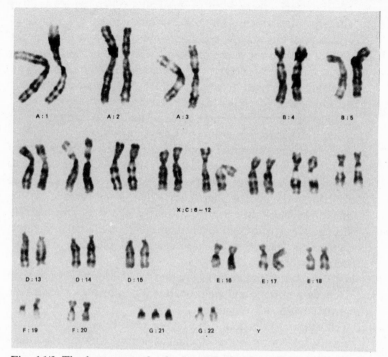

Fig. 16/3 The karyotype of a female with Down's syndrome. *Note* the 3 chromosomes at position 21

Blood is taken and the chromosomes in the white cells (lymphocytes) are analysed. It takes a minimum of 4–5 days for the result and 10 days for a complete analysis (Giemsa banding).

Is he (she) a mild case?

This is one of the first questions parents ask me. There is no correlation between the physical features and the severity of the handicap. Although there is no proof it is often said that mosaics have a higher mental ability and fewer physical features. My usual answer to the question is, 'he (she) may be a mild case but it is impossible to tell until he (she) gets older'.

What problems is the Down's child likely to encounter?

It must be emphasised that many of the problems I am about to list may *never* occur. They are only listed because some parents do want to know about them.

1. Heart defects – these occur in about 40%. There are a variety of abnormalities which occur, the commonest being known as an endocardial cushion defect. In its most severe form there are defects of both the small chambers (atria) and large chambers (ventricles) and heart valve abnormalities. Children with Down's syndrome and heart defects have a tendency to develop permanent lung changes (pulmonary hypertension) very early in life. It is most important that they are assessed by a children's heart specialist (paediatric cardiologist) in the first year.

2. Eye problems – common problems are squints, refractive errors (short- and far-sightedness), cataracts. Bacterial (staphylococcal) infections mainly on the eyelids at the base of the eyelashes and sometimes the eye (blepharo-conjunctivitis) are frequent.

3. Ear problems – glue ear (p. 215) is common in Down's syndrome. Hearing impairment is more common than in the general population, the reason being unclear but probably related to long-standing glue ear.

4. Feeding difficulties and constipation – both are more common in Down's syndrome and are probably caused by poor muscle tone of the mouth and abdomen.

5. Tendency to infection – the body's defence (immune system) against infection is not as efficient as in normal children so infections are more frequent and severe.

6. Duodenal atresia – some are born with an obstruction (atresia) of the duodenum. Bile-stained vomit may occur soon after birth and an operation is required to relieve the obstruction.

7. Hypothyroidism (deficiency of thyroid hormone). It is now well established that there is a tendency to develop hypothyroidism, particularly as the child gets older. Many of the features of hypothyroidism are similar to Down's syndrome making it clinically difficult to diagnose. In view of the associated impairment of intellect in hypothyroidism, children with Down's syndrome should have occasional checks of thyroid function. Only in this way can there be absolute certainty that they are not under achieving because of hypothyroidism.

8. Diabetes – there is an increased tendency to develop diabetes as they age.

9. Instability of neck vertebrae (atlanto-axial instability). Rarely the first and second neck vertebrae slide on one another so that they may impinge on the spinal cord as it leaves the base of the

skull. Although rare this may cause serious problems. Before taking part in contact sports, trampolining, diving or gymnastics an x-ray of the neck should be taken to make sure the vertebrae are firmly fixed in place.

10. Leukaemia – this is very rare in all children, but does appear to be slightly more common in those with Down's syndrome.

How long will he (she) live?

In general longevity is reduced compared with the normal population. It would seem that brain ageing occurs earlier. There are, however, adults in their sixties and seventies. The outlook for an individual depends on the general health, for example a child with a complex heart problem is unlikely to survive beyond middle age.

What will happen if we can't cope?

It is my practice to introduce the family to a social worker from the mental handicap team as soon as possible. She will keep in close contact with the family and will gradually inform them what community facilities are available for the child in their area. Should parents wish she may introduce them to another parent with a Down's child. At any point during the mother's stay in hospital or subsequently, if the parents feel they cannot cope, the social worker can arrange for the child to be placed in foster care, some eventually going for adoption should the parents so desire.

What should we tell our family and friends?

This poses a very real anxiety to parents immediately after they are told the diagnosis. The best advice I can give is to tell family and friends as much as you know, and as soon as possible. The truth must eventually come out and delays or half-truths will only create more difficulty and embarrassment later. Children will sense all is not well and should be told something. What the children are told and the manner in which they are told depends on their ages and level of maturity. Taking the children into one's confidence creates understanding and tolerance, setting the scene for happiness in the years to come. There is no evidence to suggest that having a child with Down's syndrome has an adverse effect on family life or leads to an increase in broken marriages.

What will he (she) be like?

Children with Down's syndrome like all of us will have their individual personality. In general they seem to have fewer behaviour·

problems than the average child hence the 'good baby' stereotype referred to in many books. At first he (she) will seem like any other baby but with time his (her) delay in development will become more obvious. As with all children the age at which developmental milestones are attained shows considerable variation.

What does mentally retarded really mean?

Children who attend normal school have an IQ (intelligence quotient) above 75. Almost all children with Down's syndrome have an IQ below 75. There are children with Down's syndrome in normal schools, but they are very much the exception to the rule. There is now good evidence that as a group Down's children reared at home are more intelligent than those reared in institutions. As yet there is no firm proof that starting an intensive stimulation programme in early infancy will improve the IQ, but most psychologists and paediatricians feel this is beneficial. Most parents like to get involved with these community-based early intervention programmes. It helps them learn about their child and they benefit from the social contact with other parents with a similar problem. The social worker from the mental handicap team will make the arrangements for admission to the programme.

Most children with Down's syndrome learn to walk and develop communication and social skills. They play sport, dance, partake in recreational activities and some get married. In general those that eventually do find employment are able to obtain only sheltered employment. The few who live or work independently in the community are the exception.

What will happen to the child when we die?

It is quite natural for elderly parents to consider this. Those who are not able to live independently will be found accommodation in sheltered housing, community homes and hostels. Society's attitude to mental handicap has undergone a great transformation in recent years; the days of putting a child in a large institution and forgetting about him (her) are fortunately a thing of the past.

Will a Down's child have children?

Males are sterile. Females can have children, however, about a third of the children born will also have Down's syndrome. The number who do have children is indeed small. While adults do enjoy cuddles and experience love very few have an active sex drive.

Can he (she) be immunised?
There is no reason why he (she) should not be immunised.

Is Down's syndrome related to the mother's age?
It has been known for many years that trisomy 21 shows an increased incidence as mothers get older. Most Down's children are now born to young mothers, the reason being that most women are having their families when they are younger. In Britain only about 6% of women give birth after 35. Other types of Down's syndrome are not related to maternal age.

Why is trisomy 21 related to the mother's age and not the father's?
In view of the fact that the extra chromosome can come from either parent there does not appear to be a satisfactory answer to this question. I suspect that information about the father's age has not been as carefully documented and extensively researched as the mother's.

Is it possible to diagnose Down's syndrome in pregnancy?
Yes, this is now possible. If the fetus has Down's syndrome, the pregnancy can be terminated if required. There are now two tests for diagnosing Down's syndrome in pregnancy:

1. Amniocentesis – this is the most frequently performed test. A needle under visual screen control is inserted through the abdomen into the womb. A small volume of fluid around the fetus is then withdrawn and sent to the laboratory. Amniocentesis is performed at about 16 weeks and takes 2–3 weeks for the result so that termination, if required, is performed at an advanced stage of pregnancy. The procedure is painless and there is no risk to the mother. The risk of a miscarriage is generally given as about 1 in 200. Some mothers may wonder why all pregnancies are not screened for Down's syndrome. There are 2 reasons; first, before 35 the risk of miscarriage is greater than the risk of having a Down's child, second, when the costs of screening all women are weighed against the amount saved by preventing Down's syndrome, routine amniocentesis is only economically viable above age 35.
2. Chorion biopsy – this is a relatively new test. A small segment of the chorion which is part of the developing placenta (afterbirth) is removed and analysed. The chromosomes in the cells of the chorion are identical to those in the fetus. Chorion biopsy may either

be performed through the abdomen as in amniocentesis or by passing a catheter (long fine flexible tube) through the vagina and monitoring its movement on a visual screen. Both methods cause minimal discomfort and carry little risk to the mother. The main advantage of chorion biopsy is that diagnosis and termination, if required, can take place between the eighth and eleventh weeks of pregnancy. This is much more acceptable to most women. The risk to the fetus has not been accurately determined. Part of the difficulty in assessing the risk has been the high number of miscarriages which normally occur quite naturally at such an early stage of pregnancy. Nevertheless, the risk is regarded as acceptably low and chorion biopsy is now widely performed throughout the world.

Chapter 17

Miscellaneous Problems

ACCIDENTAL POISONING

After falls the most common domestic accident in children is poisoning. In young children it is often difficult to know how much, if any, has been swallowed. The ensuing uncertainty is the cause of much panic and many false alarms. Each year about 20 000 children in Britain are admitted to hospital with poisoning, about 20% of all paediatric admissions. Most require no more than an overnight stay. Almost all children are under 5, most being 2 or 3. Unlike other home accidents where boys are more often affected, the frequency of poisoning is similar in boys and girls.

What are the poisons?
About 60% are medicines (tablets, capsules or liquid), the most common being painkillers. A further 30% are substances found in the home, garage and garden. The remaining 10% are poisonous plants, berries and 'mushrooms'. About 10–20 children die in Britain from poisoning each year. Deaths are rarely due to substances about the home (about 1–2 a year), most are caused by medication. Of the medicines, antidepressants account for the largest group, about a third. In most cases they have been prescribed in the previous month for the mother.

Each summer about 2–3000 children are admitted to hospital with laburnum poisoning. Although given much publicity in the media, laburnum is relatively innocuous; no child has ever died from laburnum. Admission to hospital is not necessary; symptoms (abdominal pain and vomiting), if present, usually settle within 12 hours.

How can poisoning be prevented?
The simplest way is to 'childproof' your home. It is not sufficient .

337

to do this only in your home, but it should be done in any home where your child goes. Many children are accidentally poisoned while the child is at the grandparents' home. This is not surprising as many grandparents have long forgotten the risks facing small children. Some simple measures for 'childproofing' your home are:

1. Keep all medication, poisonous household chemicals, pesticides and weedkillers out of sight and reach of children and stored away from food.
2. Never store poisons or inflammable materials (e.g. paraffin, white spirit or turpentine) in bottles or containers used for food.
3. Lock up all dangerous substances.
4. Never tell children that medicine is sweets. You may convince them in which case they may act accordingly.
5. Try to shop with safety in mind. Read the label on containers and where possible purchase the household product which is least toxic. Buy those products which are in safety containers or fitted with safety closures. Always re-seal safety closures, and never transfer the contents into other bottles or containers.

What shall I do?

This is the question the panicking parent asks when it is discovered that the child may have swallowed something. What is done depends firstly on the quantity and secondly the nature of the substance swallowed. For example, no action is required if 2 aspirins are swallowed, but swift action is required if a full bottle is swallowed.

It may be harmful to vomit certain poisons, hence a knowledge of the poison is required. As a rule children should be made to vomit the following poisons:

1. medication (tablets, capsules, liquid, suppositories, creams or ointments)
2. poisonous plants and 'mushrooms'
3. weedkillers and pesticides
4. antifreeze (ethylene glycol).

It is *not* recommended that children be made to vomit household products; vomiting is usually not necessary and, furthermore, may on occasion be harmful.

How can I make him vomit?

The child should be made to vomit by giving him ipecacuana syrup which is given with water or an orange drink. Do not give him milk as it will delay the vomiting. Almost all children vomit in 30 minutes (average 20). Unfortunately, unlike America, in Britain ipecacuana syrup cannot be purchased over the counter but can only be obtained on prescription. Despite the best preventive efforts many poisonings do still occur. If you have young children ask your family doctor to let you have a small bottle of ipecacuana syrup. The syrup has a shelf life of 5 years and should be stored with your plasters and bandages and other first-aid equipment.

Is ipecacuana syrup safe?

Yes, it is very widely used by parents in the USA with complete safety. Indeed, health education programmes endorse its use in the home and advertise it. After a child has had ipecacuana he usually vomits about 3 times over the next hour, after which he can eat normally.

How soon should the ipecacuana be given?

The sooner the better; much more poison is removed when it is given early. This is the main reason for keeping it at home. Before giving ipecacuana it is always worthwhile obtaining medical advice by telephoning your family doctor or nearest hospital accident and emergency department, provided there is no more than a few minutes delay.

Generally, it is not beneficial giving ipecacuana more than 4 hours after the poison is swallowed. Exceptions are drugs which are absorbed slowly from the stomach or those which delay stomach emptying. Drugs for which ipecacuana may be given after 4 hours are aspirin, antidepressants, tranquillisers, certain epileptic and asthmatic drugs. Your family doctor or nearest casualty department will give you advice about this.

How much ipecacuana syrup should he have?

The child should be given 15ml which should be repeated after 20 minutes if he has not vomited. (5ml is roughly equal to 1 teaspoon.) This should be followed by about 200ml (1 or 2 glasses) of water or orange squash. In very young children there are often problems in getting them to take the syrup and, surprisingly, it may be even more difficult getting them to take the liquid. Best results are achieved by not showing your panic or irritation, but by dealing calmly and firmly with the child.

Ipecacuana syrup should *only* be given to a child who is awake and alert.

What next?

Both children who have been given ipecacuana and those who have not should be taken to the nearest accident and emergency department, where the child will be examined and further action taken if necessary. In Britain if you do not have transport, dial 999 and ask for an ambulance. Always take the remains and the container of the swallowed poison with you. If there is any doubt about the nature of the poison these will help identify it, moreover they may also provide information about the amount swallowed.

In the past parents have tried to make children vomit by giving salt water drinks or sticking a finger down the child's throat. Not only are these methods relatively ineffective, but they are potentially dangerous and should never be used.

The manufacturers of some household products give first aid advice on the container about the procedure to be followed in the event of an accident. It is always important to read the label carefully before taking any action. As a rule if the child has swallowed anything corrosive give a few glasses of milk before proceeding to the nearest accident hospital. Common household products which are usually corrosive are bleaches, disinfectants, detergents, dishwashing powders and liquids and oven cleaners.

What is activated charcoal?

In Britain activated charcoal is available as Medicoal. It is available in sachets which when added to water forms a fizzy charcoal drink. After the child has vomited any poison remaining in the bowel can be mopped up by giving Medicoal; the poison is prevented from being absorbed by sticking to the charcoal which is excreted. Medicoal is very effective and safe and can be kept at home if necessary. The only major drawback is that it is extremely difficult to get the child to take it. Not surprisingly, most children do not like drinking a tasteless, black, fizzy drink. Even when a sweetener is added the reaction is not much different.

Medicoal should never be given before vomiting has occurred; the reason being that Medicoal binds with the ipecacuana and may prevent vomiting.

What is a poison centre?

There are numerous potentially harmful substances which children may swallow. Information about these poisons may not be readily available to your doctor or the casualty department doctor. For this reason so-called poison centres have been established in Britain. At each poison centre, information about any potentially toxic substance is carefully recorded and catalogued. Poison centres are available 24 hours a day by telephone; advice is given to any medical practitioner who seeks information.

Problems with button (miniature) batteries

Since the introduction of these batteries in watches, calculators, photographic equipment and children's toys, there have been reports of young children swallowing batteries or pushing them into the nose or ear. This seems to be a more common problem in the USA than in Britain.

When a child swallows a battery you should *not* try to make him vomit. Although there is no immediate risk the battery should never be ignored. The child should be taken to a hospital accident and emergency department. Before you go try to remember if the battery was new or old and see if you can find the battery code number; this may be found on the blister packaging, the appliance instruction leaflet or you may have an identical battery in the home. Some batteries may cause more harm than others; the code number helps the hospital or poison centre identify the type. New batteries are more likely to cause harm than old ones.

At the hospital an *x*-ray is done to determine the site of the battery. If the battery is stuck in the oesophagus (page 137) it is removed under general anaesthetic by passing a fine tube (endoscope) through the mouth. Batteries which have passed through the oesophagus generally do not cause any problems. Depending on where the battery is located, *x*-rays are usually done every 1–4 days to monitor its progress through the bowel. The child need not be kept in hospital until the battery is passed. Antacids to protect the bowel may be given, drugs or laxatives which facilitate progress by speeding up the bowel may also be prescribed. Most batteries are passed within a week but may take as long as a month.

Batteries which have been inserted into the nose or ear should be removed promptly; if left they cause severe tissue damage. Ear or nose drops should never be used before the battery is removed, they could make the injuries much worse.

COT (CRIB) DEATH

The sudden and unexpected death of a normal baby is one of the most distressing experiences that can occur in a family. The shock, guilt and bewilderment are traumatic and long lasting. Parents often feel that they were in some way to blame and repeatedly go over in their minds whether there was anything they could have done to prevent the tragedy. These guilt feelings are common and perfectly natural but are quite unfounded. Cot death is not a new phenomenon but it has recently gained prominence as a result of widespread and often sensational media attention. Media attention has flourished because of the highly emotive issues involved in a tragedy lacking explanation. There are many myths surrounding cot death and it is hoped that this information will dispel some of them.

What is a cot death?

The term 'cot death' was first coined by Dr A. M. Barratt, a pathologist at Cambridge University, in 1954. In *Recent Advances in Paediatrics*, he wrote 'The term "cot death" is used here to include all cases in which an apparently healthy infant is unexpectedly found dead in its sleeping quarters whether in a cot, pram or any other kind of bed.' Originally, therefore, the term included unexpected deaths which were later explained at post-mortem as well as those for which no adequate explanation could be found.

In 1965, R. G. Carpenter and C. W. Shaddick, then joint secretaries of the British Ministry of Health Enquiry into Sudden Death in Infancy, in an article in the *British Journal of Preventive and Social Medicine* adopted the term 'cot death' but narrowed its definition to 'those cases in which the information available does not reveal the cause or causes of death.'

This narrower use of the term 'cot death' corresponded closely with the definition of the term 'sudden infant death syndrome' proposed in the USA by Dr J. Bruce Beckwith at the 1969 second international conference in Seattle, USA, on the causes of sudden death in infants: 'The sudden death of any infant or young child which is unexpected by history, and in which a thorough post-mortem examination fails to demonstrate an adequate cause of death.' This diagnosis is reached by exclusion of explained deaths from the sudden unexpected deaths.

Throughout the world the term cot death has come to be used

synonymously with sudden infant death syndrome (SIDS) to describe sudden unexpected infant deaths which remain unexplained after post-mortem (autopsy) examination. The finding of an explanation will obviously depend on both the expertise of the person (pathologist) performing the post-mortem and the assiduous way an explanation is sought. Without wishing to be unkind to my colleagues it would seem that large numbers of post-mortems are performed in a perfunctory way with no attempt being made to obtain previous medical information about the child. It is for this reason that the Foundation for the Study of Infant Deaths is lobbying for all post-mortems on infants in Britain to be performed by a paediatric pathologist, a pathologist who has specialised in children's diseases. Moreover, some very rare hereditary children's conditions may cause more than one 'cot death' in a family and a paediatric pathologist would be in a better position to recognise these. In my view parents who experience the unlikely event of more than one cot death should make every attempt to have the post-mortem performed by a paediatric pathologist.

What is the Foundation for the Study of Infant Deaths (FSID)?

FSID is a registered charity, which was formed by parents and doctors in 1971. It sponsors research into the causes and prevention of sudden infant deaths, encourages support for the bereaved families, and acts as a centre for information about cot death for both professionals and parents. It is entirely dependent on voluntary contributions and has a small staff.

At what age does SIDS occur?

About 80% occur between 1–6 months, most occurring between 2–4 months. By convention the term SIDS is used only when referring to children under 2. It is uncommon but does occur in the first 2 weeks and less than 1% occur after a year.

How common is SIDS?

The incidence in Britain, USA and Australasia is about 2/1000 live births (1 in 500). The number in Britain each year is between 1000 and 2000, while in the USA the numbers are estimated at between 6000 and 8000. The incidence does seem to vary between countries; it is particularly low in Sweden and Israel (about 0.6/1000). In Britain it is the most common cause of death in infancy after the first week. It is the third most common cause of death in childhood.

Is the incidence the same for twins and triplets?

The risk for twins is more than twice that for single births, while the risk for triplets is more than twice that for twins. The incidence does not appear to be affected by whether or not they are identical.

Are boys and girls equally affected?

No, almost all studies show a greater number of SIDS boys. A recent survey of cot death in Scotland revealed an incidence of 3.3/ 1000 for boys and 2.1/1000 for girls.

Is it more common in first, or subsequent children?

It appears more common in the 2nd and 3rd child than the 1st.

What time of the year do most occur?

It is apparent in both the northern and southern hemispheres that almost two-thirds occur in the winter months. Their pattern of distribution throughout the year is very similar to deaths from respiratory causes.

Do most occur in the day or night?

It is very difficult to be precise about the time of death. We do know that most deaths are discovered in the day time between 9 a.m. and 9 p.m.

Where do most SIDS occur?

Most do actually occur in the cot, but by no means all. They may occur anywhere, for example in the perambulator, a motor car or even in the mother's arms. I have known a few to occur on the children's or maternity ward of a hospital.

What is the cause?

The proposed causes for SIDS are innumerable; some are plausible while others border on the preposterous. The answer to the question is that we do not know. Most experts believe that there is no single cause but probably multiple causes.

Are there any other risk factors associated with SIDS?

SIDS can occur in *any* family, but looking at large numbers in detail certain factors do stand out. It is important to bear in mind that these factors are more commonly associated with SIDS, but are not necessarily contributory. They can be divided into infant, maternal and paternal.

1. Infant – it is well known that premature and low birth-weight (less

than 2.5kg) infants are at increased risk. In Britain there are about 7% low birth-weight births whereas among SIDS infants 15% are of low birth-weight.

2. Maternal – maternal risk factors are if she is under 20, unmarried, poor, if she has delayed or failed to seek antenatal care, been ill during pregnancy, had short intervals between pregnancies, had miscarriages, or if she smokes heavily or takes drugs during pregnancy.

3. Paternal – the risk is increased if the father is under 20 or if he is unemployed or earns a low wage.

Work from the USA and Australia does suggest that even when social and economic factors are taken into account certain races have a greater risk than others. In the USA, where the overall risk is about 2/1000 the Asian risk is lowest at 0.51 per 1000.

Can SIDS be prevented?

There is no way of accurately predicting or preventing SIDS. In Sheffield a high risk index has been compiled and certain high risk families have been identified and visited frequently by health visitors and infants regularly weighed. This community-orientated programme appears to have been associated with a fall in the number of SIDS. Unfortunately, this experience appears unique to Sheffield as it has not been reproduced elsewhere.

There is much written in the lay press about breast feeding and sleeping position. It needs to be emphasised that SIDS occurs in all sleeping positions and in both breast and bottle fed infants.

Are all the infants completely well before they die?

It has been shown that some do have respiratory or gastrointestinal symptoms in the week preceding death.

Does the child suffer?

Most die in their sleep. Even if not asleep, it appears they become unconscious and die rapidly. As far as we are aware none of these children suffer pain or distress.

Could he have suffocated?

This is a frequent question parents ask. There is much mumbo-jumbo written about suffocation as the cause of SIDS; probably the most cogent reason for this is the very close similarity of post-mortem changes in some SIDS infants and those who suffocate. Other than rare reports of deliberate suffocation there is not a shred of evidence that external suffocation causes SIDS. Almost all bedding is made of fabrics which will admit sufficient air through the weave for the child to breathe. In any case, even the smallest infant would move his head in search of air if it were possible for his nose and mouth to become obstructed. Most child care books recommend not placing a pillow in the child's cot. It would seem that this recommendation is based more on custom than proof that there is a risk of suffocation. There is, however, no need to put a pillow in an infant's cot.

Could vomiting and choking on the vomit cause SIDS?

This is possible but unlikely. Vomit or blood-tinged froth may be found around the mouth or on the bedding. This probably occurs during or even after death and is not the cause.

Why do the police and coroner need to be involved?

In all countries unexpected deaths are required by law to be reported to some authority, who acts as the public guardian. In England this person is called the coroner who is a lawyer or doctor (Scotland has a Procurator-Fiscal). It is the duty of the coroner to distinguish death from natural causes from unnatural death. As part of his routine investigation he may instruct the police to visit the parents to make enquiries into events surrounding the death. The police may remove the child's bedding. Although a visit from the police is merely a formality, it may be very distressing but cannot be circumvented as it is the law. The fact that the coroner and the police have looked into the death is also a safeguard for the parents.

What are the effects on the family?

Each family is different. We all have our way of coping with grief, the various family members will grieve in their individual way. Relationships may be strained by feelings of guilt and misplaced blame. The mother having recently been through pregnancy will be emotionally vulnerable. If the shock does not suppress lactation she will require some advice or medication from her family doctor. Some weeks after the death the mother may become depressed when allowed to brood at home while her husband is out at work all day. Parents can best be helped by talking about the death among themselves and to others. It should never become a taboo subject. Many find talking to a parent who has been through a similar experience very helpful. This can easily be arranged through FSID or the

Society of Compassionate Friends (address on page 350). Some parents find it helpful to talk to the pathologist who performed the post-mortem or a paediatrician. This can usually be arranged through the family doctor.

Children's reactions to death, like adults, vary widely and these may be influenced by the child's temperament, his relationship to the baby as well as to his parents, and his perception of death which will depend upon his age and experience. It is important for parents despite their own desolation to listen to and observe their other children to give them the opportunity to express their feelings vocally and/or in behaviour. Parents who feel they require help with their children should consult their family doctor or health visitor.

What about the next child?

Should another child be planned the emotional well-being of the family as a whole would best be served by waiting some months rather than rushing into another pregnancy. Mourning can be best described as an illness which must run its course before recovery ensues. An interruption of the 'illness' through the anticipated new arrival will only delay recovery or make it more difficult to achieve.

The risk of SIDS in the next child is 3 times higher. This is very much a statistical risk and one which for practical purposes should be ignored. Another way of putting this risk into perspective is to point out that for every 500 infants born, 497 will not have SIDS.

What are apnoea monitors?

These are devices which measure breathing movements of the chest or abdomen and alarm when breathing ceases. None of the alarms currently available is entirely satisfactory. False alarms do occur and these can be very frightening for parents. There is no evidence that they have helped to prevent SIDS. Furthermore, they create a false sense of security as infants have died during their use.

Alarms are widely used by paediatricians often at great expense to the health service. In Britain, unlike the USA, it is not possible for parents to hire these alarms. The recommended use of these alarms by the medical profession is in my view a means of treating anxious parents and not preventing SIDS. There are occasional very special circumstances in which an alarm is helpful, but in general, support, reassurance and close supervision are more appropriate. The issue of an alarm should always be accompanied by a demonstration of infant resuscitation technique. There is no point in having an apnoea monitor if one does not know what to do when it alarms.

What is a 'near miss'?

A child in the first months of life is occasionally discovered to be pale or blue and not breathing. The panic stricken parent immediately attempts to revive him following which he is admitted to hospital. While in the hospital he is perfectly well and all investigations are normal. The term 'near miss' cot death has arisen in the belief that if the child had not been found in the nick of time a cot death would have occurred. There is no factual basis for this supposition. Large population studies of SIDS reveal that it is exceptionally rare for a SIDS infant to have had a 'near miss'.

ENLARGED GLANDS (NODES)

Enlarged glands are frequent in children and usually present as a lump or lumps in the neck or armpits. As a result of much of the publicity given to the detection of cancer, and breast cancer in particular, many parents become acutely anxious on suddenly finding a lump in the child. They immediately fear the worst and seek an urgent consultation with the family doctor. The family doctor usually takes a reassuring attitude and the parents calm down and expectantly wait for the lump to go. After a few weeks the lump may still be present when the parents once again become anxious and consult the family doctor who may then refer the child to a paediatrician. Neck lumps are a frequent cause for referral to a paediatrician.

Most superficial lumps are caused by glands (lymph nodes) which are situated in various parts of the body. There are about 500 glands in the body, the size varying between 1mm and 1–2cm depending on the age of the child. Glands enlarge in response to infections. A generalised infection such as glandular fever may cause glands in many sites to enlarge, while a local infection such as tonsillitis may cause local gland enlargement in the neck; these enlarged glands commonly being referred to as the 'tonsillar glands'.

When a paediatrician sees a child with enlarged glands an examination will be made to determine whether the glandular enlargement is generalised or localised. The abdomen may also be examined to check whether there is any enlargement of the liver or spleen. Enlargement of these organs commonly occurs in viral illnesses but may also occur in other rare illnesses. On well over 90% of occasions small, soft, non-tender, mobile lumps are found in a single area such as the neck, armpit or groin of an otherwise healthy child. When such lumps are found parents are reassured and no investigations or treatment are required. Enlarged neck glands are very common and are usually caused by viral throat infections. Parents are told that the lumps are likely to persist for many months and sometimes years, getting bigger and smaller from time to time with each repeated infection. Very occasionally a gland may need to be removed for cosmetic reasons.

Big, firm, non-mobile lumps in one site or an unusual site; lumps in many sites, particularly in an unwell child, all require further investigation. Liver or spleen enlargement may also require further investigation. The tests commonly done are a chest x-ray and a microscopic examination of the blood (a count and film). Tests for glandular fever and other viral infections and skin tests for tuberculosis are sometimes done. A small piece of the lump may be removed surgically (a biopsy) so that it can be examined in the laboratory. The further management will depend on what the cause for the lump might be. Bacteria similar to tuberculosis (non-tuberculous mycobacteria) commonly cause a large firm neck gland or abscess. The child is usually well and the swelling is not tender. In contrast to tuberculosis these lumps are commonly on one side of the neck. Because of the close similarity to tuberculosis bacteria, tuberculosis skin tests may be positive. Most of these non-tuberculous infections can be diagnosed by special skin tests, others by culturing (growing bacteria from) a segment of the gland or abscess fluid. The importance of recognising non-tuberculous infections is that unless recognised children may be unnecessarily treated for many months on antituberculous drugs. The only treatment of these infections is to remove the affected glands completely. If glands are partly removed or the abscess incompletely drained, the wound may continue to discharge for many months, leaving the child with an ugly scar.

In conclusion, the only precise way of diagnosing the cause of a superficial lump is by removing it for examination in a laboratory. However, this is neither practical nor indeed desirable when examination by a paediatrician can predict with almost 100% certainty the benign nature of the lump.

Useful Addresses

Of necessity it is only possible to list some of the many agencies and organisations which offer help, advice and counselling not only to parents but also to professionals. Most of the selected organisations relate to the areas covered in this book. It is divided into countries with the general addresses given first, followed by those of specific conditions arranged alphabetically.

UNITED KINGDOM

General

The Health Education Authority
78 New Oxford Street
London WC1A 1AH   01-631 0930

The Scottish Health Education Group
Health Education Centre, Woodburn House, Caraen Lane
Edinburgh EH10 4SG   031-447 8044

The British Dental Health Foundation
88 Gurnards Avenue, Fishermead
Milton Keynes, Bucks MK6 2BL   0908 66763

Compassionate Friends
5 Lower Clifton Hill
Bristol BS8 1BT   0272 292778

Medic-Alert Foundation
11–13 Clifton Terrace
London N4 3JP   01-263 8597

SOS Talisman, Talman Limited
21 Grays Corner, Ley Street
Ilford, Essex IG2 7RQ   01-554 5579

The Priory Centre, 11 Priory Road (Anorexia Nervosa)
High Wycombe, Bucks HP13 6SL   0494 21341

Arthritis and Rheumatism Council
41 Eagle Street, London WC1R 4AR   01-405 8572

The Asthma Society, 300 Upper Street
London N1 2XX   01-226 2260

The National Society for Autistic Children
276 Willesden Lane, London NW2 5RB   01-451 3844

Royal National Institute for the Blind
224 Great Portland Street, London W1N 6AA   01-388 1266

Spastics Society
12 Park Crescent, London W1N 4EQ   01-636 5020

Cleft Lip and Palate Association, Dental Department
Hospital for Sick Children
Great Ormond Street, London WC1H 3JH

Coeliac Society
PO Box 181, London NW2 2YA   01-459 2440

The Foundation for the Study of Infant Deaths
(Cot Death Research and Support), 5th Floor
4 Grosvenor Place, London SW1X 7HD   01-235 1721

Cystic Fibrosis Research Trust
5 Blythe Road, Bromley, Kent BR1 3RS   01-464 7211

National Deaf Children's Society
45 Hereford Road, London W2 5AH   01-229 9272

British Diabetic Association
10 Queen Anne Street, London W1M 0BD   01-323 1531

Down's Children's Association
12–13 Clapham Common Southside
London SW4 7AA   01-720 0008

British Dyslexia Association
Church Lane
Peppard, Oxon RG9 5JN   0491 7699

National Eczema Society
Tavistock House North, Tavistock Square
London WC1H 9SR   01-388 4097

British Epilepsy Association, Crowthorne House
New Wokingham Road
Wokingham, Berks RG11 3AY   0344 773122

Haemophilia Society
123 Westminster Bridge Road
London SE1 7HR   01-928 2020

The Chest and Heart Association
Tavistock House North, Tavistock Square
London WC1H 9JE   01-387 3012

Hyperactive Children's Support Group
59 Meadowside, Angmering,
Sussex BN16 4BW   0903 725182

British Kidney Patients Association
Bordon, Hants   04203 2022

Leukaemia Society
PO Box 82, Exeter, Devon   0392 218514

Royal Society for Mentally Handicapped Children
& Adults (MENCAP)
123 Golden Lane, London EC1Y 0RT   01-253 9433

The British Migraine Association
178a High Road, Byfleet
Weybridge, Surrey KT14 7ED   09323 52468

The Migraine Trust
23 Great Ormond Street, London WC1N 3HD   01-278 2676

Muscular Dystrophy Group of Great Britain
35 Macaulay Road, London SW4 0QP   01-720 8055

Sickle Cell Society
c/o Brent Community Health Council, 16 High Street
Harlesden, London NW10 4LX   01-451 3293

Association for all Speech Impaired Children (AFASIC)
347 Central Markets
Smithfield, London EC1A 9NH   01-236 3632

Association for Spina Bifida & Hydrocephalus (ASBAH)
22 Upper Woburn Place
London WC1H 0EP   01-388 1382

Thalassaemia Society
107 Nightingale Lane, London N8 7QY   01-348 0437

Voluntary Council for Handicapped Children
National Children's Bureau
8 Wakley Street, London EC1V 7QE   01-278 9441

UNITED STATES OF AMERICA

General

American Academy of Pediatrics
141 Northwest Point Road, PO Box No. 927
Elk Grove Village, IL 60007

Specific

Anorexia Aid Inc., 101 Cedar Lane
Teaneck, New Jersey 07666

Arthritis Foundation
1212 Avenue of the Americas, New York, NY 10036

Allergy Foundation of America
801 Second Avenue, New York, NY 10017   212-684 7875
(All allergic diseases are served including asthma)

National Society for Autistic Children
306 31st Street
Huntingdon, WV 25702   304-697 2638

American Council for the Blind
1211 Connecticut Avenue NW
Washington DC 20036   202-833 1251

American Foundation for the Blind
15 West 16th Street, New York, NY 10011

American Cancer Society
777 Third Avenue, New York, NY 10017   212-371 2900

United Cerebral Palsy Association Inc
66 East 34th Street, New York, NY 10016

American Cleft Palate Association
331 Salt Hall, University of Pittsburgh
Pittsburgh, PA 15261   412-681 9620

American Celiac Society
45 Gifford Avenue, Jersey City, NJ 07304

Cystic Fibrosis Foundation
3379 Peachtree Road NE, Atlanta, GA 30326   404-262 1100

National Cystic Fibrosis Research Foundation
521 Fifth Avenue, New York, NY 10017

Alexander Graham Bell Association for the Deaf
1537 35th Street NW, Washington DC 20007   202-337 5220

American Diabetes Association
600 Fifth Avenue, New York, NY 10020   212-541 4310

Juvenile Diabetes Foundation
25 East 26th Street, New York, NY 10010   212-689 7868

Epilepsy Foundation of America
1828 L Street NW, Washington DC 20036   202-293 2930

American Genetic Association
1028 Connecticut Avenue NW, Washington DC 20036

National Hemophilia Foundation
25 West 39th Street, New York, NY 10018

National Kidney Foundation
116 East 27th Street, New York, NY 10016   202-889 2210

Leukemia Society of America
211 East 43rd Street, New York, NY 10017   212-573 8484

American Academy on Mental Retardation
916 64th Avenue East, Tacoma, WA 98424   206-922 5859

Muscular Dystrophy Association of America Inc
810 Seventh Avenue, New York, NY 10019   212-586 0808

Centre for Sickle Cell Disease
2121 Georgia Avenue NW, Washington DEC 20059   202-636 7930

American Speech and Hearing Association
10801 Rockville Pike
Rockville, MD 20852   301-897 5700

Spina Bifida Association of America
104 Festone Avenue
Newcastle, Delaware 19720

National Tay-Sachs and Allied Diseases Association
122 East 42nd Street
New York, NY 10017   212-661 2780

Cooley's Anemia Blood and Research Foundation
   for Children Inc
647 Franklin Avenue, Garden City, NY 11530   516-747 2155

Tourette Syndrome Association
41/02 Bell Boulevard
Bayside, Queens, New York   718-224 2999

AUSTRALIA

General

Department of Health, McKell Buildings
Rawson Place, Sydney 2000, NSW   217 6666

Department of Health, State Health Building
147–163 Charlotte Street
Brisbane 4000, Queensland   224 0515

Public Health Promotion Services
Saving Bank Buildings, 158 Rundle Mall
Adelaide 5000, South Australia   218 3211

Health Department of Western Australia
Curtis House, 60 Beaufort Street
East Perth 6000, Western Australia   328 0241

Health Commission of Victoria
555 Collins Street, Melbourne 3000, Victoria   616 7777

Specific

Advisory Council for Children with Impaired Hearing
Treetops, Morach Road
Vermont 3133

Association for Children with Learning Difficulties
PO Box 52, Burwood 2134

Association for the Pre-school Education of Deaf Children
8 O'Loan Street, Yeronga, Queensland 4104

Australian Arthritis and Rheumatism Foundation
GPO Box 1444, Sydney, NSW 2000

Australian Association for the Mentally Retarded
Room 3 Block F, Mutton Street
Canberra City, ACT 2601

Australian Association of Toy Libraries for the Handicapped
PO Box 103, Manuica, ACT 2603

Australian Cerebral Palsy Association
5 Blake Street, North Perth, WA 6006

Australian Council for the Rehabilitation of Disabled (ACROD)
Bedford and Buckingham Streets, Surry Hills, NSW 2010

The Blind Association
12 Hubert Street, Wooloongabba
Queensland 4102

Cystic Fibrosis Association of NSW
21–22 Belmore Street, Burwood, NSW 2134

Darwin and District Spastic Paralysis Association Inc
Darwin Hospital, PO Box 147, Darwin 5790

Epileptic Welfare Association
158 Pacific Highway, North Sydney 2060

Exceptional Parents Group
c/o PO Box 340, Pymble, NSW 2073

Federation of Autistic Children's Association
c/o 545 Pacific Highway, Artarmon, NSW 2064

Handicapped Persons Bureau
Department of Youth and Community Service
323 Castlereagh Street, Sydney NSW

Mothers of Disabled
c/o 34 Liverpool Street, Sydney, NSW 2001

Multiple Handicapped Association of Queensland
303 Padstow Road, Eight Mile Plain 4123

Torrens Toy Library and Parents Advisory Centre
Special Education Department, Torrens College of Adult Education,
70 South Road, Torrensville 5031

Victorian Society for Crippled Children & Adults
79 Buckhurst Street, South Melbourne 3205

Autistic Children's Society of Tasmania
Derwent Avenue, Lindisfarne 7015

Helping Hands Club
276 Elizabeth Street, Hobart 7000
(support group of mothers of young retarded children)

Tasmanian Spastic Association Inc
Collins Street, Hobart 7000

The following will supply addresses of relevant societies and self-help
groups:

EUROPE

International Information Centre on Self-Help and Health
E van Evenstraat 2C, B-3000 Leuven, Belgium

NEW ZEALAND

The Director General
Department of Health, PO Box 5013
Wellington, New Zealand

SOUTH AFRICA

The Director General
The Department of Health and Welfare, Private Bag X63
Pretoria 0001, Transvaal, South Africa

Selected Reading

For parents, teachers, doctors, nurses and others who read or dip into this book, I offer a selection of further reading. This is divided into two lists: the first suitable for all readers, but particularly for the parent or non-medical person, and the second for others with a medical background.

GENERAL READERSHIP

Albery, E. H., Hathorn, I. S. and Pigott, R. W. (1986). *Cleft Lip and Palate: A Team Approach*. John Wright, Bristol.

Angus, R. M., Todd, L., Smith, A. and Kinmonth, A-L. (1984). *An Introduction to Diet in the Care of Children with Diabetes*. Ames Division, Miles Laboratories Limited, Slough.

Atherton, D. J. (1984). *Your Child with Eczema: A Guide for Parents*. William Heinemann Limited, London.

Baum, J. D. and Kinmonth, A-L. (1986). *Care of the Child with Diabetes*. Churchill Livingstone, Edinburgh.

*Bevan, R. G. (1982). *Learning About Epilepsy*. Medical Education Services, Oxford.

Bruch, H. (1978). *The Golden Cage*. Open Books, Somerset, England. Anorexia Nervosa.)

*Bruna, D. (1980). *Children's Haemophilia Book*. Concept Publications, Northampton.

Cunningham, C. (1982). *Down's Syndrome: An Introduction for Parents*. Souvenir Press, London.

Douglas, J. and Richman, N. (1984). *My Child Won't Sleep*. Penguin Books, Harmondsworth.

Ericksen, A. (1985). *Anorexia Nervosa: The Broken Circle*. Faber and Faber, London.

359

Finnie, N. (1974). *Handling the Young Cerebral Palsied Child at Home*. 2nd edition. William Heinemann Medical Books Limited, London.

Glasspool, M. G. (1984). *Eyes: Their Problems and Treatment*. Martin Dunitz, London.

Golding, J., Limerick, S. and Macfarlane, A. (1985). *Sudden Infant Death: Patterns, Puzzles and Problems*. Open Books, Somerset, England.

Haslam, D. (1984). *Sleepless Children: A Handbook for Parents*. Judy Piatkus Publishers, London.

Hopkins, A. (1981). *Epilepsy – The Facts*. Oxford University Press, Oxford.

Hornsby, B. (1984). *Overcoming Dyslexia*. Martin Dunitz, London.

Horrobin, J. M. (1975). *To Give an Edge*. Colwell Press, Minneapolis. (Down's syndrome.)

Hull, D. (1985). *The Macmillan Guide to Child Health*. Macmillan, London.

Illingworth, R. S. (1981). *The Normal Child*. Churchill Livingstone, Edinburgh.

Illingworth, R. S. (1981). *Your Child's Development in the First Five Years*. Churchill Livingstone, Edinburgh.

Jeavons, P. M. and Aspinall, A. (1985). *The Epilepsy Reference Book*. Harper and Row, London.

Jeffree, D. M. and McConkey, R. (1976). *Let Me Speak*. Souvenir Press, London.

Jeffree, D. M., McConkey, R. and Hewson, S. (1985). *Let Me Play*. Souvenir Press, London.

Jolly, H. (1981). *Book of Child Care: The Complete Guide for Today's Parents*. George Allen and Unwin, London.

Jones, P. D. (1984). *Living with Haemophilia*. MTP Press, Lancaster.

Kirkland, J. (1985). *Crying and Babies: Helping Families Cope*. Croom Helm, London.

Knight, B. (1983). *Sudden Death in Infancy: The 'Cot Death Syndrome'*. Faber and Faber, London.

Laidlaw, M. V. and Laidlaw, J. (1984). *Epilepsy Explained*. Churchill Livingstone, Edinburgh.

Lane, D. J. and Storr, A. (1979). *Asthma – The Facts*. Oxford University Press, Oxford.

Lask, B. (1985). *Children's Problems: A Parents' Guide to Understanding and Tackling Them*. Martin Dunitz, London.

Leach, P. (1983). *The Parents' A–Z: A Guide to Children's Health, Growth and Happiness*. Allen Lane, London.

Meadow, R. (1980). *Help for Bed Wetting*. Churchill Livingstone, Edinburgh.

Milner, A. D. (1984). *Asthma in Childhood*. Churchill Livingstone, Edinburgh.

Purser, A. (1981). *You and Your Handicapped Child*. George Allen and Unwin, London.

Rogan, P. and Hollomby, D. (1986). *Asthma – the Detective Story*. Roby Education, Merseyside.

*Rogan, P. and Hollomby, D. (1985). *Epilepsy – the Detective Story*. Roby Education, Merseyside.

Rose, C. F. and Gawel, M. (1979). *Migraine – The Facts*. Oxford University Press, Oxford.

Ryan, M. (1981). *Feeding Can be Fun*. Spastics Society, London.

Schaefer, N. (1979). *Does She Know She's There?* Harper and Row, London.

Sheridan, M. D. (1981). *From Birth to Five Years*. NFER-Nelson Publishing Co Ltd, Windsor.

Slade, R. (1984). *The Anorexia Nervosa Reference Book*. Harper and Row, London.

Smith, D. W. and Wilson, A. C. (1973). *The Child with Down's Syndrome*. W. B. Saunders Co, Philadelphia.

Stone, J. and Taylor, F. (1977). *A Handbook for Parents with a Handicapped Child*. Arrow Books, London.

Taylor, E. A. (1985). *The Hyperactive Child*. Martin Dunitz, London.

Valman, B. (1985). *Keeping Babies and Children Healthy*. Martin Dunitz, London.

Wilkinson, M. (1982). *Migraine and Headaches*. Martin Dunitz, London.

Young, H. (1980). *What Difference does it Make, Danny?* Andre Deutsch, London. (Physical Handicap.)

PROFESSIONAL MEDICAL READERSHIP

Avery, M. E. and Taeusch, W. H. (eds.) (1984). *Schaeffer's Diseases of the Newborn*. W. B. Saunders Co, Philadelphia.

Behrman, R. E. and Vaughan, V. C. (eds.) (1983). *Nelson Textbook of Pediatrics*. W. B. Saunders Co, Philadelphia.

Forfar, J. O. and Arneil, G. (eds.) (1984). *Textbook of Paediatrics*. Churchill Livingstone, Edinburgh.

Krugman, S. and Katz, S. L. (1985). *Infectious Diseases of Children*. C. V. Mosby, St Louis.

Roberton, N. R. C. (1986). *Textbook of Neonatology*. Churchill Livingstone, Edinburgh.

Rudolf, A. M. (ed.) (1982). *Pediatrics*. Appleton Century Crofts, Norwalk, Connecticut.

The Red Book. Report of the Committee on Infectious Diseases, 1986. Publications Department, American Academy of Pediatrics, Elk Grove Village, Illinois.

*Specifically for children.

Index

absent tears 230
activated charcoal (Medicoal) 340
acute epiglottitis *see* bacterial croup
allergic rhinitis/conjunctivitis 232–5
   diagnosis 233
   symptoms 232
   treatment 233–5
amblyopia *see* 'lazy eye'
amniocentesis 335
anaemia, iron deficiency 89–91
   diagnosis 90
   treatment 91
anal fissure 145–6
anaphylactoid/allergic purpura *see*
   Henoch Schönlein syndrome
anatomy:
   ear 214
   lungs and airways 190
   stomach and oesophagus 137
   urinary system 162
ankyloglossia *see* tongue tie
ankylosing spondylitis 264
anorexia nervosa 96–102
   cause 97
   physical effects 98
   psychological effects 98–9
   support groups 101–2
   treatment/management 99–101
antinuclear factor (ANF) 259, 261
apnoea monitors 347
appendicitis 155–6

arthritis 257–64
   acute 257–8
   chronic 259–64
     juvenile 259–63
       pauci-articular 259
       polyarticular 260
       systemic onset 260–1
aspirin 288
asthma 189–205
   causes 191–2
   diagnosis 193
   exercise and 203
   immunisation for child with 81
   monitoring 201, 202
   physiotherapy and 204
   positions of relaxation for use in
     205
   treatment 194–203
     drugs 195–200
       action of 197
       methods of giving 196,
         198–200
atopic dermatitis *see* eczema
autism 55–7

BCG 81
Becker muscular dystrophy 306
bed-wetting *see* nocturnal enuresis
behaviour problems (common)
   36–43
   breath-holding attacks 39–41

behaviour problems
  cot/crib rocking 42
  feeding 36–8
  head banging 41
  head rolling/nodding 41
  masturbation 42
  nail biting 42
  stammering/stuttering 42–3
  temper tantrums 38–9
  thumb/finger sucking 42
  tooth grinding 42
benign paroxysmal vertigo 278
biliary atresia 310
bilirubin 308
  raised conjugated 310
  raised unconjugated 309–10
blood group incompatibility 309
blood sugar, level in diabetes 104,
    105, 110, 113
  low 115
  meter 114
  'pricking' device to measure 114
'bone age' 10
breast, development 22
  feeding 85–7
  milk jaundice 309
breath-holding attacks 39–41
  blue type 39, 40
  white type 40
    atropine, use in 41
bronchiolitis 206–9
  causes 207
  diagnosis 208
  symptoms 207
  treatment 208
bruxism 42
bulimia 101
button batteries, poisoning by 341

capillary haemangioma *see*
  strawberry mark
cardiac catheterisation 185
centiles 1

cerebral palsy (CP) 297–302
  additional problems 299
  causes 297
  diagnosis 299
  drugs used for 301–2
  management 300–1
  types 298
chicken pox 65–6
  sequence of events 66
chilblains 250
Chinese Restaurant syndrome 290
chorion biopsy 335–6
Christmas disease 312
chronic non-specific diarrhoea
    syndrome *see* toddlers'
    diarrhoea
chronic uveitis 263
circumcision 170
cleft lip/palate 321–7
  additional problems 325–6
  feeding 323, 324, 325
  surgery 323
  treatment 322
club foot 267–8
  postural 268
  treatment 267
coeliac disease 121–4
  diagnosis 122
  treatment 122–3
'cold sores' *see* herpes labialis
colic drops 149
'comma shaped' foot 270
congenital laryngeal stridor 225
conjunctivitis 231
  allergic 232–5
constipation and encoporesis 142–6
  cause 143
  treatment 144
conversion scale (thermometer) 60
convulsions, febrile 285–9
  management 282, 287
cot/crib death 342–8
cover test (for squint) 229

cow's milk protein intolerance
(CMPI) 87–9
diagnosis 88
treatment 89
craniotabes 92
croup 222–5
bacterial 223–4
spasmodic 224
viral 222
curly toes 272
cystic fibrosis 124–9
diagnosis 125
inheritance of 125–6
screening tests 126–7
treatment 127

daytime wetting *see* diurnal enuresis
decimal age 15
dehydration 130–1
treatment 132
volume of fluid required 133
dental, development 23–4
extractions in heart conditions
185–7
hygiene 255
Denver Developmental Screening
Test 26
desensitisation 233
developmental charts 25–35
diabetes 103–20
complications 104
diet 110–12
driving and 118
holidays and 117
illness and 116
monitoring 113–15
schooling and 117–18
treatment 104, 105–10
diarrhoea and vomiting *see*
gastroenteritis
diet, in anorexia nervosa 100
for coeliac disease 122–3
for diabetes 110–12

in eczema 241
in obesity 94–5
diphtheria 74
immunisation for 75, 76
dislocated/unstable hip 264–7
cause 265
diagnosis 265
treatment 266
divarication of the recti 158–9
DNA probe test 126–7
for Duchenne muscular
dystrophy 306
Down's syndrome 327–36
associated problems 332–3
causes 329
characteristics 328
diagnosis 329–31
family problems 333–5
drugs/medicines used in/for:
acute otitis media 214
allergic conjunctivitis 234–5
allergic rhinitis 234–5
anorexia nervosa 101
asthma 195–200
breath-holding attacks 41
eczema 237–9
enuresis 177
epilepsy 280–2
fever 61
growth hormone, stimulate rise in
10
haemophilia 313
herpes infections 71
hyperactivity 51–2
incompletely descended testis 168
iron deficiency anaemia 91
juvenile chronic arthritis 263
lice 247
meningitis 295, 296
migraine 292
nappy rash 249–50
nephrotic syndrome 160
pneumonia 211

drugs/medicines used in/for
poisoning 338–9
scabies 244
sore throat 221
spasticity 302
steroids to stimulate growth spurt
11
teething 24
thalassaemia 314–15
threadworms 154
Tourette syndrome 48
urine infections 165
vaginal discharge 171
VSD 185
warts 253
whooping cough 68
Duchenne muscular dystrophy
(DMD) 302–7
clinical features 303
diagnosis 304
genetic factors 306
management 304–6
outlook 303
dyslexia 54–5

echocardiogram 185
eczema 236–42
distribution 237
foot 254
management 237–40
egg allergy, contra-indication for
vaccines 79, 82
electro-encephalograph (EEG) 279
drugs and 280
enlarged glands (nodes) 348
Enterobius vermicularis 152
enuresis 173–81
diurnal 178–81
management 179–81
nocturnal 173–8
alarm systems for 174
drugs 177
enuretic alarms 174–7

double bed mat 174
'in pants' detector alarm 174, 176
mechanism of 174
single bed mat 174, 175
epilepsy 276–85
causes 277
driving licence 284
drugs 280–2
investigations 279
school and 284
types 277–8
work and 284
epistaxis *see* nosebleeds
Epstein-Barr virus 69
erythema infectiosum 64
erythema multiforme 251
erythema toxicum 248
'exchanges' (in diabetes) 111

feeding problems 36–8
Feingold diet 52
fever 58–61
cause from infectious diseases
61–73
treatment 60–1
fifth disease *see* erythema
infectiosum
flat feet 271–2
fluoride supplementation 187
fontanelles 17

gamma globulin 72
gastroenteritis 129–34
dehydration in 130–1
treatment 131–4
gastro-oesophageal reflux 136–41
complications 136
investigations 138
management 138–40
posture 139
genital development (boys) 21
genu valgum *see* knock knee
German measles 63–4

immunisation against 63, 75, 76, 80
  sequence of events 64
glandular fever 69–70
  blood tests for 69
glucagon 116
glue ear *see* chronic otitis media
glycosylated haemoglobin 114
Gowers' sign 303
grand mal 277
gripe water 148
grommets 217
  swimming with 218
'growing pains' 256–7
growth and development 1–35
  dental development 23–4
  failure to thrive 11–16
  mental development 24–35
    milestones 27–35
  physical development 16
  sexual development 17, 20–3
  the short child 1–11
growth charts 1, 2–8
  height, boys 1, 4, 7
    girls 2, 5, 8
  preterm, boys 13
    girls 14
growth hormone, tests 10
  treatment 11
growth spurt 9
  drugs to bring on 11
growth velocity 9

habit spasm 47–9
haemoglobin 90
  in infants 91
haemophilia 312–14
  treatment 313
  types 312
Haemophilus influenza vaccine (USA) 75, 76, 81–2
halitosis 254
head banging 41

head louse 245–8
  treatment 247–8
head rolling/nodding 41
heart murmurs 182–9
  innocent 182–3
  patent ductus 187–9
  ventricular septal defect (VSD) 183–7
height charts:
  boys 2
    allowing for parents' height 4
    height velocity chart 7
  girls 3
    allowing for parents' height 5
    height velocity chart 8
Henoch Schönlein syndrome 251, 258
hepatitis 310
hepatitis B vaccine 82
hernia 157–8
  inguinal 157
  treatment 158
  umbilical 158
herpes 70–1
  gingivostomatitis 70
  labialis 70–1
hives 252
hydrocele 159
hydrocephalus 318
  treatment 320
hyperactive child 49–52
  cardinal symptoms of 50
  drugs for 51–2
  Feingold diet, use for 52
  management 51
'hypo' 115
hypoglycaemia 112, 115–16
hypospadias 169–70

idiopathic thrombocytopaenia 311–12
immunisations 74–84
  in cases of asthma/eczema 81

immunisations
  for premature babies 81
  reasons for 76
  scheme of, in UK 75
    in USA 76
  side-effects 77
infantile colic 146–9
infectious disease 61–73
  chicken pox 65–6
  erythema infectiosum 64
  German measles 63–4
  glandular fever 69–70
  herpes 70–1
  incubation 73
  infectivity 73
  measles 61–3
  mumps 68–9
  roseola infantum 64
  scarlet fever 72–3
  viral hepatitis 71–2
  whooping cough 66–8
infectious mononucleosis *see*
    glandular fever
influenza vaccine 82
inhalers (for asthma) 198–200
injection, aids 110
  sites for insulin 106, 107, 108
insulin 104, 105–10
  injection sites for 106, 107, 108
  'pen' 110
  syringes for 109
  types 105–6
intestinal biopsy 16
  in CMPI 89
  in coeliac disease 122
in-toeing 268–70
intravenous urogram (IVU) 164
intussusception 156
ipecacuana syrup, use in poisoning
    338–9
iron, dose required in anaemia 91
irritable colon of childhood *see*
    toddlers' diarrhoea

'irritable hip' 258

jaundice 308–11
  cause 308
  non-physiological 309–10
  physiological 308–9
  treatment 310–11
juvenile chronic arthritis 259–63
  categories 259–61
  diagnosis 261
  eye complications 263
  management 261–3
    medical 263
    physiotherapy 262
juvenile plantar dermatosis 253–4

karyotype 329, 330, 331
kernicterus 310
ketones 113
knock knee 271
Koplick's spots 61–2

labia minora, adherent 171
laryngomalacia *see* congenital
    laryngeal stridor
'late developer' 9
'lazy eye' 226
light treatment (for jaundice)
    310–11
light reflex test (for squint) 229
liver, inflammation of *see* viral
    hepatitis
lumbar puncture 286, 294
luteinising releasing hormone
    (LHRH) 168

masturbation 42
measles 61–3
  immunisation for 75, 76, 79–80
  sequence of events 62
meconium ileus 125
meningismus 294
meningitis 293–7
  causes 293
  diagnosis 294

outlook 295
symptoms 294
treatment 294–5
of contacts 296
meningococcal vaccine 83
mesenteric adenitis 156
micturating cysto-urethrogram
(MCU) 164
migraine 289–93
causes 290–1
management 291–2
'trigger' factors 290, 291
milestones of child's development
25–35
6 weeks 27
3 months 27–8
6 months 28
9 months 29–30
12 months 29–30
15 months 30
18 months 30–1
2 years 31–2
2½ years 32–3
3 years 33
4 years 34
5 years 34–5
milia 248
miliaria 248
molluscum contagiosum 252
Monospot test 69
mosaic 329
mumps 68–9
immunisation for (USA) 69, 76
muscular dystrophy 302
myringotomy 217

nappy rash 249–50
infantile seborrhoeic dermatitis
250
irritant dermatitis 249
thrush 249–50
nephrotic syndrome 160–1
nosebleeds 218

NSAIDS 263
nutrition 85–102
anorexia nervosa 96–102
infant feeding 85–9
breast feeding 85–7
cow's milk protein intolerance
87–9
formula feeding 87
solids, when to start 87
iron deficiency anaemia 89–91

obesity 93–5
rickets 91–2
nystagmus 42
obesity 93–5
cause 93–4
management 94–5
orchitis 69
otitis media:
acute 213–15
treatment 214
chronic 215–18
cause 215
diagnosis 215–16
treatment/surgery 217
out-toeing 270

pagophagia 90
'pallid syncope' 40
parotid gland, in mumps 68
patent ductus 187–9
Paul Bunnell test 69
peak flow meter 193
pediculosis capitis see head louse
periodic syndrome 149–52
management 151
perniosis see chilblains
pertussis see whooping cough
petit mal 278
pharyngitis see sore throat
physical development 2–3, 16–17,
18–19
pica 90
Pierre Robin syndrome 326–7

pigeon toes *see* in-toeing
pilonidal dimple *see* sacrococcygeal
  dimple
pneumococcal vaccine 82–3
pneumonia 209–12
  causes 209
  diagnosis 210
  management 210–11
  symptoms 210
poisoning, accidental 337–42
  activated charcoal, use in 340
  due to button batteries 341
  ipecacuana syrup, use in 338–9
poliomyelitis 74
  immunisation for 75, 76, 80
pseudohypertrophy 303
pseudo-squint 226, 227
psychogenic cough 48
puberty, events in 20
pubic hair development, boys 21
  girls 22, 23
pyloric stenosis 141–2
  treatment 142

Ramstedt's pyloromyotomy 142
red eye *see* conjunctivitis
reflex anoxic seizures 40
reflux (of urine) 163–4
'reflux board' 139
respiratory syncitial virus (RSV)
  207, 209
Reye's syndrome 288
rheumatoid factor (RF) 259, 260,
  261, 264
rickets 91–2
roseola infantum 64
  sequence of events 65
rubella *see* German measles
rubeola *see* measles

sacrococcygeal dimple 250
salmon patches 249
Sarcoptes scabei 242

scabies 242–5
  cause 243
  diagnosis 243
  management 243–5
scarlet fever 72–3
school refusal 52–4
scoliosis 274
Sellotape test (for threadworms) 153
Senokot, use in constipation 144
serum immunoreactive trypsin 125
sexual development 17, 20–3
  in boys 21
  in girls 22–3
  in a short child 9
shoes, choosing children's 273
short child 1–11
  comparable height with parents 6
  home conditions, state of 10
  stage of sexual development 9
sickle cell anaemia 315–16
sinusitis 219–20
'slapped cheek appearance' 64
sleep problems 43–6
  night terrors 46
  nightmares 46
  sleep walking 46
  use of drugs 45
snuffles 219
soiling *see* constipation and
  encoporesis
sore throat 220–2
  investigations 220
  tonsillectomy for 221–2
  treatment 221
spasmus nutans 42
spina bifida 317–21
  management 318–20
  surgery 319
squint 225–30
  cause 226–8
  diagnosis 228, 229
  treatment 228–30
stammering/stuttering 42–3